Clinical Manual of Psychosomatic Medicine

A Guide to
Consultation-Liaison Psychiatry

Clinical Manual of Psychosomatic Medicine

A Guide to Consultation-Liaison Psychiatry

Michael G. Wise, M.D.

Clinical Professor of Psychiatry
University of California, Davis
Adjunct Professor of Psychiatry
Uniformed Services University of the Health Sciences
F. Edward Hébert School of Medicine
Bethesda, Maryland

James R. Rundell, M.D.

Professor of Psychiatry
Uniformed Services University of the Health Sciences
F. Edward Hébert School of Medicine
Bethesda, Maryland

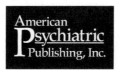

American Psychiatric Publishing, Inc.

Washington, DC
London, England

Note: The authors have worked to ensure that all information in this book is accurate at the time of publication and consistent with general psychiatric and medical standards, and that information concerning drug dosages, schedules, and routes of administration is accurate at the time of publication and consistent with standards set by the U.S. Food and Drug Administration and the general medical community. As medical research and practice continue to advance, however, therapeutic standards may change. Moreover, specific situations may require a specific therapeutic response not included in this book. For these reasons and because human and mechanical errors sometimes occur, we recommend that readers follow the advice of physicians directly involved in their care or the care of a member of their family.

Manufactured in the United States of America on acid-free paper
09 08 07 06 05   5 4 3 2 1
First Edition

Typeset in AGaramond and Formata.

American Psychiatric Publishing, Inc.
1000 Wilson Boulevard
Arlington, VA 22209-3901
www.appi.org

Library of Congress Cataloging-in-Publication Data
Wise, Michael G., 1944–
    Clinical manual of psychosomatic medicine : a guide to consultation-liaison psychiatry / by Michael G. Wise, James R. Rundell.—1st ed.
        p. ; cm.
    Includes bibliographical references and index.
    ISBN 1-58562-201-X (alk. paper)
    1. Consultation-liaison psychiatry. 2. Medicine, Psychosomatic.
    [DNLM: 1. Psychophysiologic Disorders—diagnosis. 2. Psychophysiologic Disorders—therapy. 3. Diagnosis, Differential. 4. Mental Disorders—diagnosis. 5. Mental Disorders—Therapy. 6. Psychology, Medical—methods. 7. Psychotherapy—methods. 8. Referral and Consultation. WM 90 M813c 2005] I. Rundell, James R., 1957– II. Title.
    RC455.2.C65W568 2005
    616.89′14—dc22   2004026969

British Library Cataloguing in Publication Data
A CIP record is available from the British Library.

Contents

Preface

In 1987, we wrote the first edition of the *Concise Guide to Consultation Psychiatry.* The second edition was published in 1994 and the third in 2000. This book, across all three editions, was practical and clinically focused and became one of the most popular in the Concise Guide series, finding its way into the lab coat pockets of many psychiatrists, psychiatric fellows and residents, nonpsychiatric physician colleagues, and medical students. The *Clinical Manual of Psychosomatic Medicine: A Guide to Consultation-Liaison Psychiatry* follows in the footsteps and spirit of the many editions of our concise guide.

Clinical Manual of Psychosomatic Medicine is a primary resource for psychiatrists who perform consultation, liaison, and psychosomatic work; see patients with concurrent psychiatric and medical-surgical conditions; or use a medical model in their psychiatry practice. Psychiatrists who consult on medical-surgical patients with psychiatric symptoms must understand how to evaluate and treat medically ill patients in a wide variety of clinical settings. Knowledge about the diagnosis and differential diagnosis of psychiatric syndromes, as well as the context of care delivery, improves the psychiatrist's ability to render effective recommendations in a language and manner relevant to the clinical setting. For example, a clinician who consults on a disoriented posttransplant patient may refer to chapters on mental status examination, delirium, and transplantation. Psychiatrists working in primary care will find this manual as useful as psychiatrists consulting on or managing patients in tertiary-care subspecialty settings.

We firmly believe that long-established principles of psychosomatic medicine/consultation-liaison psychiatry hold the key to psychiatrists' continued role as physicians and valued members of the medical field. These principles view the psychiatrist as 1) an expert in the administration and interpretation of the mental status examination, 2) knowledgeable about medical conditions and treatments, 3) expert at identifying toxic and medical causes for psychiatric signs and symptoms, 4) able to communicate with other physicians using the vocabulary and metaphors of medicine, 5) skilled at forming a comprehensive biopsychosocial differential diagnosis, 6) comfortable working with medical-surgical colleagues, 7) skilled in both psychopharmacology and psychotherapy, 8) cost-effective, and 9) able to work comfortably in a variety of different and unique medical and surgical settings.

Special thanks goes to Tina Marshall, who helped keep us organized. Finally, we thank our families for their patience and forbearance during the time we worked on this manual. Somehow they understood that this work was an effort to do the right thing for all of those medical-surgical patients we see who experience undiagnosed psychiatric conditions and untreated or inappropriately treated psychiatric illnesses.

Effective Psychiatric Consultation in a Changing Health Care Environment

History

Psychosomatic medicine and consultation-liaison psychiatry began in the 1920s–1930s with the development of general hospital psychiatry units and the psychosomatic medicine movement (Lipowski and Wise 2002). Rockefeller Foundation grants in 1934 and 1935 aided this developmental process by establishing closer collaboration between psychiatrists and other physicians. The number of consultation-liaison psychiatry services grew, and by the 1960s–1970s, a subspecialty scientific literature had developed. In 1974, the Psychiatry Education Branch of the National Institute of Mental Health (NIMH) decided to support the development and expansion of consultation-liaison services throughout the United States (Eaton et al. 1977). By 1980, NIMH supported 130 programs and materially contributed to the training of more than 300 consultation-liaison psychiatry fellows (Lipowski and Wise 2002). Federal budget cuts in the 1980s dramatically decreased the number of stipends. Nevertheless, consultation-liaison psychiatry continued to grow and develop during the 1980s (Lipowski and Wise 2002).

More recently, as primary care has expanded its scope of practice and influence, consultation-liaison psychiatrists have found themselves well suited to teach and consult with primary care physicians. The years since 2000 have seen a focus on achieving added qualifications status by the American Board of

Table 1–1.   Recent trends affecting the practice of psychosomatic medicine/consultation-liaison psychiatry

Managed health care's limitations and reallocation of health care resources

Direct reimbursement for psychiatric consultations is limited.

"Carve outs" of psychiatric services separate physical from mental health.

Psychiatrists must justify psychiatric services by showing cost-offset.

Shift of medical care and psychiatric consultation from inpatient to outpatient settings

Psychiatric consultation is conducted directly in primary care settings.

Shorter hospital stays limit the goals of inpatient psychiatric consultation and necessitate follow-up and transfer of treatment to the outpatient setting.

Multidisciplinary teams

Psychosomatic medicine/consultation-liaison psychiatrists increasingly work on multidisciplinary teams (e.g., with neuropsychologists, medical social workers, behavioral health psychologists, developmental pediatricians, behavioral neurologists, and psychiatric nurse practitioners).

Subspecialty units now often include psychiatrists (e.g., transplantation, physical medicine and rehabilitation, pain clinics).

Combined residency training

The number of combined residency training programs in psychiatry–internal medicine or psychiatry–family practice has increased. The effect of this increase on psychosomatic medicine training programs is not yet clear.

Subspecialty certification

The American Board of Medical Specialties has approved added qualifications certification; developmental activities (e.g., board certification examination) are under way.

Medical Specialties. Fellowship training guidelines and certification examination development are necessary steps toward that goal. Several significant historical trends affected consultation-liaison psychiatry during the 1990s and the early years of the new decade (Table 1–1).

Cost-Effectiveness of Psychiatric Consultation

As many as 30%–60% of general hospital inpatients have diagnosable psychiatric disorders (Hall et al. 2002). Depression, anxiety, and cognitive dysfunction each has been shown to predict longer hospital stays and greater hospitalization costs, even after accounting for demographics, degree of physical impairment, type of hospital unit, medical diagnosis, and circumstances of admission (Levenson et al. 1990; Saravay and Lavin 1994). Medical-psychiatric comorbidity predicts poorer outcomes and increased health care use and cost. For example, self-reported depressive symptoms or substance abuse is estimated to increase annual health care costs by more than $1,700 (Druss and Rosenheck 1999). Psychiatric consultation in general hospital patients and medical-surgical outpatients reduces mortality, morbidity, length of stay, and hospital costs (Hall et al. 2002).

Maintaining the financial viability of psychosomatic medicine services is essential in sustaining these cost-effective operations. Because centralized billing departments often place a lower priority on psychiatric billing than on more lucrative surgical and procedure-based reimbursements, a psychiatric consultation service must have direct input into its billing process. For each consult, the consultant should list all appropriate medical and psychiatric diagnoses and provide specific diagnostic criteria for each major psychiatric diagnosis. In addition, he or she should rate the level of complexity of the case. The complexity of the case, number of diagnoses, amount of time spent, and amount of information included in the note all may significantly alter the level of billing submitted for an initial consult. Finally, the consultation-liaison chief should work closely with the hospital administration to define and document sources of cost savings produced by the consultation-liaison service.

Approach to the Consultation

Consultation Style

The relative merits of an open-ended interview compared with a structured clinical examination are debated (Shakin Kunkel et al. 2002). The two styles are not mutually exclusive, and both are necessary to obtain valuable longitudinal and cross-sectional information. Structured examination is necessary for some historical data and for parts of the mental status examination. However, most information needed to make a diagnosis and a biopsychosocial formulation is obtained by simply listening. Many data are gained from patients' responses to open-ended questions, such as "What brings you into the clinic?,"

Table 1–2.   Characteristics of effective psychiatric consultation

Respond promptly to consultation requests; do today's work today.

Establish the level of urgency—emergent, urgent, or routine.

Wear a white coat—on your shoulders and in your brain.

Determine the central question—time to address comprehensively all biopsycho-social issues a patient may have, especially in inpatient settings, is rare.

Be flexible—perform consultations in medical-surgical inpatient and outpatient settings.

Respect patients' rights to know that the identified "customer" is the consulting physician.

Review medical data and collect essential information—from family, friends, or caregivers, as appropriate.

Use the biopsychosocial model—consider predispositions, precipitants, and strengths.

Make a well-reasoned differential diagnosis—consider medical, neurological, and psychiatric syndromes.

Make specific recommendations that are brief, goal oriented, and free of psychiatric jargon.

Discuss findings and recommendations with consultees in person whenever possible.

Follow up a patient in the hospital, and arrange outpatient care.

Recognize the value and role of medical psychotherapy for outpatient consultations.

Do not take over aspects of the patient's medical care unless asked to do so.

Read medical journals, and remain part of the medical community.

Educate medical administrators about cost-offset advantages of psychiatric consultation.

Work with the business office and staff to optimize reimbursement.

"How has this illness affected your life?," and "Why do you think your doctor asked the psychiatrist to see you?" Several personal and professional attributes are important to being an effective consultation-liaison psychiatrist. These attributes are summarized in Table 1–2.

Patient Confidentiality

Most patients seen in psychiatric consultation have never seen a psychiatrist before, did not request the consultation, and have not been informed about the consultation. Maintaining absolute doctor-patient confidentiality is not possible for a psychiatric consultant (Simon and Walker 2002). The physician requesting the consult is the identified "customer" and expects an answer to the consultation, even if the patient benefits from the consultation. It is best to explain this dual relationship to the patient from the start.

The primary care outpatient or inpatient record is a relatively public document. Notes regarding inpatient consultation visits are available not only to the referring primary care physician but also to other medical providers in the health care system. The Health Insurance Portability and Accountability Act (HIPPA) increased document protection requirements in health care settings. It is particularly important to satisfy these requirements when considering transmitting patient information via fax or electronic means.

Patient Follow-Up

Psychiatric consultants generally should follow up patients until they are discharged from the hospital or clinic or until the goals of the consultation are achieved. This is necessary for three reasons. First, urges to "sign off" on patients are frequently related more to negative reactions toward patients than to resolution of the presenting symptoms. Second, symptoms can recur, and a premature sign-off creates a potential loss of credibility and may lead to reconsultation. Finally, follow-up instills confidence that the consultation-liaison psychiatrist is available and willing to help.

Frequency and duration of psychiatric follow-up will vary widely depending on patient needs and financial circumstances (Simon and Walker 2002). Many patients receive maximum benefit from one or two consultation visits followed by management recommendations to the consulting physician. Some patients need a brief intervention, followed by referral back to the primary care physician. Other patients need immediate transfer to specialty mental health care clinics or units. In many situations, a period of shared follow-up with the outpatient primary care physician allows his or her continued involvement and learning.

Consultation or Liaison Psychiatry?

Liaison work is distinguished from consultation work in that the liaison psychiatrist casts an earlier and wider net, proactively seeking out psychiatric and medical comorbidity in a clinic or ward, and does not wait to see if the patient is identified and referred (Strain 2002). As Strain (1988) noted, "Liaison psychiatry attempts to deal with the **denominator** of the prevalence of psychiatric morbidity in the medical setting, whereas consultation psychiatry, by the nature of the referral process, is involved only with the **numerator**" (p. 76). Detection screening of hospitalized medical-surgical inpatients can result in less depression and cognitive impairment at time of discharge, decreased length of stay, fewer rehabilitation days, and decreased rehospitalization rates (Strain et al. 1991). For example, Hammer and colleagues (J.S. Hammer, H.T.C. Lam, and J.J. Strain, unpublished data, September 1993) screened all hospital admissions and showed that psychosocial assessment and treatment at the time of admission led to earlier discharges in patients with psychiatric comorbidity. For each dollar spent on this screening program, the hospital reported savings of $48. Unfortunately, many health care payers are less willing to pay for psychiatrists to identify new patients than to assess and treat identified patients.

Outpatient Psychosomatic Medicine

Changes in the U.S. health care system over the past 15 years have had profound effects on the delivery of medical and psychiatric care. The sites of care continue to shift away from inpatient settings to outpatient settings and away from specialty settings to primary care settings. When inpatient specialty medical-surgical care occurs, the duration of that care is shorter than ever, limiting the amount of time that inpatient psychiatric consultation can be effective. These phenomena have, of necessity, shifted much of the focus of psychosomatic medicine to the outpatient and primary care settings. Consultation psychiatrists have had to change practice patterns to adapt to these new realities. For example, lengthy diagnostic assessments are giving way to rapid, focused assessments (Simon and Walker 2002). Treatment recommendations are briefer, more focused, and practical—accommodating the practice patterns and limitations of outpatient primary care providers.

Epidemiology of Psychiatric Disorders in Primary Care

Fewer than 25% of the patients with psychiatric disorders see specialty mental health providers; most are seen in primary care settings (Regier et al. 1993). Anxiety or depressive disorders are diagnosed in 10%–15% of primary care patients (Spitzer et al. 1994; Ustun and Sartorius 1995). Half of the visits to physicians by patients with clear psychiatric diagnoses occur in primary care clinics (Schurman et al. 1985). Primary care physicians write most prescriptions for antidepressant (Simon et al. 1993) and antianxiety medications (Mellinger et al. 1984).

Medical conditions, particularly chronic illnesses, significantly increase the likelihood that a person will develop a mood disorder, an anxiety disorder, or a substance-related disorder (Hall et al. 2002).

Outpatient Psychiatric Consultation-Liaison Program Structure

Conducting psychiatric consultation in the primary care (or specialty care) clinic has the advantages of convenience and destigmatization for the patient (Simon and Walker 2002). Working alongside primary care providers provides professional credibility and an understanding of the primary care culture for the consultant. Patients and the consulting psychiatrist need to clearly understand the reason for the consultation; goals and expectations should be clarified. Sometimes, the consulting provider may participate in the consultation appointment.

For primary care physicians, it is usually important that care have as much continuity as possible. It is important not only for the same psychiatrist to see the patient during follow-up appointments but also for the patient's care to revert to the primary care clinician when the patient's condition has improved enough to fall within the scope of that provider's capabilities.

Consultation is therefore more likely to emphasize brief and focused psychiatric treatment that can be followed up by the primary care provider as soon as possible. As collaborative relationships evolve over time, the psychiatric consultant will often find that his or her relationship to the outpatient clinic will evolve from direct clinical service to patients to include more liaison activities, such as seminars, case conferences, and staff education.

Financing

The type of reimbursement or financing that exists in a health delivery setting will drive the extent to which a consulting psychiatrist can participate in a collaborative care model with outpatient primary care or medical-surgical specialty clinics. In a national health system (e.g., the military health system) or a large prepaid health plan, collaborative practice models can and do flourish. Health plan managers in these systems are more likely to understand the cost-offset and cost-benefit of providing effective mental health care to medical-surgical and primary care patients. However, fee-for-service payment systems create few incentives for providers to participate in nonbillable activities. In "carve-out" arrangements, medical and mental health care are deliberately segregated, making collaborative care models a challenge. Finally, in some settings, one single primary care physician may be responsible for patients from several different managed care organizations, each of which has its own panel of psychiatric consultants (Simon and Walker 2002).

References

Druss BG, Rosenheck RA: Patterns of health care costs associated with depression and substance abuse in a national sample. Psychiatr Serv 50:214–218, 1999

Eaton JS Jr, Goldberg R, Rosinski E, et al: The educational challenge of consultation-liaison psychiatry. Am J Psychiatry 134 (March suppl):20–23, 1977

Hall RCW, Rundell JR, Popkin MK: Cost-effectiveness of the consultation-liaison service, in The American Psychiatric Publishing Textbook of Consultation-Liaison Psychiatry: Psychiatry in the Medically Ill, 2nd Edition. Edited by Wise MG, Rundell JR. Washington, DC, American Psychiatric Publishing, 2002, pp 25–32

Levenson JL, Hamer RM, Rossiter LD: Relation of psychopathology in general medical inpatients to use and cost of services. Am J Psychiatry 47:1498–1503, 1990

Lipowski ZJ, Wise TN: History of consultation-liaison psychiatry, in The American Psychiatric Publishing Textbook of Consultation-Liaison Psychiatry: Psychiatry in the Medically Ill, 2nd Edition. Edited by Wise MG, Rundell JR. Washington, DC, American Psychiatric Publishing, 2002, pp 3–11

Mellinger G, Balter M, Uhlenhuth E: Prevalence and correlates of the long-term regular use of anxiolytics. JAMA 251:375–379, 1984

Regier D, Narrow WE, Rae DS, et al: The de facto US mental and addictive disorders service system: Epidemiologic Catchment Area prospective 1-year prevalence rates of disorders and services. Arch Gen Psychiatry 50:85–94, 1993

Saravay SM, Lavin M: Psychiatric comorbidity and length of stay in the general hospital: a review of outcome studies. Psychosomatics 35:233–252, 1994

Schurman RA, Kramer PD, Mitchell JB: The hidden mental health network: treatment of mental illness by nonpsychiatric physicians. Arch Gen Psychiatry 42:89–94, 1985

Shakin Kunkel EJ, Monti DA, Thompson TL II: Consultation, liaison, and administration of a consultation-liaison psychiatry service, in The American Psychiatric Publishing Textbook of Consultation-Liaison Psychiatry: Psychiatry in the Medically Ill, 2nd Edition. Edited by Wise MG, Rundell JR. Washington, DC, American Psychiatric Publishing, 2002, pp 13–23

Simon GE, Walker EA: The primary care clinic, in The American Psychiatric Publishing Textbook of Consultation-Liaison Psychiatry: Psychiatry in the Medically Ill, 2nd Edition. Edited by Wise MG, Rundell JR. Washington, DC, American Psychiatric Publishing, 2002, pp 917–925

Simon G, VonKorff M, Wagner EH, et al: Patterns of antidepressant use in community practice. Gen Hosp Psychiatry 15:399–408, 1993

Spitzer RL, Williams JB, Kroenke K, et al: Utility of a new procedure for diagnosing mental disorders in primary care: the PRIME-MD 1000 study. JAMA 272:1749–1756, 1994

Strain JJ: Liaison psychiatry, in Modern Perspectives in Clinical Psychiatry. Edited by Howells JG. New York, Brunner/Mazel, 1988, pp 76–101

Strain JJ: Liaison psychiatry, in The American Psychiatric Publishing Textbook of Consultation-Liaison Psychiatry: Psychiatry in the Medically Ill, 2nd Edition. Edited by Wise MG, Rundell JR. Washington, DC, American Psychiatric Publishing, 2002, pp 33–48

Strain JJ, Lyons JS, Hammer JS, et al: Cost offset from a psychiatric consultation-liaison intervention with elderly hip fracture patients. Am J Psychiatry 148:1044–1049, 1991

Ustun TB, Sartorius N: Mental Illness in General Health Care. New York, Wiley, 1995

Additional Readings

Borus JF, Barsky AJ, Carbone LA, et al: Consultation-liaison cost offset: searching the wrong grail (editorial). Psychosomatics 41:285–288, 2000

Covinsky KE, Kahana I, Chin MH, et al: Depressive symptoms and 3-year mortality in older hospitalized medical patients. Ann Intern Med 130:563–569, 1999

Goldberg RJ: Financial management challenges for general hospital psychiatry. Gen Hosp Psychiatry 23:67–72, 2001

Goldman L, Lee T, Rudd P: Ten commandments for effective consultation. Arch Intern Med 143:1753–1755, 1983

Lane D, Carroll D, Ring C, et al: Mortality and quality of life 12 months after myocardial infarction: effects of depression and anxiety. Psychosom Med 63:221–230, 2001

Penninx BW, Beekman AT, Honig A, et al: Depression and cardiac mortality: results from a community-based longitudinal study. Arch Gen Psychiatry 58:221–227, 2001

2

Mental Status Examination and Other Tests of Brain Function

The patient's mental status examination (MSE) results reflect mental and psychological function at a particular point in time—in this case, it is the time of the consultation—and are fully appreciated only when placed in the context of the patient's history and recent behavior, neurological and physical examination, and laboratory and other information. Cognitive impairment occurs frequently in elderly patients who are medically ill, especially those who are hospitalized. Unless it is severe, this impairment is often not recognized by nonpsychiatric physicians and medical personnel (Laurila et al. 2004). The consulting psychiatrist also may miss the cognitive impairment if he or she depends too much on conversation during the interview to identify impairments and does not formally test brain function. The lack of formal testing may endanger the patient. Just as a cardiologist uses stress testing to detect cardiac ischemia, the consultation psychiatrist must test cognitive function with the MSE. Also, tests of right-hemisphere, or nondominant, brain function are as important as more traditional tests of verbal function that are the domain of the left hemisphere. The psychiatrist who asks the patient to remember verbal items but does not have the patient draw and recall shapes succumbs to this pitfall and essentially ignores testing a major part of the brain's function (Ovsiew 1992).

Testing a patient's mental status in the hospital environment is difficult. Hospital rooms are noisy, and privacy is lacking. Interruptions and distractions, such as intravenous alarms, a roommate who is groaning or loudly talking with visitors, and a harried nurse or phlebotomist who must have immediate access to the patient, are common. In addition, the patient is ill, often frightened, and usually sleep deprived; in most cases, he or she has not seen a psychiatrist before and was not told about the consultation. Before the examination begins, the psychiatrist should ensure that the patient has his or her usual sensory aids (e.g., glasses and/or hearing aid). Whenever possible, roommates and others, including family members, should be asked to leave the room during the examination. This provides some privacy and also prevents significant others from answering for the patient when mental status questions are asked.

The MSE has both informal (less-structured portions) and formal (structured questions or tests) parts. It is also useful to divide the MSE and your report of that examination into two general categories: noncognitive and cognitive components (Table 2–1).

Table 2–1. Components of the mental status examination

Noncognitive	Cognitive
General appearance and behavior	Level of consciousness
Mood and affect	Attention
Thought processes and content	Speech and language
Perceptions	Orientation
Abstracting abilities	Memory
Judgment and insight	

Source.   Reprinted from Strub RL, Wise MG: "Differential Diagnosis in Neuropsychiatry," in *The American Psychiatric Press Textbook of Neuropsychiatry,* 2nd Edition. Edited by Yudofsky SC, Hales RE. Washington, DC, American Psychiatric Press, 1992, p. 231. Copyright 1992, American Psychiatric Press. Used with permission.

Mental Status Examination

Noncognitive Components

General Appearance and Behavior

The MSE begins the instant the clinician sees the patient. The patient's physical appearance, attitude, and behaviors, such as increased or decreased body movements, posturing, pacing, tremors, and choreiform or dyskinetic movements, should be described without the use of jargon.

Mood and Affect

Mood is the patient's pervasive and sustained emotional state. Terms used to describe mood are *depressed, angry, elevated, euthymic, expansive,* and *irritable.* The parameters to describe *affect*—the patient's moment-to-moment emotional states—are *range, intensity, lability,* and *appropriateness.* Affective range may be full (the patient shows a wide range of emotional states during the interview) or restricted to a particular state, such as depressed. Affective intensity among patients also can vary greatly (e.g., from the extreme rage seen in a patient with borderline personality disorder to the flat or affectless expression typically observed in a patient with Parkinson's disease). Affective lability (i.e., extremely rapid emotional shifts) often implies a toxic or medical etiology. Affect is also described as either appropriate or inappropriate to the topics under discussion.

Thought Processes and Content

Thought processes and thought content are judged by the patient's quality and quantity of speech and his or her behavior (Strub and Wise 1992). When the clinician asks the patient a question, how does he or she respond? Is the answer given responsive to the question asked (goal directed), or does he or she ramble (tangential)? The pattern of thoughts is also an important measure of thought processes. The patient's thoughts may move extremely rapidly from one idea to another (flight of ideas), may not relate in an appropriate way (loose associations), or may stop suddenly (thought blocking). The patient's thought content or major themes reflect the patient's immediate concerns, including obsessional preoccupation, suicidal or homicidal ideation, and irrational beliefs. The patient's behavior also reflects thought content. A patient who is reluctant to talk and acts very suspiciously is usually paranoid, even if he or she denies it. The patient who denies misperceptions but is seen responding to hallucinations illustrates the importance of observed behavior in the assessment of thought content.

Perceptions

Disorders of perception include illusions (misinterpretations of a real sensory experience), hallucinations (sensory perceptions in the absence of an external stimulus), delusions (fixed false beliefs), and ideas of reference (incorrect interpretations that events have direct reference to oneself). Hallucinatory perception can be visual, auditory, tactile, olfactory (smell), gustatory (taste), or kinesthetic (body movement). Although cultural variations occur, hallucinations that occur in an awake individual are almost always symptomatic of a pathological process. Auditory hallucinations are more typically seen in primary psychiatric disorders. Visual hallucinations are typically associated with brain dysfunction, although they also occur in nonpsychiatric patients with severe recent visual loss and in some patients with schizophrenia (Bracha et al. 1989). Tactile hallucinations occur commonly in patients who have had a limb amputation or substance-induced withdrawal delirium. "Phantom limb" sensation, the feeling that the amputated limb is still present, occurs in most patients who undergo amputation. Over time, the tactile hallucinations diminish and usually completely disappear. Olfactory, gustatory, or kinesthetic hallucinations are rare and are most commonly experienced by patients with partial seizures (Lishman 1998).

Abstracting Abilities

Educational level is a strong determinant of one's ability to abstract. The clinician usually conducts bedside testing by asking the patient to interpret proverbs, such as "A stitch in time saves nine." Concrete interpretations are commonly given by individuals with less than a high school education, schizophrenia (interpretations are also often bizarre), and dementia.

Judgment and Insight

Judgment is an individual's ability to correctly anticipate the consequences of one's behavior and to behave in a culturally acceptable way. Although judgment is often inferred by the answer to a question, such as "What would you do if you found a stamped, addressed envelope lying next to a mailbox?" The fact that a patient would put the aforementioned envelope in the mailbox does not mean that judgment is unimpaired, especially if that patient has just walked into the hospital hallway naked and recently urinated in the corner of his room. Recent behavior is the best way to gauge a patient's judgment. In general, insight is present if the patient realizes that a problem exists, that his or her thinking and behavior may contribute to that problem, and that he or she may need assistance.

Cognitive Components

Level of Consciousness

Psychiatric consultation is often requested for patients who have a rapid or recent change in mental status. In many instances, these patients are either lethargic or agitated following surgery, have started taking a new medication, or have significant changes in metabolic status. In addition to changes in arousal, such patients often have hallucinations and altered thought content.

Attention

The capacity to direct and maintain one's attention while screening out extraneous and irrelevant stimuli is a fundamental yet highly complex cognitive function. Inattention (the breakdown of selective attention) and distractibility are common and clinically significant neuropsychiatric symptoms. Inattention also can complicate the entire evaluation process (Mesulam 1985). For example, an inattentive patient will frequently fail tests of memory or calculation on the basis of inattention alone. Digit span is a standard psychological test for attention.

Speech and Language

Brain disease, particularly dominant-hemisphere insults, frequently disrupts a patient's speech and language. Speech defects include the slurred speech of the intoxicated patient; the soft, trailing speech of the patient with Parkinson's disease; and the dysphonia and dysarthria of the patient with amyotrophic lateral sclerosis. Language disturbances, specifically aphasias, refer to defects in word choice, comprehension, and syntax (Table 2–2). The patient's spontaneous speech should be observed and its rate, rhythm, and fluency described. Is speech fluent, and does the patient make sense? Next, comprehension must be tested. This is particularly important when the patient is on a respirator and normal speech is not possible. The clinician can ask yes-and-no ques-

Table 2–2.   Review of aphasias

Type	Speech	Compre-hension	Repetition	Naming	Writing	Reading	Associated deficits	Emotional reaction
			Characteristic					
Broca's	Nonfluent	Relatively intact	Impaired	Impaired	Impaired	Impaired	Right hemiparesis	Despair
(Patient cannot articulate and is frustrated; speech is sparse [or absent] and telegraphic.)								
Wernicke's	Fluent	Impaired	Impaired	Impaired	Impaired	Impaired	Hemianopsia ± hemisensory loss	Unaware
(Patient articulates well but speaks nonsense and does not understand.)								
Conduction	Fluent	Relatively intact	Impaired	Impaired	±Impaired	Relatively intact	±Hemisensory loss	Frustration
(Like Wernicke's aphasia except patient can understand and is aware of deficits.)								
Anomic	Fluent	Intact	Intact	Impaired	±Impaired	Intact	Varies	±Aware
(Patient cannot name objects but describes their use; makes lame excuses for deficit.)								
Global	Nonfluent	Impaired	Impaired	Impaired	Impaired	Impaired	Right hemiparesis, hemisensory loss, hemianopsia	Unaware

(Very large lesion, marked impairment.)

Source.   Reprinted from Wise MG, Rundell JR: *Concise Guide to Consultation Psychiatry*, 2nd Edition. Washington, DC, American Psychiatric Press, 1994, p. 13. Copyright 1994, American Psychiatric Press. Used with permission.

tions, such as "Do you put on your socks before your shoes?," "Is there a tree in the room?," and "Can an elephant ride a tricycle?"

Orientation

The psychiatrist should record the patient's orientation to self, place, situational awareness, and time. Serial measurement of orientation provides valuable longitudinal and treatment outcome data. The clinician should not rely on an "oriented × 4" entry in the medical chart. That usually means that the patient is pleasant and cooperative; it does not mean that the patient's orientation was tested or that he or she is not delirious.

Memory

The clinician should ask the patient to remember four unrelated items, such as tulip, eyedropper, ball, and brown (Strub and Black 2000). The patient should immediately repeat all four words to ensure that he or she has properly heard and understood them. After about 3 minutes of conversation or examination, the clinician should ask the patient to repeat the words. If the patient cannot recall the words, the clinician should give the patient clues to determine whether the words were not encoded into memory or were encoded but are difficult to retrieve. Patients who did not learn the words are not aided by prompting, whereas patients who learned the words but have difficulty accessing them usually will recall with prompting. The patient should also be asked to copy three objects and then, after several minutes, draw them from memory.

Screening Mental Status Examinations

Several bedside examinations are used to screen patients for cognitive dysfunction. Screening examinations have advantages and disadvantages (Table 2–3). For nonpsychiatric physicians who do not typically perform a formal MSE or for medical students who are learning to treat mental status problems, screening MSEs are useful. Also, the score obtained from a screening MSE, such as the Mini-Mental State Exam (MMSE), may influence a physician who doubts that the patient is cognitively impaired but believes "hard data." However, for the consultation psychiatrist, who is (or should be) an expert in measuring cognition, a screening MSE is only one part of a more extensive cognitive examination. A screening MSE is relatively insensitive and

Table 2–3. Advantages and disadvantages of screening mental status examinations (MSEs)

Advantages

Brief (usually take only 5–10 minutes)

Structured format

Single score (uncomplicated)

Face validity (questions from traditional MSE)

Familiar (questions from traditional MSE)

Less fatiguing for medically ill patients

Used repeatedly to monitor course of cognitive function

Disadvantages

Fail to identify focal deficits (high false-negative rate)

Fail to identify mild global deficits (low sensitivity)

Fail to identify well-educated patient with significant deficits

May create false sense of security when score indicates "normal" function

Education dependent (score likely to be lower for patients with less than an eighth-grade education)

Few validation studies with outpatients

Few studies on the effect of sociodemographic factors

Source. Adapted from Wise MG, Rundell JR: *Concise Guide to Consultation Psychiatry,* 2nd Edition. Washington, DC, American Psychiatric Press, 1994, p. 18. Copyright 1994, American Psychiatric Press. Used with permission.

will often miss mild to moderate confusion and inadequately tests nondominant hemispheric brain function. In addition, serial screening MSEs are often used to follow up the clinical course of a patient with delirium or dementia, especially a response to treatment.

Folstein's MMSE (Folstein et al. 1975) is probably the most widely used and best-known screening MSE. The MMSE takes about 5 minutes to administer, can be administered serially to monitor a patient's clinical course, and is a reliable and valid test in medical patients (Nelson et al. 1986). Various MMSE cutoff scores are proposed to indicate delirium or dementia. A score of 20 or less may indicate impairment (Folstein et al. 1975); however, Mungas (1991) proposed that a score of 0–10 corresponds to severe cognitive impairment, 11–20 to moderate impairment, 20–25 to mild impairment, and 25–30 to questionable impairment or intact function. A high score on the MMSE is insufficient to declare that the patient has normal cognitive function. Many patients who had delirium according to an electroencephalogram scored in the 20–29 range out of 30 on the MMSE (M.G. Wise, unpublished data, 1989).

Other Useful Tests of Cognitive Function

The consultation psychiatrist must be an expert in selection, administration, and meaning of cognitive tests, even when the patient is bedridden or on a respirator. In this section, we describe several essential, clinically useful, tests. Lishman's (1998) classic text has an excellent detailed discussion of cognitive function and psychometric tests.

The *Bender-Gestalt Test* (Bender 1938) examines the patient's ability to copy designs. During a full protocol, nine designs are presented to the patient, one at a time, and he or she is asked to copy them. Errors suggest brain dysfunction, and error-free performance strongly supports the absence of brain disease. Visual memory can be tested by asking the patient to reproduce the figures from memory after a brief period has elapsed. One can select and carry three or four of these cards for testing at the bedside.

The *Blessed Dementia Scale* has two parts, which are used separately or together (Blessed et al. 1968). One part measures the patient's ability to perform everyday activities, and the second part measures the patient's ability to perform an information-memory-concentration test. Information about daily activities is provided by a knowledgeable family member or close friend. The Blessed Dementia Scale does not have a cutoff score to establish the diagnosis of dementia. Instead, an increasing score correlates with worsening dementia.

The *Clock Drawing Test* is a very useful bedside test and is part of a basic MSE (Lishman 1998). Many examiners prefer to hand the patient a blank sheet of paper and ask him or her to draw the entire clock, including the circle; however, patients often will draw a small circle and scribble numbers inside. This makes assessment of dyspraxia impossible, especially if the patient is mildly impaired. For this reason, we recommend that the patient be given a sheet of paper with a large circle already drawn on it and then be instructed, "Write in the numbers as if this circle is the face of a clock." After the patient is partially finished with the task, the psychiatrist should interject, "When you finish, draw in the hand of the clock so that the time says 10 until 11 o'clock." Note that the time requested can simplify the task (e.g., 3 o'clock) or make it more complicated, as in the previous example. This task is easy to administer and is very instructive, particularly for documenting construction-al apraxia and, therefore, early dementia (Esteban-Santillan et al. 1998) or de-lirium (Trzepacz and Meagher 2004). At least five methods are used to score the Clock Drawing Test (Richardson and Glass 2002). (See Figure 3–2 in Chapter 3, "Delirium," in this book for a demonstration of this test.)

The *Frank Jones story* tests the patient's ability to conceptualize a situation and to solve a problem. The patient is asked to explain the following story: "I have a friend by the name of Frank Jones whose feet are so big that he has to put on his pants by pulling them over his head." The psychiatrist should watch the patient's immediate response closely (i.e., does the patient in-stantly smile or appear puzzled and confused?). Then the psychiatrist asks the patient, "Can Mr. Jones do that?" A patient with normal cognitive function will laugh and explain in an understandable way why it is impossible. When patients with cognitive difficulties hear the story, they often do not laugh because they do not "get it." They are also unable to rationally explain their response. Patients with delirium may laugh (they seem to understand), but their explanations often are bizarre. For example, "He can't...well, maybe he can if he unzips his fly," "He just can't," or "I guess so if he takes off his shoes."

The *Marie Three Paper Test* provides a quick assessment for comprehen-sion and receptive aphasia (Lishman 1998). Three different-sized pieces of paper are placed in front of the patient. The patient is asked to take the big-gest piece and hand it to the examiner, take the smallest piece and throw it to the ground, and take the middle-sized one and place it in his or her pocket.

The *Reitan-Indiana Aphasia Screening Test* is a pocket-sized, easily admin-istered, brief aphasia screen (Reitan 1984). This test gives a reasonable survey of aphasic symptoms, including ability to copy, name, spell, write, read, cal-culate, and demonstrate the use of an object (ideomotor praxis).

The *Set Test* is a test of verbal fluency designed to screen elderly patients for dementia (Isaacs and Kennie 1973). The patient is asked to name 10 items from each of four categories. A useful mnemonic to recall the four categories is F-A-C-T (fruits-animals-colors-towns). The patient is asked to name 10 fruits, then to name 10 animals, and so on. The score is the total number of items correctly named, with a maximum score of 40. In patients aged 65 or older, scores lower than 15 are clearly abnormal and indicate impairment. (Note: this is not a timed test. It is an excellent test for frontal lobe dysfunction and is a great distraction after presenting four words to remember.)

The *Trail Making Test (Trail Parts A and B)* consists of several circles distributed on a sheet of paper (Reitan 1958). In Part A, the circles contain numbers, and the patient is asked to connect the numbers in sequence by drawing a line as quickly as possible from one circle to the next. In Part B, each circle contains either a number or a letter. The patient is asked to alternate between numbers and letters (i.e., 1, then A, then 2, then B, and so on). Trail Parts A and B are timed, and age-corrected norms are available. More than one error on either test is usually significant.

The *Vigilance Test* measures the patient's ability to sustain attention. For example, a series of letters is read at a rate of one per second, and the patient is asked to raise his or her hand each time the letter *A* is read.

Other useful bedside tests include a sheet of paper with drawings on one side for the patient to copy and a series of mathematical problems on the other side. The problems should vary from very simple (e.g., $1+7=\_$) to more complex (e.g., $9,798 \div 23 = \_\_\_$). Observing the patient while he or she attempts to draw and calculate is quite informative, both about brain function and about the patient's personality style.

Tests of Executive Function

Executive function is often used to describe mental processes used to initiate, maintain, and organize the flow of information and to coordinate actions. Examples of these processes include attention allocation, goal maintenance, and other functions that stabilize performance. Several of the tests already mentioned, such as the Trail Making Test (Part B), the Set Test, and the Clock Drawing Test, are used to test executive function (frontal lobe). Other tests used include the Stroop Test, Wisconsin Card Sorting Test (WCST), and estimation questions.

The *Stroop Test* is derived from the natural interference that occurs when a color word, such as *blue,* is written in an incongruently colored ink such as red. The patient is shown a list of such words and is asked to read them aloud. Then, the patient is shown another list and is asked to say the color of the ink used. The number of correct answers given during a set time is compared with norms.

The *WCST* consists of 64 cards. Each card has from one to four stars, triangles, crosses, or circles displayed in one of four colors. Stimulus cards are laid out, so that the subject can sort cards according to color, form, or number. The examiner responds "right" or "wrong" to the subject's trial-and-error choices. After the subject makes 10 consecutive correct color responses, the clinician should, without warning, change the organizing principle to form. After the subject makes 10 consecutive correct form responses, without warning, the clinician should change the organizing principle to number (and so on). A total score is obtained, along with the number of perseverative and nonperseverative errors.

Neurological Examination

A basic bedside neurological examination is essential in any patient with cognitive dysfunction, suspected somatoform or conversion disorder with neurological complaints, or malingering. The examination does not need to be time-consuming. Often, the patient's history suggests deficits and helps focus the examination.

In a basic neurological examination, the clinician should do the following:

1. Check deep tendon reflexes for symmetry. Check for the presence of a Babinski reflex. Some clinicians also check for primitive reflexes (snout, grasp, glabellar, and palmomental).
2. Check muscle strength for asymmetry, weakness, tone, or embellishment.
3. When possible, observe gait and associated arm movements.
4. Examine cranial nerve function.
5. Check the distribution of any sensory complaints.
6. Check for signs of meningeal irritation, such as neck stiffness, headache, or Kernig's and Brudzinski's signs.

The Consultation Psychiatrist as Neuropsychiatrist

The ability to correlate neuropsychiatric or behavioral dysfunction with cortical anatomy is difficult. It requires skill and practice and is not an exact sci-

Table 2–4. Cortical mapping of brain dysfunction

Abnormality	Frontal	Dominant temporo-parietal	Dominant parietal	Nondominant parietal	Nondominant temporo-parietal	Occipital	Corpus callosum
Motor	Motor impersistence Inertia Impaired rapid sequential movements Stimulus-bound behavior (e.g., echopraxia, gegenhalten)	Dysgraphia	Ideokinetic (ideomotor) dyspraxia Kinesthetic dyspraxia	Constructional dyspraxia Dressing dyspraxia Kinesthetic dyspraxia			Inability to tie shoes with eyes closed Ideokinetic dyspraxia in hand ipsilateral to dominant hemisphere Constructional dyspraxia in hand contralateral to dominant hemisphere Alexia without agraphia

Table 2–4.   Cortical mapping of brain dysfunction (*continued*)

Abnormality	Frontal	Dominant temporo-parietal	Dominant parietal	Nondominant parietal	Nondominant temporo-parietal	Occipital	Corpus callosum
Language	Broca's aphasia Transcortical aphasia Motor aprosody[a] Verbigeration	Wernicke's aphasia Driveling, word approximations, neologisms, stock phrases, phonemic paraphasias, private use of words Pure word deafness Dysgraphia Dyslexia Dysnomia Letter agnosia Number agnosia Sensory aprosodia	Dyslexia Dysnomia				

Table 2–4.   Cortical mapping of brain dysfunction (continued)

Abnormality	Frontal	Dominant temporo-parietal	Dominant parietal	Nondominant parietal	Nondominant temporo-parietal	Occipital	Corpus callosum
Memory	Impaired short-term memory store	Impairment of rehearsed consolidated memory			Impaired musical memory	Impaired visual memory	
Other	Impaired concentration Global disorientation Impaired judgment Impaired problem solving Impaired abstraction Right spatial neglect		Finger agnosia Dyscalculia Right-left disorientation East-west disorientation Dysstereognosis Dysgraphesthesia Impaired symbolic categorization	Dysstereognosis Dysgraphesthesia Anosognosia Prosopagnosia Paragnosia Reduplicative paramnesia Left spatial neglect			Dysstereognosis of hand ipsilateral to dominant hemisphere Dysgraphesthesia of hand ipsilateral to dominant hemisphere

[a]Nondominant frontal lobe.

Source.   Modified from Taylor MA, Sierles FS, Abrams R: *The American Psychiatric Press Textbook of Neuropsychiatry.* Edited by Hales RE, Yudofsky SC. Washington, DC, American Psychiatric Press, 1987, p. 6. Copyright 1987, American Psychiatric Press. Used with permission.

ence. Approximate cortical localization of various cognitive and behavioral functions is summarized in Table 2–4.

Knowledge of brain-behavior relationships is important for psychiatrists to function well as consultants in the hospital setting. The psychiatrist also must understand neurological terminology. The following list contains a few commonly used neurological terms. The prefix *a-* means complete loss of ability (e.g., aphasia is the loss of ability to comprehend or express speech), and the prefix *dys-* means an impaired ability, as in the following examples:

- *Dysarthria*—disturbance of articulation of speech caused by muscle dysfunction
- *Dysbulia*—decrease in willpower
- *Dyscalculia*—impaired ability to do mathematical calculations
- *Dysgnosia*—impaired ability to recognize the importance of sensory impressions
- *Dysgraphia*—impaired ability to express thought in writing
- *Dyslexia*—impaired ability to read
- *Dysphasia*—impaired ability to comprehend, elaborate, or express speech
- *Dyspraxia*—impaired ability to use objects correctly
- *Dysprosody*—disturbance of pitch, rhythm, and variation of speech
- *Dystaxia*—impaired motor coordination

References

Bender L: A Visual-Motor Gestalt Test and Its Clinical Use. New York, American Orthopsychiatric Association, 1938

Blessed G, Tomilinson BE, Roth M: The association between quantitative measures of dementia and of senile change in the cerebral grey matter of elderly subjects. Br J Psychiatry 114:797–811, 1968

Bracha HS, Wolkowitz OM, Lohr JB, et al: High prevalence of visual hallucination in research subjects with chronic schizophrenia. Am J Psychiatry 146:526–528, 1989

Esteban-Santillan C, Praditsuwan R, Ueda H, et al: Clock drawing test in very mild Alzheimer's disease. J Am Geriatr Soc 46:1266–1269, 1998

Folstein MF, Folstein SE, McHugh PR: 'Mini-Mental State': a practical method for grading the cognitive state of patients for the clinician. J Psychiatr Res 12:189–198, 1975

Isaacs B, Kennie AT: The Set Test as an aid to the detection of dementia in old people. Br J Psychiatry 123:467–470, 1973

Laurila JV, Pitkala KH, Strandberg TE, et al: Detection and documentation of dementia and delirium in acute geriatric wards. Gen Hosp Psychiatry 26:31–35, 2004

Lishman WA: Organic Psychiatry: The Psychological Consequences of Cerebral Disorder, 3rd Edition. Oxford, England, Blackwell Scientific, 1998

Mesulam M-M: Attention, confusional states, and neglect, in Principles of Behavioral Neurology. Edited by Mesulam M-M. Philadelphia, PA, FA Davis, 1985, pp 125–140

Mungas D: In-office mental status testing: a practical guide. Geriatrics 46:54–66, 1991

Nelson A, Fogel BS, Faust D: Bedside cognitive screening instruments: a critical assessment. J Nerv Ment Dis 174:73–83, 1986

Ovsiew F: Bedside neuropsychiatry: eliciting the clinical phenomena of neuropsychiatric illness, in The American Psychiatric Press Textbook of Neuropsychiatry, 2nd Edition. Edited by Yudofsky SC, Hales RE. Washington, DC, American Psychiatric Press, 1992, pp 89–126

Reitan RM: Validity of the Trail Making Test as an indicator of organic brain damage. Percept Mot Skills 8:271–276, 1958

Reitan RM: Aphasia and Sensory-Perceptual Deficits in Adults. Tucson, AZ, Neuropsychology Press, 1984

Richardson HE, Glass JN: A comparison of scoring protocol on the Clock Drawing Test in relation to ease of use, diagnostic group, and correlation with the Mini-Mental State Examination. J Am Geriatr Soc 50:169–173, 2002

Strub RL, Black FW: The Mental Status Examination in Neurology, 4th Edition. Philadelphia, PA, FA Davis, 2000

Strub RL, Wise MG: Differential diagnosis in neuropsychiatry, in The American Psychiatric Press Textbook of Neuropsychiatry, 2nd Edition. Edited by Yudofsky SC, Hales RE. Washington, DC, American Psychiatric Press, 1992, pp 227–243

Trzepacz PT, Meagher DJ: Delirium, in The American Psychiatric Publishing Textbook of Psychosomatic Medicine. Edited by Levenson JL. Washington, DC, American Psychiatric Publishing, 2004, pp 91–130

Additional Reading

Feher EP, Doody R, Pirozzolo FJ, et al: Mental status assessment of insight and judgment. Clin Geriatr Med 5:477–498, 1989

3

Delirium

Delirium is a transient, reversible, global dysfunction in cerebral metabolism that has an acute onset (more rarely, a subacute onset). Delirium has many aliases: acute brain failure, acute brain syndrome, encephalopathy, confusional state, reversible dementia, and intensive care unit (ICU) psychosis. The term *ICU psychosis* should be abandoned. It infers a cause-and-effect relation between the ICU setting and delirium and thus implies that no clinical action is necessary. No more evidence exists for ICU psychosis than for ICU arrhythmias or ICU seizures. Delirium is gradually receiving more attention from psychiatrists and other physicians, and the American Psychiatric Association (1999) has published delirium practice guidelines.

Epidemiology and Risk Factors

Delirium occurs in about 15%–18% of patients aged 65 years or older on medical and surgical wards (Trzepacz et al. 2004). Its prevalence is even higher in certain populations—30% in post–coronary artery bypass graft (CABG) surgery patients, 40% in post–hip surgery patients and patients with advanced cancer, and 81% in ICU patients on mechanical ventilators (Ely et al. 2004). The mortality associated with this psychiatric disorder is high; delirium indicates impending death in 25% of patients (Folstein et al. 1991). In addition to an increased risk of mortality, patients with delirium stay in the hospital longer than nondelirious patients (Ely et al. 2004; Marcantonio et al. 1994).

Patients who are at increased risk for delirium (Figure 3–1) include the elderly (who often also have dementia and medical morbidity), patients with central nervous system (CNS) disorders (e.g., stroke, Parkinson's disease, HIV infection), postsurgical patients (e.g., postcardiotomy, posttransplantation, post–hip surgery), burn patients, and drug-dependent patients who are experiencing withdrawal. If children are excluded, the incidence of delirium increases with the age of the patient population studied, with the highest risk group usually being patients age 60 and older (Lipowski 1990). Increasing age is also associated with increasing prevalence of dementia, which is itself an independent risk factor for delirium.

Preexisting brain damage, whether preoperative CNS neurological abnormalities (Koponen and Riekkinen 1993; Marcantonio et al. 1994) or dementia (Kolbeinsson and Jonsson 1993), lowers the patient's threshold for developing delirium. The aging brain has less "cerebral reserve" and flexibility in the face of physiological perturbations, including changes in vasculature, decreased cholinergic activity, and increased monoamine oxidase activity; all of these may increase an individual's vulnerability to delirium. Even with a relatively minor insult, such as a urinary tract infection, elderly patients are more likely than younger adults to develop delirium.

Clinical Characteristics

Diagnostic Criteria

DSM-IV-TR (American Psychiatric Association 2000) diagnostic criteria for delirium are listed in Table 3–1. The core characteristics are impairment of consciousness and reduced ability to focus or sustain attention. Other DSM-IV-TR criteria are an acute change in cognition (onset usually over hours to days) that is not better accounted for by dementia and mental status fluctuations during the day. When delirium is present, a specific diagnosis is made

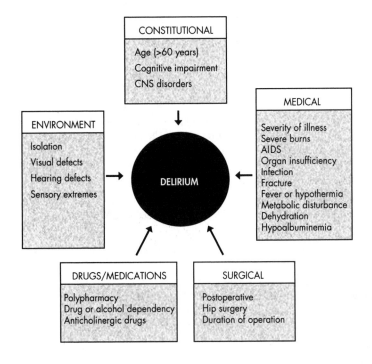

Figure 3–1.   Risk factors for developing delirium.

Note.   CNS = central nervous system.
Source.   Adapted from Trzepacz PT, Meagher DJ, Wise MG. "Neuropsychiatric aspects of Delirium," in *Essentials of Neuropsychiatry and Clinical Neurosciences.* Edited by Yudofsky SC, Hales RE. Washington, DC, American Psychiatric Publishing, 2004, pp. 141–187. Copyright 2004, American Psychiatric Publishing. Used with permission.

based on etiology. If an etiology is determined, the diagnosis is delirium due to a general medical condition (e.g., delirium due to hepatic encephalopathy or delirium due to hypoglycemia), substance-induced delirium (including medication side effects), or delirium due to multiple etiologies. If the clinician is unable to determine a specific etiology, a diagnosis of delirium not otherwise specified is made.

Table 3–1.   DSM-IV-TR diagnostic criteria for delirium due to . . .
[indicate the general medical condition]

A.   Disturbance of consciousness (i.e., reduced clarity of awareness of the environment) with reduced ability to focus, sustain, or shift attention.

B.   A change in cognition (such as memory deficit, disorientation, language disturbance) or the development of a perceptual disturbance that is not better accounted for by a preexisting, established, or evolving dementia.

C.   The disturbance develops over a short period of time (usually hours to days) and tends to fluctuate during the course of the day.

D.   There is evidence from the history, physical examination, or laboratory findings that the disturbance is caused by the direct physiological consequences of a general medical condition.

Coding note: If delirium is superimposed on a preexisting Vascular Dementia, indicate the delirium by coding 290.41 Vascular Dementia, With Delirium.

Coding note: Include the name of the general medical condition on Axis I, e.g., 293.0 Delirium Due to Hepatic Encephalopathy; also code the general medical condition on Axis III.

Source.   Reprinted from American Psychiatric Association: *Diagnostic and Statistical Manual of Mental Disorders,* 4th Edition, Text Revision. Washington, DC, American Psychiatric Association, 2000. Used with permission.

Prodrome

Some patients manifest symptoms, such as restlessness, anxiety, irritability, distractibility, or sleep disruption, immediately prior to the onset of an overt delirium. Review of the patient's hospital medical chart, particularly the nursing notes, often identifies prodromal features.

Temporal Course

Two features of the temporal course of delirium are characteristic and assist in differential diagnosis: 1) abrupt or acute onset of symptoms and 2) fluctuation of symptom severity during an episode. Waxing and waning of symptoms typically occur, with relatively lucid intervals fluctuating with more severe symptoms; careful examination usually shows continued, although more subtle, cognitive impairment even during lucid periods.

Neuropsychiatric Impairment

The patient with delirium has difficulty sustaining attention and is usually either distractible or unable to focus. Short-term memory is impaired. In the presence of impaired registration, memory difficulties may be secondary to attention deficits. After recovering from delirium, some patients are amnestic for the entire episode, others have islands of memory, and a few will recall the entire episode. Disorientation to time and place is typical in delirium. Patients often have visuoconstructional impairment and are unable to copy simple geometric designs or to draw more complex figures such as a clock face (see Figure 3–2 later in this chapter; see also Chapter 2: "Mental Status Examination and Other Tests of Brain Function"). Clock face drawing requires input from the nondominant parietal cortex for overall spatial proportions and relations, from the dominant parietal cortex for details such as numbers or hands, and from the prefrontal cortex for understanding the concept of time. Many higher-level executive functions are subserved by the prefrontal cortices, especially the dorsolateral region. These functions, including switching mental sets, abstraction, sequential thinking, verbal fluency, temporal memory, and judgment, are affected in delirium (Trzepacz 1994).

Patients with delirium often have disorganized thought patterns. The severity of the thought disturbance can range from tangentiality and circumstantiality to loose associations. At the most severe level of thought disorganization, speech may resemble a fluent aphasia (Wise and Trzepacz 1999). Language impairments range from mild dysarthria or mumbling to dysphasia or muteness. Word-finding difficulty, dysnomia with paraphasias, and reduced comprehension are common.

Perceptual Disturbances

The patient with delirium often experiences misperceptions, usually illusions or hallucinations. Illusions and hallucinations can be auditory or visual; the latter are more common. Tactile, gustatory, and olfactory hallucinations are less common.

Psychomotor Disturbances

Some patients with delirium are hypoactive, others are hyperactive, and a significant number alternate between these two states. A hyperactive delirium, such as delirium tremens (DTs), is rarely undetected. This is not the case for hypoactive delirium. The patient with hypoactive delirium often goes unnoticed or receives an incorrect label, such as depressed, unmotivated, having a character disorder, or uncooperative. On neurological examination, motor findings may include tremor, myoclonus, asterixis, and reflex or muscle tone changes. The tremor associated with delirium, particularly toxic-metabolic, is generally absent at rest but apparent during movement (action or intention tremors).

Sleep-Wake Cycle Disturbances

During delirium, the patient's normal diurnal rhythm is often reversed, with lethargy during the day and arousal during the night. Normalization of sleep is an important treatment goal. Reduction of external cues during the night may increase disorientation or paranoia and result in agitation and "sundowning."

Abnormal Electroencephalogram Findings

Electroencephalogram (EEG) changes virtually always accompany delirium. Hepatic encephalopathy is classically associated with severe slowing, including triphasic delta waves. Figure 3–2 shows the correlation among the EEG, Clock Drawing Test, and mental status; these patients all had delirium secondary to toxic-metabolic etiologies. Less typically, the EEG pattern in delirium is characterized by excess low-voltage beta waves, as seen most typically in DTs (Kennard et al. 1945). Patients with delirium caused by anticholinergic toxicity or posttraumatic brain injury show electroencephalographic slowing (Trzepacz 1994).

Unfortunately, a given individual's normal dominant posterior rhythm could be slowed but still be in the normal alpha range and, therefore, be read as "normal." For example, a patient's usual background characteristic alpha rhythm is 13 Hz; when it slows to 9 Hz, it is technically still in the normal alpha range. The only way to document this abnormality is to compare the EEG with a previous baseline EEG or with a repeat EEG done after the delirium clears.

Differential Diagnosis

The differential diagnosis of delirium is extensive, and confusional states often have multiple causes. Francis et al. (1990) found that 56% of elderly patients with delirium had a single definite or probable etiology, and the remaining 44% had an average of 2.8 etiologies per patient. Because the dif-

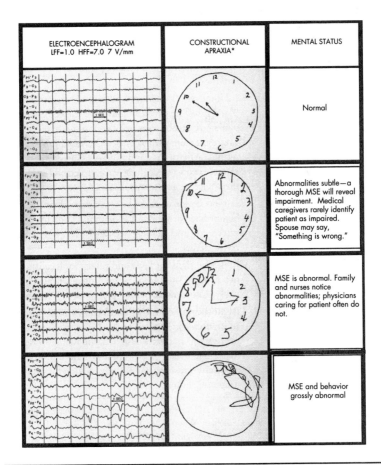

Figure 3–2.   Comparison of electroencephalogram (EEG), Clock Drawing Test, and mental status examination (MSE).

*The patient is given a sheet of paper with a large circle drawn on it and then is instructed, "Write in the numbers as if this circle is the face of a clock." After the patient is partially finished with the task, the psychiatrist should interject, "When you finish, draw in the hand of the clock so that the time says 10 until 11 o'clock."

Source.   Reprinted from Wise MG, Brandt GT: "Neuropsychiatric Aspects of Delirium," in *The American Psychiatric Press Textbook of Neuropsychiatry,* 3rd Edition. Edited by Yudofsky SC, Hales RE. Washington, DC, American Psychiatric Press, 1997, p. 454. Copyright 1997, American Psychiatric Press. Used with permission.

Table 3–2.   Differential diagnosis of delirium: emergent diagnoses—WHHHHIMP

Wernicke's encephalopathy or Withdrawal	Check for Wernicke's triad: confusion, ataxia, and ophthalmoplegia (lateral gaze paralysis most common).
Hypoxemia, Hypertensive encephalopathy, Hypoglycemia, or Hypoperfusion	Check for type 1 diabetes mellitus. Check arterial blood gases, oxygen saturation, and current and past vital signs. Hypoperfusion or hypoxemia of the brain can result from several causes: decreased cardiac output, arrhythmias, pulmonary failure, carbon monoxide poisoning, hypotension, cerebral vascular insufficiency, and severe anemia.
Intracranial bleeding or Infection	Examine for subarachnoid or intraparenchymal hemorrhage or subdural hematoma. Look for infectious processes (e.g., elevated white blood cell count, fever).
Meningitis or encephalitis	Check vital signs for fever and general or localizing neurological signs (e.g., meningismus with stiff neck). Also consider oncological and viral causes.
Poisons or medications	The most common causes of delirium are exogenous substances—prescribed and over-the-counter medications or illicit substances and toxins. Order a toxicology screen (if appropriate). Take a thorough medication history, particularly looking for drug-drug interactions.

Source.   Adapted from Wise MG, Brandt G: "Delirium," in *The American Psychiatric Press Textbook of Neuropsychiatry,* 2nd Edition. Edited by Yudofsky SC, Hales RE. Washington, DC, American Psychiatric Press, 1992, pp. 300–301. Copyright 1992, American Psychiatric Press. Used with permission.

ferential diagnosis of delirium is so broad, a two-tiered diagnostic system is clinically useful. The first tier contains the emergent items, and the second tier contains other diagnostic considerations.

Emergent diagnoses are listed using the mnemonic WHHHHIMP (Table 3–2). These diagnoses are considered emergent because failure to immediately recognize the delirium and treat the etiology may result in injury or death to the patient. Medications are an extremely common cause of delirium (Table 3–3), so a thorough review and correlation of the medication records (either administration or discontinuation) with behavioral change are

Table 3–3.   Common medications associated with delirium

Analgesics: meperidine, opiates

Antibiotics: acyclovir, ganciclovir, amphotericin B, interferon, cephalosporins, rifampin, isoniazid, tetracycline, gentamicin, ticarcillin

Anticholinergics: antihistamines, antispasmodics, atropine, benztropine, phenothiazines, scopolamine, promethazine, tricyclic antidepressants, trihexyphenidyl, belladonna alkaloids

Anticonvulsants: phenobarbital, phenytoin, valproic acid

Anti-inflammatories: Corticotropin, corticosteroids

Antineoplastic drugs: methotrexate, tamoxifen, vinblastine, vincristine, asparaginase, aminoglutethimide

Antiparkinsonian drugs: amantadine, bromocriptine, L-dopa, carbidopa

Cardiac drugs: β-blockers, captopril, clonidine, digitalis, lidocaine, mexiletine, methyldopa, quinidine, tocainide, procainamide

Sedative-hypnotics: barbiturates, benzodiazepines, glutethimide

Sympathomimetics: amphetamine, cocaine, ephedrine, epinephrine, phenylephrine, theophylline

Others: cimetidine, disulfiram, lithium, metrizamide, ranitidine, quinacrine

Source.   Adapted from Wise MG, Brandt G: "Delirium," in *The American Psychiatric Press Textbook of Neuropsychiatry,* 2nd Edition. Edited by Yudofsky SC, Hales RE. Washington, DC, American Psychiatric Press, 1992, pp. 300–301. Copyright 1992, American Psychiatric Press. Used with permission.

important. The second, somewhat less emergent, tier considers other potentially contributory diagnoses. Table 3–4 summarizes these diagnoses with the mnemonic I WATCH DEATH. This mnemonic reminds the clinician that the morbidity and mortality associated with untreated delirium are significant. Several important aspects of the physical examination, mental status examination, and laboratory examination of a patient with delirium assist with differential diagnosis. They are summarized in Table 3–5.

Making the Diagnosis

The diagnosis of delirium requires recognition of the clinical features and a thorough evaluation of the patient's mental and physical status. Administering the Mini-Mental State Exam (MMSE) alone is not a sufficient bedside mental status examination. In an unpublished study performed in an EEG laboratory (M.G. Wise 1989), all patients with global diffuse slowing on EEG

Table 3–4.   Differential diagnosis of delirium using mnemonic I WATCH DEATH

Infection	Encephalitis, meningitis, syphilis, HIV disease, sepsis
Withdrawal	Alcohol, barbiturates, sedative-hypnotics
Acute metabolic	Acidosis, alkalosis, electrolyte disturbance, hepatic failure, renal failure
Trauma	Closed-head injury, heatstroke, postoperative states, severe burns
CNS pathology	Abscess, hemorrhage, hydrocephalus, subdural hematoma, infection, seizures, stroke, tumors, metastases, vasculitis
Hypoxia	Anemia, carbon monoxide poisoning, hypotension, pulmonary failure, cardiac failure
Deficiencies	Vitamin B_{12}, folate, niacin, thiamine
Endocrinopathies	Hyper- or hypoadrenocorticism, hyper- or hypoglycemia, myxedema, hyperparathyroidism
Acute vascular	Hypertensive encephalopathy, stroke, arrhythmia, shock
Toxins or drugs	Medications, illicit drugs, pesticides, solvents (see Table 3–3)
Heavy metals	Lead, manganese, mercury

Note.   CNS = central nervous system.
Source.   Reprinted from Wise MG, Trzepacz PT: "Delirium (Confusional States)," in *The American Psychiatric Press Textbook of Consultation-Liaison Psychiatry.* Edited by Rundell JR, Wise MG. Washington, DC, American Psychiatric Press, 1996, p. 268. Copyright 1996, American Psychiatric Press. Used with permission.

(i.e., delirium) were given a series of mental status tests. Several patients who had delirium according to the EEG (global slowing) scored in the 20–29 range out of 30 on the MMSE. The most helpful bedside mental status examination for detecting mild confusion in that study was the Clock Drawing Test (see Figure 3–2). Therefore, the examiner must test a broad range of cognitive functions to document the diffuse impairment found in delirium. Cognitive functions tested should include attention and concentration, short- and long-term memory, visuoconstructional ability (see Figure 3–2), abstraction, and language, such as writing and confrontational naming.

The gold standard for diagnosis is a clinical evaluation in which DSM criteria are used, and the most useful diagnostic laboratory measure is the EEG. Several instruments are available that measure a broader range of symptoms

Table 3–5.   Assessment of the patient with delirium

Physical status

History

Physical and neurological examination

Review of vital signs and anesthesia record if postoperative

Review of medical records

Careful review of medications and correlation with behavioral changes

Mental status

Interview

Cognitive tests (e.g., Clock Drawing Test, Trail Parts A and B)

Basic laboratory tests—*consider in every patient with delirium*

Blood chemistries (electrolyte, glucose, calcium, albumin, blood urea nitrogen, creatinine, aspartate aminotransferase, bilirubin, alkaline phosphatase, magnesium, and phosphate levels; Venereal Disease Research Laboratory [VDRL] test)

Complete blood count

Serum drug levels (e.g., digoxin, theophylline, phenobarbital, cyclosporine)

Arterial blood gases or oxygen saturation

Urinalysis and collection for culture and sensitivity

Urine drug screen

Electrocardiogram

Chest X ray

Additional laboratory tests—*order as indicated by clinical condition*

Electroencephalogram

Lumbar puncture

Brain computed tomography or magnetic resonance imaging

Blood chemistries (e.g., heavy metal screen, B_{12} and folate levels, lupus erythematosus prep, antinuclear antibody test, urinary porphyrin levels, HIV test)

Source.   Reprinted from Wise MG, Trzepacz PT: "Delirium (Confusional States)," in *The American Psychiatric Press Textbook of Consultation-Liaison Psychiatry.* Edited by Rundell JR, Wise MG. Washington, DC, American Psychiatric Press, 1996, p. 267. Copyright 1996, American Psychiatric Press. Used with permission.

of delirium and can be used for screening purposes or to quantitate symptom severity. The Confusion Assessment Method (CAM; Inouye et al. 1990) is a widely used screening tool. The CAM is an algorithm of four cardinal symptoms of delirium intended for use in high-risk settings by nonpsychiatric clinicians. It can be supplemented by more intensive interviews to diagnose delirium. A recent modification of the CAM is the CAM-ICU (Ely et al. 2004), which is used in severely medically ill patients. The Delirium Rating Scale (DRS; Trzepacz et al. 1988) and the more recent, substantially revised version— the DRS-R-98 (Trzepacz et al. 2001)—require some psychiatric training to administer and rate the severity of a broad range of delirium symptoms according to explicit descriptions. The DRS-R-98 distinguishes delirium from dementia, schizophrenia, depression, and other medical conditions; it is available in many languages. The Memorial Delirium Assessment Scale is a 10-item severity rating scale (Breitbart et al. 1996) that is used after the diagnosis of delirium and is intended to be used repeatedly.

Treatment and Management

The treatment of delirium has two separate and important aspects (Table 3–6). The first is critical and bears directly on the survival of the patient—identification and reversal, when possible, of the reason(s) for the delirium. The second aspect of treatment is to reduce psychiatric symptoms of delirium with medications and environmental interventions regardless of whether psychosis or agitation is present (American Psychiatric Association 1999).

Reversal of Remediable Etiologies

The patient with delirium should be placed in a room near the nursing station, and vital signs should be checked frequently. A sitter should be employed if necessary. The medical staff must ensure good oxygenation and monitor fluid input and output. All nonessential medications must be discontinued. If an etiology for the confusional state is not identified immediately, further laboratory, radiological, and physical examinations are recommended.

Medications

Clinical experience indicates that neuroleptic medication is helpful and that haloperidol, a potent antipsychotic with virtually no anticholinergic or hy-

Table 3–6. Management of delirium

Provide medical care

Goal: find and correct, whenever possible, the etiology of the delirium

Perform physical and neurological examination

Perform laboratory evaluation

Discontinue nonessential medications

Monitor vital signs (frequently), fluid input and output, and oxygenation

Determine whether patient is in significant pain (may not be volunteered if on respirator)

Avoid interruptions in sleep, whenever possible

Prevent and manage disruptive and dangerous behaviors

Place the patient in a room near the nursing station

If dangerous behaviors occur, consider a sitter

Maintain bed in low position, and use side rails only if patient insists on getting out of bed

Use restraints only if necessary (for emergencies or if medication fails)

Avoid placement in a room with another delirious patient

Avoid a room cluttered with equipment or furniture

Use medications as needed

Use haloperidol for agitation; give intravenously whenever possible to avoid side effects and antagonizing the patient

Avoid use of benzodiazepines as sole agents, except in alcohol or sedative-hypnotic withdrawal delirium

Avoid use of narcotics unless the patient has significant pain; do not use meperidine

Avoid anticholinergic medications; effects are additive

Facilitate reality (not a stand-alone treatment)

Encourage presence of family members

Provide familiar clues (e.g., clock, calendar)

Provide adequate day and night lighting (e.g., use a night-light)

Minimize transfers (e.g., perform procedures in room whenever possible)

Maximize staff continuity

Reduce excessive environmental stimuli

Orient the patient to staff, surroundings, and situations repetitively, particularly before procedures

Table 3–6. Management of delirium *(continued)*

Facilitate reality (not a stand-alone treatment) *(continued)*

Make available sensory aids (e.g., hearing aids, glasses)

Encourage use of personal belongings

Repeatedly reassure the patient

Source. Adapted from Wise MG, Hilty DM, Cerda GM, et al.: "Delirium (Confusional States)," in *The American Psychiatric Publishing Textbook of Consultation-Liaison Psychiatry: Psychiatry in the Medically Ill,* 2nd Edition. Edited by Wise MG, Rundell JR. Washington, DC, American Psychiatric Publishing, 2002, p. 266. Copyright 2002, American Psychiatric Publishing. Used with permission.

potensive properties, is probably the drug of first choice because it does not suppress respirations, it has minimal cardiotoxicity, and it can be given intravenously. Other antipsychotic medications that have been used successfully include droperidol, olanzapine, risperidone, and quetiapine. A recently published double-blind trial of risperidone and haloperidol (given orally) for the treatment of delirium showed no significant difference in efficacy (Han and Kim 2004).

Although droperidol is used by physicians for control of nausea and vomiting, and by anesthesiologists as a preanesthetic agent, it is a potent antipsychotic. Droperidol is approved for intravenous use but has a higher potential than haloperidol for causing orthostatic hypotension. Risperidone and olanzapine have less potential than haloperidol to cause unwanted extrapyramidal symptoms but are given orally. Less potent antipsychotics, such as chlorpromazine and thioridazine, are more likely to cause hypotension and anticholinergic side effects at higher doses and are, therefore, problematic in many cases. However, in patients who are very sensitive to medications, such as patients with acquired immunodeficiency syndrome (AIDS) and delirium who are hospitalized, low-dose, low-potency antipsychotics may prove helpful. Breitbart et al. (1996) conducted a double-blind study comparing treatment of delirium with low-dose haloperidol (mean dose=2.8 mg/24 hours; range= 0.8–6.3 mg/24 hours), low-dose chlorpromazine (mean dose=50 mg/24 hours; range=10–70 mg/24 hours), or lorazepam (mean dose=3 mg/24 hours; range=0.5–10 mg/24 hours). Both antipsychotics significantly improved symptoms without inducing extrapyramidal side effects, whereas lorazepam "appeared to merely sedate patients, reducing level of consciousness and awareness of the environment, or to produce idiosyncratic or paradoxical agitation" (p. 235).

A task force of more than 40 disciplines (Shapiro et al. 1995) reviewed the literature on intravenous sedation of adult patients in the intensive care setting. They classified the recommendations in the literature into one of three levels: Level 1—convincingly justifiable on the basis of scientific evidence alone; Level 2—reasonably justifiable on the basis of available scientific evidence and strongly supported by expert critical care opinion; and Level 3—adequate scientific evidence is lacking but widely supported by available data and expert critical care opinion. Task force recommendations included haloperidol for delirium (classified as Level 1), lorazepam for anxiety (Level 2), and midazolam or propofol for sedation of less than 24 hours (Level 2).

Guidelines for haloperidol dosage are summarized in Table 3–7. Haloperidol and droperidol, especially when given in intravenous boluses at high doses, may prolong the QTc interval. Therefore, neither should be given when the patient's baseline QTc is greater than 450 msec or if a prior dose causes prolongation of the QTc interval from baseline. In a report of 1,100 consecutive ICU patients, intravenous haloperidol was implicated in inducing torsades de pointes tachyarrhythmia in 4 patients (Wilt et al. 1993). Benzodiazepines such as lorazepam have been used successfully as adjuncts to high-potency neuroleptics such as haloperidol. Small doses of intravenous lorazepam, particularly in patients whose symptoms have not responded to haloperidol alone, often help to decrease agitation and decrease the amount of haloperidol required.

Benzodiazepines are the drugs of choice in the treatment of DTs, certain other drug withdrawal states, and complex partial seizure status. Intravenous midazolam and lorazepam are frequently used emergently to treat severe agitation.

Environmental Interventions

Environmental interventions are sometimes helpful but are *not* a primary treatment for delirium. The half-life of reassurance and reorientation for a patient with delirium is usually less than a minute. Both nurses and family members can very frequently reorient the patient to date and surroundings. It may help to place a clock, a calendar, and familiar objects in the room. Adequate light in the room during the night may decrease frightening illusions or hasten reorien-

Table 3–7.   Guidelines for haloperidol dosage

Level of agitation	Starting dose (mg)
Mild	0.5–2.0
Moderate	2.0–5.0
Severe	5.0–10.0

1. If haloperidol is used intravenously, clear the intravenous line with normal saline prior to bolus infusion. Heparin can precipitate intravenous haloperidol.
2. For elderly patients, use a starting dose of 0.5–2.0 mg.
3. Allow 30 minutes between doses; *check QTc interval on the electrocardiogram before repeating dose.*
4. For continued agitation, double the previous dose.
5. If no improvement after three doses, give 0.5–1.0 mg lorazepam intravenously concurrently, or alternate lorazepam with haloperidol every 30 minutes.
6. Once the patient is calm, add the total milligrams of haloperidol required; administer the same number of milligrams over the next 24 hours.
7. Assuming the patient remains calm, reduce the dose by 50% every 24 hours.
8. To convert intravenous to oral dosage, double the intravenous dose (divide oral dose into two or three doses).

Source.   Adapted from Wise and Terrell 1998, p. 973.

tation during awakenings. Rooms with windows may help the patient retain orientation. A private room for the patient with delirium is not recommended unless adequate supervision is provided. Returning aids such as eyeglasses or hearing aids to patients who normally use them may improve the quality of sensory input and help patients better understand their surroundings.

Course (Prognosis)

The clinical duration of delirium ranges from less than 1 week to 2 months; the typical duration is 10–12 days (American Psychiatric Association 1999). The outcome possibilities are full recovery; progression to stupor, coma, or death; seizures; chronic brain syndromes; and injuries, such as fracture or subdural hematomas from falls. Most patients who experience delirium have a full recovery (Lipowski 1990), but only 4%–40% of patients have a full recovery by the time of hospital discharge; the rate of recovery at discharge is closer to 15% for elderly patients (American Psychiatric Association 1999). Persistent cognitive deficits are common, particularly in AIDS patients, with only 27% having full recovery of cognition (American Psychiatric Association 1999). Cognitive deficits also may be due to previously unrecognized dementia that was exposed by the delirium. Seizures that can accompany delirium are more likely to occur with drug withdrawal, particularly alcohol withdrawal and burn encephalopathy (Antoon et al. 1972).

Several clinical researchers have studied systematic interventions to improve outcome for patients who develop delirium. Unfortunately, with exceptions (Marcantonio et al. 2001), most studies show little or no effect of systematic interventions on outcome (Bogardus et al. 2003; Cole et al. 2002).

References

American Psychiatric Association: Practice guideline for the treatment of patients with delirium. Am J Psychiatry 156 (suppl):1–20, 1999

American Psychiatric Association: Diagnostic and Statistical Manual of Mental Disorders, 4th Edition, Text Revision. Washington, DC, American Psychiatric Association, 2000

Antoon AY, Volpe JJ, Crawford JD: Burn encephalopathy in children. Pediatrics 50:609–616, 1972

Bogardus ST Jr, Desai MM, Williams CS, et al: The effects of a targeted multicomponent delirium intervention on postdischarge outcomes for hospitalized older patients. Am J Med 114:383–390, 2003

Breitbart W, Marotta R, Platt MM, et al: A double-blind trial of haloperidol, chlorpromazine, and lorazepam in the treatment of delirium in hospitalized AIDS patients. Am J Psychiatry 153:231–237, 1996

Cole MG, McCusker J, Bellavance F, et al: Systematic detection and multidisciplinary care of delirium in older medical inpatients: a randomized trial. CMAJ 167:753–759, 2002

Ely EW, Shintani A, Truman B, et al: Delirium as a predictor of mortality in mechanically ventilated patients in the intensive care unit. JAMA 291:1753–1762, 2004

Folstein MF, Bassett SS, Romanoski AJ, et al: The epidemiology of delirium in the community: the Eastern Baltimore Mental Health Survey, in International Psychogeriatrics. Edited by Miller NE, Lipowski ZJ, Lebowitz BD. New York, Springer, 1991, pp 169–176

Francis J, Martin D, Kapoor W: A prospective study of delirium in hospitalized elderly. JAMA 263:1097–1101, 1990

Han CS, Kim YK: A double-blind trial of risperidone and haloperidol for the treatment of delirium. Psychosomatics 45:297–301, 2004

Inouye SK, van Dyck CH, Alessi CA, et al: Clarifying confusion: the Confusion Assessment Method: a new method for detection of delirium. Ann Intern Med 113:941–948, 1990

Kennard MA, Bueding E, Wortis WB: Some biochemical and electroencephalographic changes in delirium tremens. Q J Stud Alcohol 6:4–14, 1945

Kolbeinsson H, Jonsson A: Delirium and dementia in acute medical admissions of elderly patients in Iceland. Acta Psychiatr Scand 87:123–127, 1993

Koponen HJ, Riekkinen PJ: A prospective study of delirium in elderly patients admitted to a psychiatric hospital. Psychol Med 3:103–109, 1993

Lipowski ZJ: Delirium: Acute Confusional States. New York, Oxford University Press, 1990

Marcantonio ER, Goldman L, Mangione CM, et al: A clinical prediction rule for delirium after elective noncardiac surgery. JAMA 271:134–139, 1994

Marcantonio ER, Flacker JM, Wright RJ, et al: Reducing delirium after hip fracture: a randomized trial. J Am Geriatr Soc 49:516–522, 2001

Shapiro BA, Warren J, Egol AB, et al: Practice parameters for intravenous analgesia and sedation for adult patients in the intensive care unit: an executive summary. Society of Critical Care Medicine. Crit Care Med 23:1596–1600, 1995

Trzepacz PT: Neuropathogenesis of delirium: a need to focus our research. Psychosomatics 35:375–391, 1994

Trzepacz PT, Baker RW, Greenhouse J: A symptom rating scale for delirium. Psychiatry Res 23:89–97, 1988

Trzepacz PT, Mittal D, Torres R, et al: Validation of the Delirium Rating Scale—Revised–98: comparison with the Delirium Rating Scale amd the Cognitive Test for Delirium. J Neuropsychiatry Clin Sci 13:229–242, 2001

Trzepacz PT, Meagher DJ, Wise MG: Neuropsychiatric aspects of delirium, in Essentials of Neuropsychiatry and Clinical Neurosciences. Edited by Yudofsky SC, Hales RE. Washington, DC, American Psychiatric Publishing, 2004, pp 141–187

Wilt JL, Minnema AM, Johnson RF, et al: Torsades de pointes associated with the use of intravenous haloperidol. Ann Intern Med 119:391–394, 1993

Wise MG, Terrell CD: Neuropsychiatric disorders: delirium, psychotic disorders, and anxiety, in Principles of Critical Care, 2nd Edition. Edited by Hall JB, Schmidt GA, Wood LDH. New York, McGraw-Hill, 1998, pp 965–978

Wise MG, Trzepacz PT: Delirium (confusional states), in Essentials of Consultation-Liaison Psychiatry. Edited by Rundell JR, Wise MG. Washington, DC, American Psychiatric Press, 1999, pp 81–93

Additional Readings

Berrios GE: Delirium and confusion in the 19th century: a conceptual history. Br J Psychiatry 139:439–449, 1981

Ely EW, Stephens RK, Jackson JC, et al: Current opinions regarding the importance, diagnosis, and management of delirium in the intensive case unit: a survey of 912 healthcare professionals. Crit Care Med 32:106–112, 2004

Fernandez F, Holmes V, Adams F, et al: Treatment of severe, refractory agitation with a haloperidol drip. J Clin Psychiatry 49:239–241, 1988

Frye MA, Coudreaut MF, Hakeman SM, et al: Continuous droperidol drip infusion for management of agitated delirium in an ICU. Psychosomatics 36:301–305, 1995

Liptzin B, Levkoff SE: An empirical study of delirium subtypes. Br J Psychiatry 161:843–845, 1992

Metzger E, Friedman R: Prolongation of the corrected QT and torsades de pointes cardiac arrhythmia associated with intravenous haloperidol in the medically ill. J Clin Psychopharmacol 13:128–132, 1993

Platt MM, Breitbart W, Smith M, et al: Efficacy of neuroleptics for hypoactive delirium (letter). J Neuropsychiatry Clin Neurosci 6:66–67, 1994

Riker RR, Fraser GL, Cox PM: Continuous infusion of haloperidol controls agitation in critically ill patients. Crit Care Med 22:433–440, 1994

Tune L, Carr S, Cooper T, et al: Association of anticholinergic activity of prescribed medications with postoperative delirium. J Neuropsychiatry Clin Neurosci 5:208–210, 1993

Wise MG, Brandt G: Delirium, in The American Psychiatric Press Textbook of Neuropsychiatry, 2nd Edition. Edited by Hales RE, Yudofsky SC. Washington, DC, American Psychiatric Press, 1992, pp 300–301

4

Dementia

Dementia is a syndrome of acquired persistent impairment characterized by deficits in at least three areas of mental activities such as memory, language, visuospatial skills, emotion or personality, and cognition (Cummings and Mega 2003). An early review reported that as many as one-third of dementia patients who initially present for evaluation have at least partially reversible dementia (Rabins 1983); however, a more recent meta-analysis suggested that potentially reversible dementias occur in 9% of patients, but only 0.6% of cases are actually reversed (0.3% partially and 0.3% fully) (Clarfield 2003). The principal causes of dementia are degenerative, vascular, demyelinating, traumatic, neoplastic, inflammatory, infectious, toxic-metabolic, and dementia syndromes associated with psychiatric disorders (see Gray and Cummings 2002).

Epidemiology

The most commonly occurring dementia is dementia of the Alzheimer's type (DAT), accounting for approximately 50%–70% of the patients evaluated for progressive cognitive decline. Perhaps another 10%–20% show a combination of Alzheimer's disease with either vascular pathology or diffuse Lewy body disease. Vascular dementia, or Lewy body disease (depending on the writer), is reportedly the second most common cause of dementia (Gray and Cummings 2002). In the autopsy study by Fu et al. (2004), 5.9% of cases were pure vascular dementia, and 6.4% of cases were diffuse Lewy body disease. A small percentage of patients, 4% in the Fu et al. (2004) study, have frontotemporal dementia. Added together, DAT, vascular dementia, Lewy body disease, and frontotemporal dementias usually account for 80%–90% of dementias. The largest cause of potentially reversible dementias is psychiatric disorders. Other causes of potentially reversible dementias include alcohol, metabolic disturbances, hydrocephalus, and neoplasms.

Clinical Characteristics

The Concept of Cortical and Subcortical Dementia

A clinically useful way to conceptualize degenerative dementias is to divide them into cortical, subcortical, and mixed dementias. *Cortical dementias* are disorders producing dysfunction predominantly of the cerebral cortex and are characterized by the four *A's:* amnesia, aphasia, apraxia, and agnosia (Gray and Cummings 2002). DAT is the classic example of a cortical dementia. *Subcortical dementias* are disorders primarily involving the deep gray and deep white matter structures, including the basal ganglia, thalamus, and frontal lobe projections of these subcortical structures. Examples of predominantly subcortical dementias are dementias associated with Parkinson's disease, Huntington's disease, and striatonigral degeneration. Table 4–1 presents clinical features that help to distinguish cortical and subcortical dementias. *Mixed dementias* can produce clinical syndromes with cortical and/or subcortical features. Vascular dementia is the most common type of mixed dementia.

Degenerative Dementias

Cortical Dementia

DAT.   The diagnosis of DAT requires the gradual, progressive development of multiple cognitive deficits, including memory impairment and nonmemory cognitive disturbances (American Psychiatric Association 2000). The typical language disturbance is a fluent aphasia with anomia. Naming and compre-

Table 4–1.   Distinguishing features of cortical and subcortical dementias

	Subcortical	Cortical
Language	No aphasia	Aphasia early
Memory	Recall impaired; recognition is better preserved than recall	Amnesia: recall and recognition impaired
Visuospatial skills	Impaired	Impaired
Calculation	Preserved until late	Involved early
Frontal systems	Disproportionately affected	Impaired to the same degree as other abilities
Cognitive processing speed	Slowed early	Response time normal until late in disease course
Personality	Apathetic, inert	Unconcerned or disinhibited
Mood	Depressed	Euthymic
Speech	Dysarthric	Normal articulation[a]
Posture	Bowed or extended	Normal, upright[a]
Coordination	Impaired	Normal[a]
Gait	Abnormal	Normal[a]
Motor speed	Slowed	Normal[a]
Movement disorders	Common (chorea, tremor, tics, rigidity)	Absent[a]

[a]Motor system involvement occurs late in the course of the cortical dementias.
Source.   Reprinted from Gray KF, Cummings JL: "Dementia," in *The American Psychiatric Publishing Textbook of Consultation-Liaison Psychiatry: Psychiatry in the Medically Ill,* 2nd Edition. Edited by Wise MG, Rundell JR. Washington, DC, American Psychiatric Publishing, 2002, p. 276. Copyright 2002, American Psychiatric Publishing. Used with permission.

hension are progressively impaired, whereas the ability to repeat is relatively preserved (Cummings and Benson 1986). Disturbances in executive cognitive functions include impaired abstracting, sequencing, planning, and organizing. Apathy, distractibility, overreliance on environmental cues, agitation, and a tendency to perseverate also may result from disturbed executive cognitive systems (Gray and Cummings 2002; Royall et al. 1992). The DSM-IV-TR (American Psychiatric Association 2000) diagnostic criteria for DAT are listed in Table 4–2. If the patient's symptoms meet DSM criteria for DAT, the

Table 4–2. DSM-IV-TR diagnostic criteria for dementia of the Alzheimer's type

A. The development of multiple cognitive deficits manifested by both

    (1) memory impairment (impaired ability to learn new information or to recall previously learned information)

    (2) one (or more) of the following cognitive disturbances:

        (a) aphasia (language disturbance)

        (b) apraxia (impaired ability to carry out motor activities despite intact motor function)

        (c) agnosia (failure to recognize or identify objects despite intact sensory function)

        (d) disturbance in executive functioning (i.e., planning, organizing, sequencing, abstracting)

B. The cognitive deficits in Criteria A1 and A2 each cause significant impairment in social or occupational functioning and represent a significant decline from a previous level of functioning.

C. The course is characterized by gradual onset and continuing cognitive decline.

D. The cognitive deficits in Criteria A1 and A2 are not due to any of the following:

    (1) other central nervous system conditions that cause progressive deficits in memory and cognition (e.g., cerebrovascular disease, Parkinson's disease, Huntington's disease, subdural hematoma, normal-pressure hydrocephalus, brain tumor)

    (2) systemic conditions that are known to cause dementia (e.g., hypothyroidism, vitamin B_{12} or folic acid deficiency, niacin deficiency, hypercalcemia, neurosyphilis, HIV infection)

    (3) substance-induced conditions

E. The deficits do not occur exclusively during the course of a delirium.

F. The disturbance is not better accounted for by another Axis I disorder (e.g., Major Depressive Disorder, Schizophrenia).

Source. Reprinted from American Psychiatric Association: *Diagnostic and Statistical Manual of Mental Disorders,* 4th Edition, Text Revision. Washington, DC, American Psychiatric Association, 2000, pp. 157–158. Copyright 2000, American Psychiatric Association. Used with permission.

diagnosis is very likely correct; however, if the patient who has dementia does not meet DAT criteria, the clinician who indicates that "this is not Alzheimer's disease" according to DSM criteria will be wrong 38%–61% of the time when compared with postmortem pathological diagnoses (Nagy et al. 1998).

Table 4–3.   Consensus criteria for dementia with Lewy bodies

A.   Progressive cognitive decline sufficient to cause social and occupational impairment (note: memory impairment may not occur in early stages). Deficits in attention, executive function, and visuospatial ability may be especially prominent.

B.   One (possible dementia with Lewy bodies) or two (probable dementia with Lewy bodies) of the following core features:

   1.   Fluctuating cognition with pronounced variation in attention and alertness
   2.   Recurrent visual hallucinations that are typically well formed and detailed
   3.   Spontaneous motor feature of parkinsonism

C.   Features that support the diagnosis

   1.   Repeated falls
   2.   Syncope
   3.   Transient loss of consciousness
   4.   Neuroleptic sensitivity[a]
   5.   Systematized delusions
   6.   Hallucinations in other modalities
   7.   Rapid eye movement behavioral disorder
   8.   Depression

[a]Typical and atypical neuroleptics can precipitate severe reactions, irreversible parkinsonism, or impaired consciousness or induce autonomic disturbances in 40%–50% of DLB patients; mortality is also increased severalfold (McKeith 2002). Cholinesterase inhibitors are often helpful.
Source.   Adapted from McKeith et al. 1996.

Table 4–4.   Clinical criteria for frontotemporal dementia

A.   Behavioral and cognitive decline manifested by either of the following:

   1.   Progressive personality or behavioral change
   2.   Progressive expressive and naming impairment

B.   Deficits significantly impair social or occupational functioning

C.   Gradual significant decline

D.   No other central nervous system or systemic disease is responsible

E.   The deficits do not occur exclusively during delirium

F.   The disturbance is not due to a psychiatric diagnosis

Source.   Adapted from McKhann GM, Albert MS, Grossman M, et al.: "Clinical and Pathological Diagnosis of Frontotemporal Dementia: Report of the Work Group on Frontotemporal Dementia and Pick's Disease." *Archives of Neurology* 58:1803–1809, 2001.

Dementia with Lewy bodies.   About 15%–25% of elderly patients with dementia may have Lewy bodies in their brain stem and cortex (McKeith et al. 1996). DSM-IV-TR does not include diagnostic criteria for dementia with Lewy bodies; consensus guidelines for the clinical and pathological diagnosis were published elsewhere and are listed in Table 4–3.

Frontotemporal dementia.   Frontotemporal dementia affects primarily cortical structures and is usually difficult to differentiate from DAT in the early stages. The most prominent neuropsychiatric features are apathy and disinhibition, and features of Klüver-Bucy syndrome (e.g., hyperorality, hypersexuality, placidity, sensory agnosia, dietary changes) can occur early (Cummings and Mega 2003). The clinical criteria for frontotemporal dementia are listed in Table 4–4.

Subcortical Dementia

Parkinson's disease.   Assessment of dementia in Parkinson's disease is complex because the effects of aging, depression (in perhaps half of all Parkinson's disease patients), and chronic disability must be considered in addition to profound motor deficits (Gray and Cummings 2002). Parkinson's disease patients may show either mild, spontaneous extrapyramidal features or exaggerated sensitivity to standard doses of neuroleptic medications. The illness progresses, often rapidly, and long-term follow-up indicates that up to 78% of these patients develop dementia (McKeith and Mosimann 2004). Although dementia in Parkinson's disease is considered a subcortical dementia, the presentation and course can vary. This likely occurs because DAT can occur in patients with Parkinson's disease, and dementia with Lewy bodies also can produce a cortical-type dementia in association with Parkinson's disease.

Huntington's disease.   The clinical triad of dementia, chorea, and a positive family history define Huntington's disease. Huntington's disease patients have diminished cognitive speed, a memory retrieval deficit (characterized by poor spontaneous recall but preserved recognition memory), poor executive functions, and motor symptoms (Gray and Cummings 2002). The absence of aphasia and other cortical features distinguishes Huntington's disease from DAT (Folstein et al. 1990). Personality changes such as irritability or apathy are common and may antedate the onset of chorea. Depression is common in Huntington's disease.

Mixed Dementia

Vascular dementia. Chronic ischemic vascular disease, hemorrhage, and anoxia are the most common causes of vascular dementia. The accumulation of cerebral infarctions produces the progressive cognitive impairment termed *multi-infarct dementia*. In contrast to cortical dementias, vascular dementia is characterized by an abrupt onset, a stepwise progression, a fluctuating course, depression, pseudobulbar palsy, a history of hypertension, a history of strokes, evidence of associated atherosclerosis, and focal neurological symptoms and signs on examination. Table 4–5 lists the DSM-IV-TR diagnostic criteria for vascular dementia.

Table 4–5. DSM-IV-TR diagnostic criteria for vascular dementia

A. The development of multiple cognitive deficits manifested by both

   (1) memory impairment (impaired ability to learn new information or to recall previously learned information)

   (2) one (or more) of the following cognitive disturbances:

      (a) aphasia (language disturbance)

      (b) apraxia (impaired ability to carry out motor activities despite intact motor function)

      (c) agnosia (failure to recognize or identify objects despite intact sensory function)

      (d) disturbance in executive functioning (i.e., planning, organizing, sequencing, abstracting)

B. The cognitive deficits in Criteria A1 and A2 each cause significant impairment in social or occupational functioning and represent a significant decline from a previous level of functioning.

C. Focal neurological signs and symptoms (e.g., exaggeration of deep tendon reflexes, extensor plantar response, pseudobulbar palsy, gait abnormalities, weakness of an extremity) or laboratory evidence indicative of cerebrovascular disease (e.g., multiple infarctions involving cortex and underlying white matter) that are judged to be etiologically related to the disturbance.

D. The deficits do not occur exclusively during the course of a delirium.

Source. Reprinted from American Psychiatric Association: *Diagnostic and Statistical Manual of Mental Disorders,* 4th Edition, Text Revision. Washington, DC, American Psychiatric Association, 2000, p. 161. Copyright 2000, American Psychiatric Association. Used with permission.

Alcoholic dementia. The relation between alcohol and dementias is somewhat complicated. In general, the association appears to be U shaped, especially with wine. When compared with abstinence, the association between alcohol and dementias declines somewhat with alcohol consumption of 1 drink or less per week; declines further with 1–6 drinks per week; and at 7–13 alcoholic drinks per week, the association is still lower than with abstinence but more than with 1–6 drinks per week. At 14 drinks or more per week (heavier alcohol consumption), the risk for alcohol-induced dementia, Alzheimer's disease, and vascular dementia is increased compared with abstinence (Mukamal et al. 2003), especially in men who carry the apolipoprotein E ε4 allele. When compared with other dementias, patients with alcohol-induced dementia are often less cognitively impaired, unmarried, and do not have further cognitive and functional deterioration after abstinence (Oslin and Cary 2003).

Alcoholic dementia is found in approximately 3% of alcoholic patients, and subtle deficits occur in 50% (Cummings and Mega 2003); 45% of alcoholic patients who are older than 65 have dementia (Cummings and Benson 1992). Physicians tend to misdiagnose the alcoholic patient's dementia as Korsakoff's psychosis (Cutting 1982). The atrophy seen on computed tomographic scan will reverse in some alcoholic patients with abstinence (Cummings and Mega 2003). Neuropsychological abnormalities associated with alcoholic dementia also can partially reverse with abstinence.

Dementia Associated With Psychiatric Disorder: Pseudodementia

Pseudodementia implies a deceptive or false dementia, which may not be accurate (Cummings and Benson 1992). The term *dementia syndrome of depression* is more accurate in a subset of patients with depression and cognitive dysfunction (see Chapter 5, "Depression," in this volume for a more detailed discussion of cognitive function in major depression). Pseudodementia is associated with several psychiatric disorders; of these, depression is by far the most common psychiatric disorder that produces intellectual impairment. Cognitive abnormalities frequently occur in the elderly depressed patient and less commonly occur in the young depressed patient. Depressive pseudodementia usually has the following characteristics:

- Personal and/or family history of mood disorder
- Sudden onset of symptoms

- Complaints about cognitive deficits, and halfhearted efforts or "I don't know" responses to questions that test cognitive function by the patient
- Equal impairment of recent and remote memory
- Inconsistent results on tests of cognitive function

In contrast, the patient with dementia usually does not have a psychiatric history, attempts to conceal disabilities, tries hard to perform cognitive tasks but fails, has memory loss for recent events greater than that for remote events, and consistently performs poorly on neuropsychiatric tests. Psychiatric disorders that are associated less commonly with dementia-like symptoms include somatization disorder, conversion disorder, malingering, factitious disorder, Ganser's syndrome, mania, and obsessive-compulsive disorder.

Differential Diagnosis and Evaluation

The differential diagnosis of dementia syndromes is summarized in Table 4–6.

Mental Status Examination

An accurate diagnosis cannot be established without a careful mental status examination (MSE). The MSE serves as a probe of brain function but must be conceptualized as a structure built on a solid foundation of intact attentional systems (Gray and Cummings 2002). The consultant must first confirm that attention is undiminished, then the other major cognitive domains are assessed in a logical sequence. (The MSE is described in Chapter 2, "Mental Status Examination and Other Tests of Brain Function," in this volume.)

History

The clinical history should be obtained and corroborated through reliable caregivers. The clinician should investigate the type of onset (gradual vs. sudden) and pattern of progression (relentless vs. stepwise). The clinician also should ask about important associated health issues such as hypertension, history of strokes, transient ischemic attacks, or arrhythmias (especially atrial fibrillation), alcohol intake, drug abuse (especially injection drug use), and prescribed and over-the-counter medications. The consultant must understand the typical features of a dementia syndrome to address potentially reversible etiologies and management strategies.

Table 4–6.   Differential diagnosis of dementia syndromes

Alzheimer's disease
Dementia with Lewy bodies
Vascular dementia   } 80%–90% of patients with dementia have one or a combination of these diagnoses
Frontotemporal dementia

Parkinsonian syndromes with dementia (e.g., Parkinson's disease, progressive supranuclear palsy)

Huntington's disease

Infection-related dementias

Prion diseases

Toxic and metabolic
   dementias

Myelinoclastic dementias

Traumatic dementias

Neoplastic dementias

Hydrocephalic dementias

Inflammatory conditions (e.g., systemic lupus erythematosus, antiphospholipid antibody syndrome)

Dementias associated with psychiatric disorders (e.g., depression, schizophrenia)

Source.   Adapted from Gray and Cummings 2002.

Laboratory Assessment

Laboratory assessment is an important part of a dementia evaluation. Table 4–7 lists a battery of tests necessary during the initial assessment of a patient with a dementia syndrome. If specific clinical evidence for the potential cause of the dementia is present (e.g., history of injection drug abuse), then appropriate tests are ordered (i.e., human immunodeficiency virus test). A structural imaging study is important when dementia is diagnosed to identify reversible causes, focal lesions, and other potential diagnoses.

Table 4–7. Tests in the assessment of dementia

Required screening battery
Complete blood count
Erythrocyte sedimentation rate
Blood glucose
Blood urea nitrogen
Electrolytes
Liver function tests
Serum calcium and phosphorus
Structural imaging study (initial assessment)
Thyroid-stimulating hormone
Vitamin B_{12} and folate levels
Fluorescent treponemal antibody absorption (FTA-ABS)

If unexplained fever or urinary symptoms present
Urinalysis
Urine culture and sensitivity

If unexplained fever or pulmonary symptoms present
Chest X ray

If cardiovascular symptoms present or evidence of vascular dementia
Electrocardiogram

If risk factors for HIV present
Serum HIV test

If drug intoxication suspected
Serum drug levels or toxic screen

Tests selected on the basis of specific symptoms or history
Blood gases
Heavy metals
Disease-specific tests (e.g., serum copper and ceruloplasmin for Wilson's disease)
Lumbar puncture (usually after computed tomography or magnetic resonance
    imaging) if evidence of infection, demyelinating disease, inflammatory disease,
    or neoplasm

Source. Reprinted from Gray KF, Cummings JL: "Dementia," in *The American Psychiatric Publishing Textbook of Consultation-Liaison Psychiatry: Psychiatry in the Medically Ill,* 2nd Edition. Edited by Wise MG, Rundell JR. Washington, DC, American Psychiatric Publishing, 2002, p. 293. Copyright 2002, American Psychiatric Publishing. Used with permission.

Neuroimaging

Atrophy is present on computed tomography (CT) and magnetic resonance imaging (MRI) in most patients with DAT. Patients with DAT also usually have significantly larger ventricles than do age-matched control subjects. In general, correlations between ventricular enlargement and cognitive function are stronger than those between cortical atrophy and cognition (Giacometti et al. 1994). Areas of decreased lucency in the white matter are seen on head CT in most patients with vascular dementia. MRI is the most sensitive structural imaging technique for diagnosing vascular dementia (Gray and Cummings 2002).

Neuropsychological Testing

Neuropsychological testing is much more sensitive and specific than screening MSEs such as the Mini-Mental State Exam (see Chapter 2) and can 1) distinguish between mild dementia and normal aging in elderly individuals, 2) differentiate mild dementia from the effects of low educational level or limited natural cognitive capacities, 3) provide detailed quantitative information that may help distinguish different types of dementia, and 4) establish a baseline description of cognitive function that may be followed over time to determine whether the patient is undergoing progressive decline (Gray and Cummings 2002).

Treatment and Management

The treatment and management of dementia have several objectives (Table 4–8):

1. *Treat reversible diagnoses.* These diagnoses include medical and psychiatric disorders that can present with an apparent dementia (e.g., hypothyroidism, depressive pseudodementia). In addition, depression often accompanies and amplifies the cognitive dysfunction of dementias. In such cases, an antidepressant trial is recommended. If alcohol-induced dementia is diagnosed, abstinence can reverse or stabilize cognitive impairment and atrophy on CT.
2. *Treat coexisting medical conditions.* If the patient is hypertensive, optimal blood pressure control (systolic 135–150 mm Hg) may help stabilize a

Table 4–8. Treatment and management of dementia

Treat reversible diagnoses (e.g., hypothyroidism, depressive pseudodementia, abstinence in alcohol-induced dementia)

Treat or optimally manage coexisting medical conditions (e.g., hypertension)

Consider treatments that restore cognitive function or delay decline

Trial of cholinesterase inhibitors in Alzheimer's disease, dementia with Lewy bodies, vascular dementia, and Parkinson' disease with dementia

Alzheimer's dementia

Delay progression (e.g., vitamin E, selegiline, memantine)

Use memantine in moderate to severe disease, either alone or in combination with cholinesterase inhibitors

Manage and treat behavior problems

Use nonpharmacological interventions whenever possible

When medications are required (extreme caution with antipsychotics in dementia with Lewy bodies):

Choose target symptoms

Start at a low dose and increase slowly

Monitor target symptoms and side effects closely

Provide a consistent environment and legal arrangements (e.g., powers of attorney, wills)

Support caregivers and monitor caregivers for depression

---

vascular dementia; daily aspirin therapy (325 mg/day) can be used to inhibit platelet aggregation (Meyer et al. 1989). Ticlopidine may ameliorate progressive ischemic injury in patients who fail to tolerate or respond to aspirin.

3. *Consider treatments that restore cognitive function or delay decline.* Patients who have Alzheimer's dementia, vascular dementia, dementia with Lewy bodies, and Parkinson's disease with dementia can potentially benefit from cholinesterase inhibitors (i.e., donepezil, galantamine, or rivastigmine) (Cummings and Mega 2003). Thus, an adequate trial is warranted in the vast majority of patients.

In addition, several treatments may delay or slow the progression of DAT: vitamin E, selegiline, possibly statins and cholinesterase inhibitors, and memantine. Memantine was approved by the Food and Drug Administration for treatment of moderate to severe Alzheimer's disease in October 2003. Memantine is a low-affinity, uncompetitive N-methyl-D-aspartate antagonist that improved cognition and slowed decline in patients with Alzheimer's disease; it can be combined with cholinesterase inhibitors (van Dyck 2004).

4. *Manage and treat behavior problems.* Nonpharmacological interventions should be used whenever possible. Exercise training increases physical and cognitive function (Heyn 2004). The clinician should use simple vocabulary and repeat communications frequently. When medications are required, the physician should choose target symptoms, start medications at a low dose, increase the dosage slowly, and monitor target symptoms and side effects closely. If a major tranquilizer is necessary, an atypical antipsychotic should be started at a low dosage (e.g., olanzapine 2.5–5.0 mg/day; risperidone 0.25–1.0 mg/day). Low-potency neuroleptics such as thioridazine and chlorpromazine should be avoided because of their potent anticholinergic and hypotensive side effects. Caution is necessary when treating dementia with Lewy bodies or Parkinson's disease with dementia. Patients with these dementias are extraordinarily sensitive to antipsychotic medications, and severe adverse reactions are not uncommon. Propranolol may help control aggressive behavior in some patients. Clonazepam (0.5 mg) can be used to maintain sleep in patients with frequent awakening or nocturnal wandering; trazodone (25–100 mg) is useful for agitation and for patients with difficulty falling asleep (Pinner and Rich 1988).

5. *Provide a consistent environment.* The patient with dementia needs a safe, consistent, familiar, predictable environment. Early in the course of a dementing illness, the patient is usually most comfortable at home. If the patient has to leave home for unfamiliar surroundings, it may precipitate anxiety and/or deterioration in the patient's condition. When the diagnosis of dementia is made, the clinician should encourage the patient and his or her family immediately to make legal arrangements (e.g., powers of attorney, wills) before the patient becomes incompetent. Adequate nutrition, hydration, and vigilance for infections and other medical illnesses are important as well.

6. *Support caregivers.* The family and other caregivers of the patient with dementia require support, especially a caregiving spouse. The emotional strain and time demands placed on the caregivers of a person with dementia are often overwhelming. In a recent large multicenter study,

32% of the caregivers were classified as depressed (Covinsky et al. 2003). Caregivers need respites from these demands. Alzheimer's Family Support Group, a nationwide organization, offers such assistance. Two books are "required" reading for caregivers: *The 36-Hour Day* (Mace and Rabins 2001) and *Understanding Alzheimer's Disease* (Aronson 1988).

References

American Psychiatric Association: Diagnostic and Statistical Manual of Mental Disorders, 4th Edition, Text Revision. Washington, DC, American Psychiatric Association, 2000

Aronson MK: Understanding Alzheimer's Disease: What It Is, How to Cope With It, Future Directions. New York, Scribner's, 1988

Clarfield AM: The decreasing prevalence of reversible dementias: an updated meta-analysis. Arch Intern Med 163:2219–2229, 2003

Covinsky KE, Newcomer R, Fox P, et al: Patient and caregiver characteristics associated with depression in caregivers of patients with dementia. J Gen Intern Med 18: 1006–1014, 2003

Cummings JL, Benson DF: Dementia of the Alzheimer's type: an inventory of diagnostic clinical features. J Am Geriatr Soc 34:12–19, 1986

Cummings JL, Benson DF: Dementia: A Clinical Approach. Boston, MA, Butterworth-Heinemann, 1992, pp 95–152, 217–265, 345–364

Cummings JL, Mega MS: Neuropsychiatry and Behavioral Neuroscience. New York, Oxford University Press, 2003

Cutting J: Alcoholic dementia, in Psychiatric Aspects of Neurologic Disease, Vol 2. Edited by Benson DF, Blumer D. New York, Grune & Stratton, 1982, pp 149–165

Folstein SE, Brandt J, Folstein MF: Huntington's disease, in Subcortical Dementia. Edited by Cummings JL. New York, Oxford University Press, 1990, pp 87–107

Fu C, Chute DJ, Farag ES, et al: Comorbidity in dementia: an autopsy study. Arch Pathol Lab Med 128:32–38, 2004

Giacometti AR, Davis PC, Alazraki NP, et al: Anatomic and physiologic imaging of Alzheimer's disease. Clin Geriatr Med 10:277–298, 1994

Gray KF, Cummings JL: Dementia, in The American Psychiatric Publishing Textbook of Consultation-Liaison Psychiatry: Psychiatry in the Medically Ill, 2nd Edition. Edited by Wise MG, Rundell JR. Washington, DC, American Psychiatric Publishing, 2002, pp 273–306

Heyn P, Abreu BC, Ottenbacher KJ: The effects of exercise training on elderly persons with cognitive impairment and dementia: a meta-analysis. Arch Phys Med Rehabil 85:1694–1704, 2004

Mace NL, Rabins PV: The 36-Hour Day, Revised Edition: A Family Guide to Caring for Persons With Alzheimer's Disease, Related Dementing Illness and Memory Loss in Later Life. New York, Warner Books, 2001

McKeith IG: Dementia with Lewy bodies. Br J Psychiatry 180:144–147, 2002

McKeith IG, Mosimann UP: Dementia with Lewy bodies and Parkinson's disease. Parkinsonism Relat Disord 10 (suppl 1):S15–S18, 2004

McKeith IG, Galasko D, Kosaka K, et al: Consensus guidelines for the clinical and pathologic diagnosis of dementia with Lewy bodies (DLB): report of the Consortium on DLB International Workshop. Neurology 47:1113–1124, 1996

McKhann GM, Albert MS, Grossman M, et al: Clinical and pathological diagnosis of frontotemporal dementia: report of the Work Group on Frontotemporal Dementia and Pick's Disease. Arch Neurol 58:1803–1809, 2001

Meyer JS, Rogers RL, McClintic K, et al: Randomized clinical trial of daily aspirin therapy in multi-infarct dementia: a pilot study. J Am Geriatr Soc 37:549–555, 1989

Mukamal KJ, Kuller LH, Fitzpatrick AL, et al. Prospective study of alcohol consumption and the risk of dementia in older adults. JAMA 289:1405–1413, 2003

Nagy Z, Esiri MM, Hindley NJ, et al: Accuracy of clinical operational diagnostic criteria for Alzheimer's disease in relation to different pathological diagnostic protocols. Dement Geriatr Cogn Disord 9:219–226, 1998

Oslin DW, Cary MS: Alcohol-related dementias: validation of diagnostic criteria. Am J Geriatr Psychiatry 11:441–447, 2003

Pinner E, Rich CL: Effects of trazodone on aggressive behavior in seven patients with organic mental disorders. Am J Psychiatry 145:1295–1296, 1988

Rabins PV: Reversible dementia and the misdiagnosis of dementia: a review. Hosp Community Psychiatry 34:830–835, 1983

Royall DR, Mahurin RK, Gray KF: Bedside assessment of executive cognitive impairment: the Executive Interview. J Am Geriatr Soc 40:1221–1226, 1992

van Dyck CH: Understanding the latest advances in pharmacologic interventions for Alzheimer's disease. CNS Spectrum 9 (suppl 5):24–28, 2004

Additional Readings

Bliwise DL: What is sundowning? J Am Geriatr Soc 42:1009–1011, 1994

Carlyle W, Ancill RJ, Sheldon L: Aggression in the demented patient: a double-blind study of loxapine versus haloperidol. Int Clin Psychopharmacol 8:103–108, 1993

De Deyn PP, Carrasco MM, Deberdt W, el al: Olanzapine versus placebo in the treatment of psychosis with or without associated behavioral disturbances in patients with Alzheimer's disease. Int J Geriatr Psychiatry 19:115–126, 2004

Jones BN, Reifler BV: Depression coexisting with dementia: evaluation and treatment. Med Clin North Am 78:823–840, 1994

Lishman AW: Senile dementias, presenile dementias and pseudodementias, in Organic Psychiatry: The Psychological Consequences of Cerebral Disorder, 3rd Edition. Oxford, England, Blackwell Scientific, 1998, pp 428–506

Otto M, Cepek L, Ratzka P, et al: Efficacy of flupirtine on cognitive function in patients with Creutzfeld-Jacob disease: a double-blind study. Neurology 62:714–718, 2004

Petersen RC, Smith GE, Ivnik RJ, et al: Memory function in very early Alzheimer's disease. Neurology 44:867–872, 1994

Rabinowitz J, Katz IR, De Deyn PP, et al: Behavioral and psychological symptoms in patients with dementia as a target for pharmacotherapy with risperidone. J Clin Psychiatry. 65:1329–1334, 2004

Victor M: Alcoholic dementia. Can J Neurol Sci 21:88–99, 1994

Wise MG, Gray KF, Seltzer B: Delirium, dementia, and amnestic disorder, in The American Psychiatric Press Textbook of Psychiatry, 3rd Edition. Edited by Hales RE, Yudofsky SC, Talbott JA. Washington, DC, American Psychiatric Press, 1999, pp 317–362

5

Depression

Epidemiology

The lifetime prevalence rate for major depressive disorder is 5%–12% for men and 10%–25% for women. The point prevalence rate is 2%–3% for men and 5%–9% for women (American Psychiatric Association 2000). Almost 80% of the individuals with a major depressive disorder did not receive "minimally adequate" treatments (i.e., at least four outpatient visits with a physician and an antidepressant or a mood stabilizer for a minimum of 30 days, or at least eight outpatient psychotherapy visits for 30 minutes or more with a mental health specialist) (Kessler et al. 2003).

The point prevalence for a major depressive disorder in the medically ill is considerably higher: 10%–36% for general medical inpatients and 9%–16% for general medical outpatients (Rouchell et al. 2002). Mood disorders are present in 26% of the patients seen in outpatient primary care settings and account for more impairment than common medical disorders (Spitzer et al. 1995).

Interrelations Between Depression and Other Medical Illnesses

The interplay between major or minor depression and other medical illnesses is complex. The patient who has a medical illness is more likely to develop depression. Once depressed, the patient has increased morbidity and mortality and a worse prognosis. The reverse is also true. Depression may cause other medical illnesses, such as cardiovascular disease, stroke, cancer, and epilepsy. The potential components in this bidirectional relation are listed in Table 5–1.

Table 5–1.   Increased morbidity and mortality: interrelation between medical illnesses and depression

Noncompliance—increases mortality in medical illness and is more likely to occur in depressed individuals.

Shared risk factors (e.g., smoking, hypertension, diabetes, hypercholesterolemia, obesity)—for example, smoking is associated with several medical diseases (including depression); depressed individuals are much more likely to smoke.

Hypothalamic-pituitary-adrenocortical axis and sympathoadrenal activation—cause elevated cortisol and norepinephrine.

Decreased heart rate variability and low baroreflex sensitivity—both increase the relative risk of cardiac mortality; individuals with depression have a significant decrease in heart rate variability and reduction in baroreflex sensitivity.

Chronic inflammation—baseline levels of inflammation are implicated in cardiovascular disease; patients who are depressed have elevated inflammatory markers.

Platelet activation—plays a role in ischemic heart disease, and aspirin improved long-term survival; untreated patients who are depressed have a variety of platelet abnormalities that lead to platelet activation, and selective serotonin reuptake inhibitors normalize platelet function.

Increased stress—risk factor for adverse cardiovascular events and depression.

Source.   Adapted from Joynt KE, Whellan DJ, O'Conner CM: "Depression and Cardiovascular Disease: Mechanisms of Interaction." *Biological Psychiatry* 54:248–261, 2003.

Medical illness and mood disorders each individually decrease quality of life and productivity and increase health care use, but what are the combined effects when a patient has a medical illness and depression? Simon (2003) reported that depression and chronic medical illness produce differing patterns of impairments, and those impairments are additive. In addition, data on health care costs indicate a strong association between depression and increased cost at all levels of medical comorbidity; however, the relation is closer to multiplicative than additive (Simon 2003).

Clinical Characteristics

Diagnostic Criteria

The mnemonic Sig:E Caps (Prescribe Energy Capsules) is a useful way to remember and is a tool to teach primary care physicians the diagnostic criteria for major depressive episode (Table 5–2). To diagnose major depressive episode, DSM-IV-TR (American Psychiatric Association 2000) requires at least five of nine depressive symptoms, and one of the symptoms must be either depressed mood or loss of interest or pleasure during the same 2-week period. Of importance, DSM-IV-TR also states that symptoms are excluded from the diagnosis if they are due to the direct physiological effects of a substance…or a general medical condition (American Psychiatric Association 2000). These exclusions present a conundrum for the consulting psychiatrist. Constitutional features of medical illnesses and side effects of treatments often produce neurovegetative symptoms, such as fatigue, insomnia, and poor appetite. How are neurovegetative complaints handled in a patient who is medically ill and taking several medications? Should these symptoms be excluded when diagnosing depression? This is a challenging and potentially frustrating issue. Many consultation psychiatrists do not use DSM-IV-TR's exclusive approach to diagnose major depressive disorder in medical-surgical patients. Cohen-Cole and Stoudemire (1987) recommended an inclusive approach to the diagnosis of depression in the medically ill; that is, count all symptoms toward the diagnosis of depression regardless of whether they might be secondary to another medical illness or medications. This approach may lead to some false-positive diagnoses, but that is preferable to withholding treatment to medically ill patients who are depressed and could benefit from treatment.

Table 5–2. Mnemonic for diagnostic criteria for major depressive episode

Sig:E Caps (Prescribe Energy Capsules)

Sleep	Insomnia or hypersomnia
Interests	Loss of interest or pleasure in activities
Guilt	Excessive guilt, worthlessness, hopelessness
Energy	Loss of energy or fatigue
Concentration	Diminished concentration ability, indecisive
Appetite	Decreased appetite, >5% weight loss or gain
Psychomotor/physical symptoms	Psychomotor retardation or agitation Physical and painful symptom associated with depression
Suicidality	Suicidal thought, ideation, plan, or attempt

Some experienced psychiatrists use another approach: they substitute psychological symptoms for the neurovegetative symptoms that confound the diagnosis. For example, Endicott (1984) replaced change in appetite or weight with tearfulness or depressed appearance, sleep disturbance with social withdrawal, indecisiveness with lack of reactivity to events, and loss of energy or fatigue with brooding pessimism.

The diagnosis of dysthymic disorder (three Sig:E Caps symptoms present; one must be depressed mood) in the medically ill is restricted in DSM-IV-TR by the same exclusion criteria that complicate the diagnosis of major depressive disorder and also requires a duration of 2 years. In the medical-surgical setting, dysthymia is often used to mean either 1) a chronic characterological mood syndrome (i.e., essentially equivalent to depressive personality disorder) or 2) minor depression (i.e., depression that is significant but falls short of the full criteria for major depression and the time criteria for dysthymia).

Acute illness and hospitalization are stressful events that can precipitate a depressive reaction. This depressive reaction can meet the criteria for the diagnosis of adjustment disorder with depressed mood, which is one of the most common diagnoses made by psychiatrists in the general hospital or clinic setting (Rouchell et al. 2002). Patients with adjustment disorder are often good candidates for psychotherapy.

Primary and Secondary Etiologies

The psychiatric consultant in the general hospital frequently suspects that a major depressive episode is due to a specific medical or toxic etiology; however, the consultant should avoid the functional versus organic dichotomy that is often applied to psychiatric diagnoses in medical settings. A functional label implies that no biological component exists. The functional–organic split fosters the belief that psychiatric disorders are not medical, or even real. We recommend that clinicians use the neutral terms secondary and primary instead, which are already widely used in medicine. The term secondary refers to a psychiatric syndrome that occurs after a medical event or ingestion of a neuroactive substance; primary implies an autonomous psychiatric disorder that is unrelated to other medical events.

Depression as a Neurodegenerative Disorder

A growing body of evidence suggests that depression, in at least some individuals, is a neurodegenerative disorder (MacQueen et al. 2003). Young patients who are depressed show deficits in executive function and memory that seem to worsen in older patients who are chronically depressed (Fossati et al. 2002; Porter et al. 2003). Numerous studies report reduced brain volumes (Pantel et al. 1997) and/or decreased hippocampal volumes in older depressed patients (MacQueen et al. 2003); this atrophy seems to progress with duration of depressive illness and may be secondary to glucocorticoid excess or toxicity seen in depression (Sheline et al. 1996). An alternative hypothesis for cell loss or atrophy is that stress reduces brain-derived neurotrophic factors; this effect is blocked by antidepressants (Duman 2004).

The accumulating evidence should give pause to clinicians who label the cognitive dysfunction seen in depressed older patients as pseudo- or reversible dementia. It might more accurately be called the dementia syndrome of depression. When Alexopoulus et al. (1993) conducted a controlled study of geriatric depression and "reversible dementia," reversible cognitive impairment was a prodrome of irreversible dementia in nearly 50% of patients.

Differential Diagnosis

The clinician must try to determine whether a medically ill patient has a mood disorder and, if so, whether it is primary or secondary. First, to help establish the presence of major depression in a patient with severe medical illness, the clinician should look for psychological symptoms, such as anhedonia, guilt, worthlessness, helplessness, hopelessness, and suicidal ideation, rather than rely purely on neurovegetative symptoms, such as fatigue, weight loss, and poor sleep. Second, the clinician should review the history of depression in the patient and his or her family. Patients with primary unipolar depression typically have a history of multiple depressive episodes, with an average of five or six episodes over 20 years (Winokur 1986). First-degree relatives of unipolar depressed patients experience major depression seven times more frequently than do control subjects. Third, the clinician should look for potentially reversible medical and toxic causes of the depressive syndrome. Medical conditions and several neuroactive agents are associated with the onset of depressive syndromes. Many of the substance-related associations are anecdotal and are based on a temporal relation between the event and the subsequent depressive episode. A temporal association does not mean that a cause-and-effect relation exists; however, studies link some toxic or metabolic factors to the onset of major depressive syndromes. Table 5–3 is a list of conditions and toxic agents associated with secondary depressive disorders.

Other neuropsychiatric disorders, such as delirium, dementia, psychoactive substance use disorders, anxiety disorders, schizophrenia, somatoform disorders, and personality disorders, can resemble or accompany depression. The distinction between early dementia and depression is often difficult; clinically helpful considerations are summarized in Table 5–4. Remember, dementia and depression often coexist, and cognitive dysfunction often accompanies depression (see section "Depression as a Neurodegenerative Disorder" earlier in this chapter). (See Chapter 4, "Dementia," in this volume for a more detailed discussion of the diagnosis of dementia.)

Treatment and Management

Reversal of Etiology

After the diagnosis of depression is established, the clinician must identify etiologies of the depressive syndrome that may be reversed or ameliorated (see Table 5–3). If the etiology is found but cannot be reversed, if no remediable etiology is found, or if the depression does not resolve after the offending agent is removed, the patient may need antidepressant treatment.

Response Versus Remission

The current standard of treatment is remission (i.e., absence of depressive symptoms, often defined as a 17-item Hamilton Rating Scale for Depression [Ham-D$_{17}$] score$\leq$7), not just a response to treatment (usually defined as a 50% or greater reduction in the Ham-D$_{17}$ score). In other words, a depressed patient may "feel much better" with treatment (i.e., responds to treatment), but lingering or residual depressive symptoms mean a much higher risk of relapse, continued impairments, and increased use of medical services (Doraiswamy et al. 2001; Simon 2003).

Remission is easily measured in a clinical research setting, in part because patients with other medical illnesses are excluded and because well-established measurement tools such as the Ham-D are used. The definition and measurement of remission in depressed patients who have one or several other medical illnesses are not as simple. For example, a 50-year-old woman with severe de-

Table 5–3. Medical conditions and toxic agents associated with secondary depressive disorders

Endocrine disorders
Addison's disease
Cushing's disease
Diabetes mellitus
Hyperparathyroidism
Hypopituitarism
Hypothyroidism

Infections
Encephalitis
Epstein-Barr virus
Hepatitis
HIV
Pneumonia
Postinfluenza
Tertiary syphilis
Tuberculosis

Tumors
Central nervous system
Lung
Pancreas

Neurological disorders
Cerebrovascular disease
Dementia (particularly subcortical)
Epilepsy (particularly with a
  temporal lobe focus)
Huntington's disease
Multiple sclerosis
Parkinson's disease
Postconcussional disorder
Progressive supranuclear palsy
Sleep apnea
Stroke
Subarachnoid hemorrhage

Medications
Amphetamine withdrawal
Antihypertensives: methyldopa, clonidine,
  guanethidine, reserpine, diuretics
Barbiturates
Benzodiazepines
β-Blockers
Cholinesterase inhibitors
Cimetidine
Cocaine withdrawal
Corticosteroids
Disulfiram
Gonadotropin-releasing hormone agonists
Levodopa
Mefloquine
Metoclopramide
Chemotherapeutic agents: vinblastine,
  vincristine, procarbazine, L-asparaginase,
  interferon alfa
Interleukin-2
Opiates
Progesterone-releasing implanted
  contraceptives

Others
Alcoholism
Anemia
Electrolyte abnormalities
Heavy metal poisoning
Hypertension
Systemic lupus erythematosus

Table 5–4.   Differentiating depression and dementia

	Depression	Dementia
Insidious onset	Weeks–months	Months–years
Psychological distress present	Yes	No
Frequently answers "I don't know"	Yes	No
Higher cortical function deficits (dysphasia, dyspraxia)	No	Yes
Remote memory less impaired than recent memory	No	Yes
Inconsistent mental status examination findings on repeated examinations	Yes	No
Past or family history of mood disorder	Yes	No
Aware of cognitive deficits	Yes	No
Neuroimaging study results usually abnormal	No	Yes

Note.   Depression and dementia can occur together, especially in subcortical dementias. When a patient with dementia also has comorbid major depression, his or her cognitive deficits are greatly magnified.

pression and type 1 diabetes mellitus is admitted to the hospital. After she is medically stabilized, psychiatry consultation is requested. Assuming that the patient was euthymic prior to this depressive episode, which is often not the case, remission might be defined as regaining predepression levels of function and physical symptoms. In a more difficult-to-judge case, a 70-year-old man is admitted to the hospital after a Broca's area stroke and develops a severe depression during rehabilitation. How will remission or optimal treatment be defined? In clinical practice, it usually means that the patient begins to progress like others in rehabilitation who have had a similar insult. In any case, well-established measurement tools and definitions for remission are less available in patients with chronic or debilitating medical illness.

Pharmacological Management

Table 5–5 lists antidepressants, dosage ranges, and receptor affinities, which also determine side effects. For example, sedative potency and appetite stimulation are related to central nervous system (CNS) histamine$_1$ (H$_1$) receptor affinity, anticholinergic potency is related to peripheral muscarinic receptor affinity, and orthostatic hypotension is related to peripheral α_1 receptor affinity.

Table 5–5. Cyclic and related antidepressants

Generic name	Trade name	Alternative modes of administration†	Initial dose (mg)^b	Usual therapeutic dose range (mg)^b	Effect^a					
					NE reuptake blockade	5-HT reuptake blockade	DA reuptake blockade	ACh blockade	Histamine blockade	α₁ blockade
Amitriptyline	Elavil, others	im, iv^c	25–75	150–300	2	3	1	4	3	3
Amoxapine	Asendin	—	50–150	100–600	3	1	1	1	2	2
Bupropion	Wellbutrin Wellbutrin SR Wellbutrin XL	—	100 bid 150 qd	300–450 300–400	1	0	1	1	1	1
Citalopram	Celexa	Liquid	20	20–60	0	3	0	0	0	0
Clomipramine	Anafranil	—	25	100–250	2	4	1	2	0	2
Desipramine	Norpramin, others	—	25–75	75–200	4	0	1	2	1	2
Doxepin	Sinequan, others	Liquid	25–75	150–300	2	1	0	3	4	3
Duloxetine	Cymbalta	—	30–60	40–120	4	4	1	0	0	0
Escitalopram	Lexapro	Liquid	10	10–20	0	3	0	0	0	0

Table 5–5. Cyclic and related antidepressants *(continued)*

Generic name	Trade name	Alternative modes of admin-istration†	Initial dose (mg)[b]	Usual therapeutic dose range (mg)[b]	NE reuptake blockade	5-HT reuptake blockade	DA reuptake blockade	ACh blockade	Histamine blockade	α_1 blockade
Fluoxetine	Prozac	Liquid	20	20–60	1	3	1	1	0	1
Imipramine	Tofranil, others	im, iv[c]	25–75	150–300	2	2	0	3	2	3
Maprotiline	Ludiomil	—	25–75	75–300	4	0	1	2	3	2
Milnacipran[d]	Ixel	—	25–50 bid	50–200	2	2	1	0	0	0
Mirtazapine[e]	Remeron	—	15	15–30	—[e]	—[e]	0	2	4	1
Nefazodone	Serzone	—	50 bid	300–600	2	2	1	0	0	2
Nortriptyline	Pamelor, others	—	20–40	50–200	3	1	0	2	2	1
Paroxetine	Paxil	Liquid	20	20–50	1	4	1	2	0	1
Protriptyline	Vivactil	—	10–20	20–60	3	1	0	3	2	2
Sertraline	Zoloft	Liquid	50	50–200	0	4	1	1	0	1
Trazodone	Desyrel	—	50	100–600	1	2	0	0	1	3

Effect[a]

Table 5–5. Cyclic and related antidepressants *(continued)*

Generic name	Trade name	Alternative modes of administration[†]	Initial dose (mg)[b]	Usual therapeutic dose range (mg)[b]	Effect[a]					
					NE reuptake blockade	5-HT reuptake blockade	DA reuptake blockade	ACh blockade	Histamine blockade	α_1 blockade
Trimipramine	Surmontil	—	25–75	75–300	1	2	0	3	4	3
Venlafaxine	Effexor	—	25 tid	225–375	1	3	0	0	0	1
	Effexor XR		75 qd	225–375						

Note.   ACh=acetylcholine; DA=dopamine; 5-HT=serotonin; NE=norepinephrine; im=intramuscular; iv=intravenous; bid=twice a day; qd=once a day; tid=three times a day.

[a]0=least effect; 4=most effect.

[b]Doses for elderly and medically ill patients are often lower.

[c]Not approved by the U.S. Food and Drug Administration for intravenous administration.

[d]Used as an antidepressant outside United States; undergoing clinical trials in United States for fibromyalgia indication.

[e]Mirtazapine blocks the noradrenergic α_2 auto- and heteroreceptors responsible for controlling norepinephrine and 5-HT release. In addition, mirtazapine potently blocks 5-HT$_2$ and 5-HT$_3$ receptors, which helps prevent side effects associated with nonselective 5-HT activation.

[†]Many drugs can be made into rectal suppositories or even lotions by willing pharmacists.

Source.   Adapted from Fait ML, Wise MG, Jachna JS, et al.: "Psychopharmacology," in *The American Psychiatric Publishing Textbook of Consultation-Liaison Psychiatry: Psychiatry in the Medically Ill,* 2nd Edition. Edited by Wise MG, Rundell JR. Washington, DC, American Psychiatric Publishing, 2002, p. 948. Copyright 2002, American Psychiatric Publishing. Used with permission.

Tricyclic Antidepressants

General issues.   Tricyclic antidepressants are still used in the hospital and clinic. They are used for chronic pain, headache, insomnia, anxiety, panic, and bed-wetting. Lower doses of tricyclic antidepressants are sometimes required in patients with liver disease, elderly and malnourished patients, and patients taking medications that can slow tricyclic antidepressant metabolism (e.g., paroxetine, fluoxetine). Higher antidepressant doses may be needed in patients taking medications that induce hepatic enzymes (e.g., carbamazepine, phenytoin, and barbiturates).

Adverse effects.   A premedication orthostatic blood pressure measurement that shows a decline in systolic blood pressure greater than 15 mm Hg is associated with a higher risk for significant orthostatic hypotension after starting treatment. Tricyclic antidepressants may lower seizure threshold. Maprotiline is the worst offender in this regard. In patients with cardiac illness, knowledge of the cardiac effects of tricyclic antidepressants is important. When tricyclic antidepressants are within normal therapeutic serum level ranges, they have little, if any, effect on left ventricular performance, even in patients with low ejection fractions. For patients with a history of angina, it is important to be aware that anticholinergic effects may increase the heart rate and slightly increase cardiac workload. Tricyclic antidepressants may, like type IA antiarrhythmic drugs such as quinidine, prolong ventricular depolarization by delaying conduction in the His-Purkinje cardiac conduction system. Ventricular dysrhythmias may actually improve. However, a patient who has preexisting bundle branch disease is at risk for second- or third-degree heart block (Glassman and Bigger 1981). Conduction delay will appear on the electrocardiogram as increased duration of the QTc, QRS, and PR intervals. Risk of sudden death increases if QTc is greater than 440 msec (Schwartz and Wolf 1978).

Monoamine Oxidase Inhibitors

General issues.   Depressive syndromes with prominent anxiety, phobias, panic, or obsessions have shown a better response in some studies to monoamine oxidase inhibitors (MAOIs) than to other antidepressants. MAOIs are also used when the symptoms have a poor response to another type of agent or the patient has a history of good response to an MAOI. The two MAOIs used in the United States—phenelzine (45–90 mg/day) and tranylcypromine

(30–50 mg/day)—irreversibly inhibit both MAO-A and MAO-B. Common initial daily doses are 30 mg and 20 mg, respectively. Selegiline at lower doses is a selective irreversible inhibitor of MAO-B and is indicated for the treatment of Parkinson's disease. At higher doses, it is a nonselective inhibitor of MAO and has been used to treat depression.

Adverse effects. MAOIs have the advantage in medically ill patients of having virtually no cardiac effects, relatively low sedative potential (except phenelzine), and no anticholinergic activity. However, the potential for causing orthostatic hypotension is very high, sometimes occurring up to several weeks after the drug has been started. MAOIs also can produce hypertensive crises in the presence of tyramine-containing foods; MAOI use requires dietary counseling. Other potential adverse effects of MAOIs are anorgasmia, sedation (more common with phenelzine), activation (more common with tranylcypromine), dry mouth, urinary hesitancy, constipation, weight gain, edema, and myoclonic twitches. Another source of difficulty is concomitant use of MAOIs with sympathomimetics, other psychotropic agents, and meperidine. The use of these agents with MAOIs can result in a hypertensive crisis or severe serotonin syndrome (Nierenberg and Semprebon 1993). Caution should be exercised when switching from an MAOI to another antidepressant. A 2-week drug-free period is recommended to allow time for MAO to regenerate.

Selective Serotonin Reuptake Inhibitors

General issues. The selective serotonin reuptake inhibitors (SSRIs) are generally well tolerated by the depressed medically ill patient. SSRIs differ in the presence of active metabolites and elimination half-life. For example, fluoxetine, which has an elimination half-life of 1–3 days, is converted to norfluoxetine, a potent SSRI with a half-life of 7–9 days. Therefore, steady-state plasma levels are not reached for 5–6 weeks; a similar amount of time is required to clear norfluoxetine from the patient's system after discontinuation. In contrast, sertraline and paroxetine have short elimination half-lives (Nemeroff 1993). A recent, large study of depressed patients treated in primary care clinics with one of three SSRIs (fluoxetine, paroxetine, or sertraline) showed interesting results. Depressed mood and sense of well-being improved significantly and continuously over 9 months, while physical and painful symptoms improved somewhat during the first month of treatment but showed minimal improvement and resolution thereafter (Greco et al. 2004). If these results prove true, norepinephrine reuptake inhibition or enhancement may be an essential adjunct in the treatment of painful physical symptoms (Max et al. 1992).

Patients frequently ask how long they should continue taking SSRI (and other) antidepressant medications once depression is in remission. Data suggest (Reimherr et al. 1998) that relapse rates of patients in remission who stop taking SSRI medication are about twice as high 3 months later (49% vs. 26%) and 2.5 times higher 6 months after discontinuation (23% vs. 9%).

Adverse effects. The most common side effects of SSRIs are gastrointestinal distress, nervousness, sexual dysfunction, and insomnia. Almost all SSRIs inhibit enzymes in the cytochrome P450 system and can cause accumulation of medications metabolized by this system (see Chapter 10, "Important Pharmacological Issues," in this volume for more details). Paroxetine is the most potent inhibitor of the important 2D6 enzyme, followed by fluoxetine and sertraline. Cytochrome P450 2D6 metabolizes many antiarrhythmics, antidepressants, neuroleptics, codeine, oxycodone, and hydroxycodone (Otton et al. 1993). In addition, about 7% of Caucasians are deficient in this enzyme and are therefore slow metabolizers (Otton et al. 1993).

Other Antidepressants

General issues. Several nontricyclic, non-SSRI antidepressants, including bupropion, trazodone, venlafaxine, mirtazapine, and duloxetine, are available (see Table 5–5).

Adverse effects. Bupropion can be stimulating and causes fewer anticholinergic effects than do tricyclic antidepressants, little orthostatic hypertension, and few adverse sexual side effects (Fait et al. 2002). However, bupropion may produce anxiety, agitation, insomnia, increased motor activity, gastrointestinal side effects, and headache. It is commonly used for treatment-resistant cases and as an adjunct to other antidepressants.

Trazodone's sedating properties and lack of anticholinergic side effects make it a widely used medication in lower doses for sleep. However, its association with priapism and orthostatic hypotension limits its use as an antidepressant. Trazodone is sometimes combined with an SSRI to address different sets of target symptoms. Trazodone has fewer cardiac effects than do other cyclic antidepressants and apparently does not slow conduction. However, it may exacerbate ventricular irritability, so it should be used with caution in patients with heart disease.

Venlafaxine blocks reuptake of serotonin at lower doses and norepinephrine at higher doses; its dual action at higher doses, usually thought to occur in the 150–225+ mg/day range, appears to benefit some patients whose condition has not responded to SSRIs or other antidepressants and is effective in reducing the pain of diabetic neuropathy. Venlafaxine has a dose-related risk of hypertension; it also causes high rates of sexual dysfunction in men and women.

Mirtazapine is moderately anticholinergic and very antihistaminic; therefore, it is associated with increased appetite, weight gain, and significant sedation. Mirtazapine is well suited for certain patients (e.g., a patient with advanced cancer who is depressed, has no appetite, and cannot sleep).

Duloxetine is a dual-action antidepressant that differs from venlafaxine. Even at low doses, duloxetine is a potent inhibitor of both serotonin and norepinephrine. Initial data show low rates of sexual dysfunction, no dose-related hypertension, and a mild discontinuation syndrome; dual-action antidepressants (SNRIs) show efficacy in painful syndromes (e.g., diabetic neuropathy).

Psychostimulants

General issues. Psychostimulant medications, such as methylphenidate (plasma half-life = 1–2 hours) and dextroamphetamine (plasma half-life = 6–8 hours), are useful in the treatment armamentarium. Table 5–6 lists situations in which psychostimulants are an important treatment option. Psychostimulants are fast acting, well tolerated, and safe among elderly and medically ill patients (Massand et al. 1991). Usual dosage ranges are 5–20 mg/day for both methylphenidate and dextroamphetamine. Because these medications have short half-lives, two doses per day are usually given, one in the morning and one at noon or early afternoon. Doses later than 3:00 P.M. should be avoided so that sleep is not disturbed. When effective, the onset of action is usually within 2–3 days.

Adverse effects. Psychostimulants have few side effects; potential adverse effects include sinus tachycardia and other arrhythmias, blood pressure elevation, psychosis, insomnia, anorexia, and exacerbation of spasticity in patients with upper motor neuron disease. These side effects usually occur at doses much higher than those recommended. Physicians have a bias against psycho-

Table 5–6.   Clinical situations in which psychostimulants are an important treatment option

When neurovegetative features of depression threaten health or life and a rapid response is needed

When cardiac and other adverse effects of other antidepressants should be avoided

When diagnostic uncertainty exists—a good response to a trial of a stimulant often helps confirm a diagnosis of depression

In terminally ill patients with profound psychomotor retardation

For treatment-resistant depression

For adult attention-deficit disorder

For late-stage HIV disease (AIDS)–associated secondary mood disorders

For poststroke depression

For depression associated with subcortical dementias (e.g., dementia associated with Parkinson's disease)

---

stimulant medications because of their potential for abuse. At the doses recommended for the treatment of depression in the medical setting, the risk is negligible.

Electroconvulsive Therapy

Electroconvulsive therapy (ECT) is a first-line treatment for depressed patients who are severely malnourished or dehydrated, who have catatonia, who have a previously documented good response to ECT, and who have delusional depression (Welch 1991). The percentage of patients who respond (79%) and achieve full remission (75%) is very impressive when compared with medications; treatment response to ECT is rapid, with 65% achieving remission at or before week 4 (ECT treatment #10) (Husain et al. 2004). ECT's main adverse effect is anterograde and retrograde memory loss. This memory loss is usually mild and transient and disappears within a few weeks. Unilateral nondominant electrode placement decreases memory loss.

There are no absolute contraindications to ECT; however, some medical conditions increase the morbidity associated with ECT and require thoughtful review of the risks and benefits. These include 1) conditions that cause increased intracranial pressure, 2) conditions that increase the risk of serious hemorrhage, and 3) pathophysiological states that cause hemodynamic compromise, such as an acute myocardial infarction or malignant arrhythmias (Rouchell et al. 2002). The addition of β-blockers and antiarrhythmics before ECT reduces some of these risks. Mortality associated with ECT is less than 0.05% and is essentially the same as the risk of brief general anesthesia.

Medical Psychotherapy

The psychiatric examination is not complete without an attempt by the psychiatric consultant to understand the meaning of the illness to the patient. When past experiences or current level of psychological function is an issue, talk therapy is often helpful (see also Chapter 13, "Personality, Response to Illness, and Medical Psychotherapy," in this volume). Because most hospital stays are short, brief therapies are used. For patients seen in outpatient consultation, cognitive therapy, psychodynamic psychotherapy, and supportive psychotherapy are available treatment options.

Cognitive therapy is particularly useful for patients with false beliefs about their illness, such as patients who believe that illness represents punishment or weakness, have unrealistic or distorted fears and expectations, and have exaggerated or inappropriate responses to loss (Fava et al. 1988). Data suggest that cognitive-behavioral treatment of residual depressive symptoms may decrease the number of recurrences of full major depressive episodes (Fava et al. 1998a, 1998b). Evidence indicates that cognitive therapy may fare as well as medication for mild and moderate depression (DeRubeis et al. 1999). Cognitive therapy is a sound treatment both in addition to antidepressant medication and instead of antidepressant medication in patients who will not take medication.

Some brief psychodynamic psychotherapies can be completed in 6–10 sessions. Supportive psychotherapy is appropriate for a large portion of patients with medical illnesses who are seen by psychiatrists. The value to the patient of abreacting or "just talking" is often underestimated. Group psychotherapy promotes support, improves interpersonal relationships, models adaptive coping mechanisms, decreases loneliness, and helps the patient develop a sense of meaning in life. Spiegel (1990) used psychoeducational group therapy to treat depression in patients with metastatic breast cancer. He found that the patients in group therapy lived twice as long as the patients who received only routine oncological care. In more recent studies, psychosocial interventions have not prolonged survival but have improved mood and decreased pain perception (Goodwin et al. 2001).

Treatment Outcome

Depression can increase the likelihood of developing other medical illnesses (Evans and Charney 2003). Also, clear and convincing evidence indicates that depression increases mortality, morbidity, and health care use and impedes recovery in patients who have other medical illnesses (Evans and Charney 2003). For example, poststroke depression increased mortality 50% at 1 year (Robinson 2003). Antidepressant treatment of poststroke depression improves recovery (activities of daily living) and increases survival; antidepressants also can prevent depression following stroke and may reduce subsequent hospitalization for cardiovascular disease and perhaps mortality (Robinson 2003). Recent trials in which sertraline was used to treat depression in patients after myocardial infarction showed less consistent results, although results did show that sertraline was effective and safe.

Attempts to answer the question "Are medically ill patients who develop major depression more resistant to antidepressants than are healthier comparators?" have yielded conflicting results. Koike et al. (2002) found that depressed patients with comorbid medical illness received treatment at the same rate as depressed patients without other medical disorders, but the patients with comorbidity were more depressed at 6- and 12-month follow-up. However, Stockton et al. (2004) compared outcome and treatments among three patient groups with major depression—1) those with no medical comorbidity, 2) those with low levels of medical comorbidity, and 3) those with high levels of medical comorbidity—and found no difference in treatments received or outcomes.

References

American Psychiatric Association: Diagnostic and Statistical Manual of Mental Disorders, 4th Edition, Text Revision. Washington, DC, American Psychiatric Association, 2000

Alexopoulos GS, Meyers BS, Young RC, et al: The course of geriatric depression with "reversible dementia": a controlled study. Am J Psychiatry 150:1693–1699, 1993

Cohen-Cole SA, Stoudemire A: Major depression and physical illness: special considerations in diagnosis and biologic treatment. Psychiatr Clin North Am 10:1–17, 1987

DeRubeis RJ, Gelfand LA, Tang TZ, et al: Medications versus cognitive behavior therapy for severely depressed outpatients: mega-analysis of four randomized comparisons. Am J Psychiatry 156:1007–1013, 1999

Doraiswamy PM, Khan ZM, Donahue RM, et al: Quality of life in geriatric depression: a comparison of remitters, partial responders, and nonresponders. Am J Geriatr Psychiatry 9:423–428, 2001

Duman RS: Role of neurotrophic factors in the etiology and treatment of mood disorders. Neuromolecular Med 5:11–25, 2004

Endicott J: Measurement of depression in patients with cancer. Cancer 53:2243–2248, 1984

Evans DL, Charney DS: Mood disorders and medical illness: a major public health problem. Biol Psychiatry 54:177–180, 2003

Fait ML, Wise MG, Jachna JS, et al: Psychopharmacology, in The American Psychiatric Publishing Textbook of Consultation-Liaison Psychiatry: Psychiatry in the Medically Ill, 2nd Edition. Edited by Wise MG, Rundell JR. Washington, DC, American Psychiatric Publishing, 2002, pp 939–987

Fava GA, Sonino N, Wise TN: Management of depression in medical patients. Psychother Psychosom 49:81–102, 1988

Fava GA, Rafanelli C, Grandi S, et al: Prevention of recurrent depression with cognitive behavioral therapy. Arch Gen Psychiatry 55:816–820, 1998a

Fava GA, Rafanelli C, Grandi S, et al: Six-year outcome for cognitive behavioral treatment of residual symptoms in major depression. Am J Psychiatry 155:1443–1445, 1998b

Fossati P, Coyette F, Ergis AM, et al: Influence of age and executive function on verbal memory of inpatients with depression. J Affect Disord 68:261–271, 2002

Glassman AH, Bigger T: Cardiovascular effects of therapeutic doses of tricyclic antidepressants: a review. Arch Gen Psychiatry 38:815–820, 1981

Goodwin PJ, Leszcz M, Ennis M, et al: The effect of group psychosocial support on survival in metastatic breast cancer. N Engl J Med 345:1719–1726, 2001

Greco T, Eckert G, Kroenke K: The outcome of physical symptoms with treatment of depression. J Gen Intern Med 19:813–818, 2004

Husain MM, Rush AJ, Fink M, et al: Speed of response and remission in major depressive disorder with acute electroconvulsive therapy (ECT): a Consortium for Research in ECT (CORE) report. J Clin Psychiatry 65:485–491, 2004

Kessler RC, Berglund P, Demler O, et al: The epidemiology of major depressive disorder: results from the National Comorbidity Survey Replication (NCS-R). JAMA 289:3095–3105, 2003

Koike AK, Unutzer J, Wells KB: Improving the care for depression in patients with comorbid medical illness. Am J Psychiatry 159:1738–1745, 2002

MacQueen GM, Campbell S, McEwen BS, et al: Course of illness, hippocampal function, and hippocampal volume in major depression. Proc Natl Acad Sci USA 100:1387–1392, 2003

Massand P, Pickett P, Murray GB: Psychostimulants for secondary depression in medical illness. Psychosomatics 32:203–208, 1991

Max MB, Lynch SA, Muir J: Effects of desipramine, amitriptyline, and fluoxetine on pain in diabetic neuropathy. N Engl J Med 326:1250–1256, 1992

Nemeroff CB: Paroxetine: an overview of the efficacy and safety of a new selective serotonin reuptake inhibitor in the treatment of depression. J Clin Psychopharmacol 13 (suppl 2):18–22, 1993

Nierenberg DW, Semprebon M: The central nervous system serotonin syndrome. Clin Pharmacol Ther 53:84–88, 1993

Otton SV, Wu D, Joffe RT, et al: Inhibition by fluoxetine of cytochrome P450 2D6 activity. Clin Pharmacol Ther 53:401–409, 1993

Pantel J, Schroder J, Essig M, et al: Quantitative magnetic resonance imaging in geriatric depression and primary degenerative dementia. J Affect Disord 42:69–83, 1997

Porter RJ, Gallagher P, Thompson JM, et al: Neurocognitive impairment in drug-free patients with major depressive disorder. Br J Psychiatry 182:214–220, 2003

Reimherr FW, Amsterdam JD, Quitkin FM, et al: Optimal length of continuation therapy in depression: a prospective assessment during long-term fluoxetine treatment. Am J Psychiatry 155:1247–1253, 1998

Robinson R: Poststroke depression: prevalence, diagnosis, treatment, and disease progression. Biol Psychiatry 54:376–387, 2003

Rouchell AM, Pounds R, Tierney JG: Depression, in The American Psychiatric Publishing Textbook of Consultation-Liaison Psychiatry: Psychiatry in the Medically Ill, 2nd Edition. Edited by Wise MG, Rundell JR. Washington, DC, American Psychiatric Publishing, 2002, pp 307–338

Schwartz PJ, Wolf S: QT interval prolongation as predictor of sudden death in patients with myocardial infarction. Circulation 57:1074–1077, 1978

Sheline YI, Wang PW, Gado MH, et al: Hippocampal atrophy in recurrent major depression. Proc Natl Acad Sci U S A 93:3908–3913, 1996

Simon GE: Social and economic burden of mood disorders. Biol Psychiatry 54:208–215, 2003

Spiegel D: Can psychotherapy prolong cancer survival? Psychosomatics 31:361–366, 1990

Spitzer RL, Kroenke K, Linzer M, et al: Health-related quality of life in primary care patients with mental disorders: results from the PRIME-MD 1000 Study. JAMA 274:1511–1517, 1995

Stockton P, Gonzales JJ, Stern NP, et al: Treatment patterns and outcomes of depressed medically ill and non-medically ill patients in community psychiatric practice. Gen Hosp Psychiatry 26:2–8, 2004

Welch CA: Electroconvulsive therapy in the general hospital, in Massachusetts General Hospital Handbook of General Hospital Psychiatry, 3rd Edition. Edited by Cassem NH. St. Louis, MO, Mosby-Year Book, 1991, pp 269–280

Winokur G: Unipolar depression, in The Medical Basis of Psychiatry. Edited by Winokur G, Clayton PJ. Philadelphia, PA, WB Saunders, 1986, pp 60–79

Additional Readings

Cathebras PJ, Robbins JM, Kirmayer LJ, et al: Fatigue in primary care: prevalence, psychiatric comorbidity, illness behavior and outcome. J Gen Intern Med 7:276–286, 1992

Freedland KE, Carney RM, Lustman PJ, et al: Major depression in coronary artery disease patients with vs without a prior history of depression. Psychosom Med 54:416–421, 1992

Liberzon I, Goldman RS, Hendrickson WJ: Very brief psychotherapy in the psychiatric consultation setting. Int J Psychiatry Med 22:65–75, 1992

Mueller TI, Leon AC, Keller MB, et al: Recurrence after recovery from major depressive disorder during 5 years of observational follow-up. Am J Psychiatry 156:1000–1006, 1999

6

Mania

Clinical Characteristics

General Considerations

Patients with primary and secondary mania are seen by consultation-liaison psychiatrists, who require a thorough knowledge of medical and toxic etiologies of manic syndromes. Estimates of lifetime prevalence rates for a manic episode in the general population range from 1.2%–1.6% (Kessler et al. 1997; Weissman et al. 1996). Because bipolar disorder rarely presents after age 50, first-time manic episodes in older patients are almost always secondary.

Diagnostic Criteria

The diagnosis of a manic episode, according to DSM-IV-TR (American Psychiatric Association 2000), requires elevated, expansive, or irritable mood, lasting at least 1 week, or any duration if hospitalization is necessary because of the manic episode. In addition, at least three symptoms from a list of seven cardinal manic episode features (four if the mood is irritable) have been present, and social or occupational functioning is impaired (American Psychiatric Association 2000). The diagnostic criteria for manic episode are summarized in Table 6–1 with the mnemonic GIDDINESS. A hypomanic episode differs only in that social and occupational functioning are not impaired and may even be enhanced.

Table 6–1.   Mnemonic for diagnostic criteria for manic episode: GIDDINESS

Grandiosity
Increased activity
Decreased judgment (risky activities)
Distractibility
Irritability
Need for sleep decreased
Elevated mood
Speedy thoughts
Speedy talk

Secondary mania is due to specific, identifiable medical or toxic factors. In DSM-IV-TR, secondary mania is called "mood disorder due to a general medical condition, with manic features" or "substance-induced mood disorder, with manic features." As in primary mania, the essential feature of this syndrome is a prominent and persistent elevated or expansive mood. Secondary mania is not diagnosed if the mood disturbance occurs in the course of a delirium.

Pathophysiology

Numerous studies of patients with brain damage have found that patients who develop secondary mania have a significantly greater frequency of lesions in the right hemisphere than do patients with brain injury who become depressed or do not develop any mood disturbance at all (McDaniel and Sharma 2002). The right-hemisphere lesions associated with mania are in specific structures that are connected to the limbic system. The right basotemporal cortex is particularly important because direct lesions of this cortical region are associated with secondary mania (Starkstein and Robinson 1992).

Differential Diagnosis

As with depression, the same three principles of diagnostic inquiry apply to mania. First, the diagnosis should be established—the clinician should look for psychological and behavioral features of mania, such as grandiosity, spending sprees, and foolish investments. Second, the clinician should review the history of mania, hypomania, and depression in the patient and his or her family. The initial onset of primary bipolar manic episodes rarely occurs after age 50; the mean age at onset is 30 (Goodwin and Jamison 1990). Women are at increased risk for recurrence during the postpartum period (L. S. Cohen et al. 1995). The median lifetime number of affective (depressive plus manic) episodes in a bipolar patient is nine (Clayton 1986). Of patients with bipolar disorder, 52% have a parent with mood disorder history, and 63% have at least one family member with a mood disorder. Third, the clinician should carefully review the medical chart, laboratory values, radiographs, physical examination findings, and medication history to identify potentially reversible etiologies. Table 6–2 lists medical conditions and neuroactive substances associated with secondary mania.

Treatment and Management

General Considerations

The treatments for secondary and primary mania are similar, with two exceptions. First, in secondary mania, the etiological agent is identified and removed, whenever possible. This might include surgical procedures to remove tumors, medications to correct metabolic abnormalities, and removal of toxic agents associated with secondary mania. Second, lithium is not usually a first-line treatment for secondary mania because of increased side effects in patients who are medically ill and/or elderly. However, there are some exceptions—lithium has been used successfully in treating mania secondary to corticosteroids and brain tumors without seizures (McDaniel and Sharma 2002). Neuroleptics can help with control of acute mania symptoms; risperidone at a mean modal dose of 4 mg/day has been found effective in rapidly reducing hostility, excitement, anxiety, and disorganized thinking (Hirschfeld et al. 2004). Treating mania in pregnant women involves significant challenges—see Chapter 17, "Special Psychosomatic Medicine Settings and Situations," in this volume for a summary of important considerations in the use of mood stabilizers during pregnancy and the postpartum period.

Table 6–3 presents a summary of dosing information for the antimanic drugs: lithium, carbamazepine, valproate, gabapentin, lamotrigine, and clonazepam.

Table 6–2.   Causes of secondary mood disorder, manic

Neurological conditions	Medications *(continued)*
Focal neurological lesions	Antiretroviral agents
Tumors (gliomas, meningiomas, thalamic metastases)	Baclofen
	Bromide
Cerebrovascular lesions (temporal, right hemispheric), including stroke and head trauma	Buspirone
	Captopril
	Carbamazepine
Temporal lobe seizure	Cimetidine
Thalamotomy	Clonidine withdrawal
Right hemispherectomy	Cocaine
Huntington's disease	Corticosteroids/corticosteroid withdrawal
Wilson's disease	
Postencephalopathic parkinsonism	Cyclobenzaprine
Idiopathic calcification of basal ganglia	Cyproheptadine
	Hallucinogens
Nonfocal neurological lesions	Iproniazid
Posttraumatic encephalopathy	Isoniazid
General paresis	Levodopa
Neurosyphilis	Lorazepam
Multiple sclerosis	Methylphenidate
Viral meningoencephalitis	Metoclopramide[a]
Cryptococcal meningoencephalitis	Metrizamide
Pick's disease	Phencyclidine
Klinefelter's syndrome	Procainamide
Kleine-Levin syndrome	Procarbazine
HIV encephalopathy	Procyclidine
Post–St. Louis type A encephalitis	Propafenone
	Sympathomimetic amines
Medications	Thyroid preparations
Alcohol	Tolmetin
Alprazolam[a]	Triazolam[a]
Amantadine	Yohimbine[a]
Amphetamines	Zidovudine

Table 6–2. Causes of secondary mood disorder, manic *(continued)*

Systemic conditions	Other
Hyperthyroidism	Aspartame
Hyperthyroidism with starvation diet	L-Glutamine
Uremia	
Hemodialysis	
Cushing's syndrome	
Puerperal psychosis	
Infectious mononucleosis	
Niacin deficiency	
Vitamin B_{12} deficiency	
Carcinoid	
Use of hyperbaric chamber	
Postoperative excitement	
Premenstrual psychosis	

[a]Mania occurred in patients with history of mood disorders.
Source. Adapted from McDaniel JS, Sharma SM: "Mania," in *The American Psychiatric Publishing Textbook of Consultation-Liaison Psychiatry: Psychiatry in the Medically Ill,* 2nd Edition. Edited by Wise MG, Rundell JR. Washington, DC, American Psychiatric Publishing, 2002, p. 345. Copyright 2002, American Psychiatric Publishing. Used with permission.

Pharmacological Management

Lithium

General issues. Lithium is titrated within a rather narrow therapeutic range. Toxic effects occur at doses only moderately higher than those for therapeutic effects. Therefore, the clinician must monitor serum lithium levels carefully; the levels are typically drawn 12 hours after the last dose. Doses should generally begin at 300 mg/day and be increased gradually to achieve the generally accepted therapeutic range of serum lithium concentrations of 0.6–1.2 mEq/L. Patients in an acute manic phase are best treated with lithium doses that achieve serum concentrations at the upper end of this therapeutic range (0.8–1.2 mEq/L). However, in severely ill medical patients, in elderly patients, or in those with renal disease, lower doses are typically used. Assuming normal renal function and no drug interactions (e.g., cyclosporine inhibits the kidney's secretion of lithium), lithium's half-life is 18–36 hours. Steady-state

Table 6–3. Antimanic medications

Generic name	Trade name	Starting dosage (mg)[a]	Usual dosage or dosage range (mg)[a]	Serum level	Cautions
Lithium	Eskalith	300 bid	600–1,200	0.6–1.2 mEq/L	Increased toxicity when used with NSAIDs, selective COX-2 inhibitors, metronidazole, ACE inhibitors (e.g., enalapril, captopril, and angiotensin II receptor antagonists (e.g., losartan), calcium channel blocking agents, thiazide diuretics, and SSRIs Pregnancy category D
Carbamazepine	Tegretol	200 bid	600–1,600	8–12 µg/mL	Aplastic anemia and agranulocytosis Pregnancy category D When combined with CYP3A4 inducers (e.g., cisplatin, doxorubicin HCl) or inhibitors (e.g., ketoconazole)
Valproate	Depakote, others	250 bid	625–3,800	50–125 µg/mL	Hepatotoxicity Pregnancy category D Pancreatitis
Aripiprazole	Abilify	15 qd	30 qd	—	When combined with CYP3A4 inducers (e.g., carbamazepine) or inhibitors (e.g., ketoconazole); when combined with CYP2D6 inhibitors (e.g., quinidine, fluoxetine, paroxetine)
Olanzapine	Zyprexa	15 qd	20–30 qd[b]	—	When combined with CYP1A2 inducers (e.g., carbamazepine) or inhibitors (e.g., fluvoxamine)

Table 6–3. Antimanic medications *(continued)*

Generic name	Trade name	Starting dosage (mg)[a]	Usual dosage or dosage range (mg)[a]	Serum level	Cautions
Quetiapine	Seroquel	100 bid	400 bid	—	When combined with CYP3A4 inhibitors (e.g., ketoconazole)
Risperidone	Risperdal	2 qd	6 qd	—	When combined with CYP2D6 inhibitors (e.g., quinidine, fluoxetine, paroxetine) When combined with CYP3A4 inducers (e.g., carbamazepine) Orthostatic hypotension
Ziprasidone	Geodon	40 bid	80 bid	—	When combined with CYP3A4 inducers (e.g., carbamazepine) or inhibitors (e.g., ketoconazole) QT prolongation

Note. ACE=angiotensin-converting enzyme; COX-2=cyclo-oxygenase-2; CYP=cytochrome P450; NSAID=nonsteroidal anti-inflammatory drug; SSRI=selective serotonin reuptake inhibitor; bid=twice a day; qd=every day.

[a]Doses for elderly and medically ill patients are often lower.

[b]Safety at dosages above 20 mg qd not evaluated.

Source. Adapted from Fait ML, Wise MG, Jachna JS, et al.: "Psychopharmacology," in *The American Psychiatric Publishing Textbook of Consultation-Liaison Psychiatry: Psychiatry in the Medically Ill,* 2nd Edition. Edited by Wise MG, Rundell JR. Washington, DC, American Psychiatric Publishing, 2002, p. 958; Keck PE, Perlis RH, Otto MW, et al.: "Treatment of Bipolar Disorder 2004." *Postgraduate Medicine* (Special Report) December 2004; *Physicians' Desk Reference,* 59th Edition. Montvale, NJ, Thompson Healthcare, 2005.

serum levels take 5–8 days to achieve, and clinical effects usually begin around 10–14 days. For this reason, concomitant antipsychotic or benzodiazepine use (e.g., clonazepam) is often necessary for acute control of agitation and psychosis. Long-term lithium therapy reduces the risk of relapse in bipolar disorder, at least for the manic episodes (Geddes et al. 2004).

Lithium is dialyzable and is therefore given to patients on renal dialysis *after* their dialysis treatments; the usual dose is 300–600 mg/day (L.M. Cohen 2002). Dialysis patients do not eliminate lithium naturally, so they do not require daily lithium supplementation aside from their postdialysis dose. Serum levels of lithium are tested several hours after dialysis because plasma levels may actually rise in the postdialysis period when equilibration between blood and tissue stores occurs. Dialysis is the treatment of choice in cases of life-threatening lithium toxicity.

Adverse effects.   In healthy individuals, the side effects of lithium are usually mild, generally well tolerated, and often transient. The most common side effects are tremor, nausea, vomiting, diarrhea, polyuria, and polydipsia. Hypothyroidism, rashes, nephrogenic diabetes insipidus, interstitial nephritis, and weight gain are less frequent. Nonspecific ST segment and T-wave changes are commonly seen on the electrocardiogram (ECG); conduction defects and arrhythmias are rare. Approximately 50% of the patients taking lithium will have these benign and reversible T-wave flattenings (Cassem et al. 2004). At a minimum, the clinician should obtain a baseline ECG, electrolyte measurements, thyroid function tests, pregnancy tests in women of childbearing age, weight measurements, and renal function tests before starting lithium. Lithium use in the first trimester of pregnancy has been linked to fetal cardiac anomalies (Llewellyn et al. 1998).

Sodium and lithium are reabsorbed competitively by the kidney in the proximal tubules. However, only sodium is reabsorbed in the distal tubules. Patients taking diuretics that act on the distal tubule, such as thiazides, are at higher risk for lithium toxicity because they will excrete more sodium and retain lithium. If polyuria is distressing or clinically significant, it often can be effectively managed by lowering the dose or changing to carbamazepine. An alternative strategy to manage distressing polyuria is to add a thiazide diuretic to decrease lithium elimination, which allows a reduction in the lithium dose. Lithium dosage can be reduced as much as 50% if thiazide diuretics (usual dosage = 10–20 mg/day) are used to enhance lithium reabsorption at the proximal tubules; this may protect the distal nephron from high lithium concentrations and decrease lithium-related adverse effects. Lithium combined with risperidone or haloperidol is more effective for treatment of acute mania than lithium alone (Sachs et al. 2002).

Lithium toxicity markedly affects the central nervous system (CNS) and can be a life-threatening emergency in psychosomatic medicine settings. Symptoms of lithium-induced CNS toxicity include ataxia, slurred speech, and nystagmus and can proceed to convulsions, coma, and death if lithium levels are greater than 2.5 mEq/L. The threshold for more serious side effects is lower in predisposed or medically ill patients.

Anticonvulsant Mood Stabilizers

General issues.   Both carbamazepine and valproate are effective treatments of mania, particularly in patients with secondary mania (see Table 6–3). Carbamazepine is a compound structurally similar to tricyclic antidepressants. Although the precise mechanism of action of carbamazepine in mood syndrome amelioration is not clearly known, it inhibits norepinephrine release at synapses and appears to decrease γ-aminobutyric acid (GABA) turnover in animals (Post 1982). Although carbamazepine has shown effectiveness in treating acute mania in most trials, its side-effect profile has made it a less popular choice in psychosomatic medicine settings than valproic acid, a widely used anticonvulsant that enhances GABA activity in the brain (McDaniel and Sharma 2002).

A third generation of anticonvulsants is entering clinical use: lamotrigine, gabapentin, and topiramate (Post et al. 1998). These medications have not yet been established by randomized trials as effective treatments of secondary mania. Anecdotal case reports and open trials are encouraging. Gabapentin's mechanism of action is not well understood, but it has several qualities that make it attractive in the clinical setting. For example, it is not necessary to monitor plasma levels, and it is not bound to plasma proteins (McDaniel and Sharma 2002). Lamotrigine is believed to act by stabilizing the presynaptic neuronal membrane through blockade of sodium channels, preventing release of glutamate (McDaniel and Sharma 2002). It is generally well tolerated and can be coadministered with other anticonvulsant antimanic agents.

Adverse effects.   When prescribing carbamazepine to medically ill patients, its potential hematological toxicity, quinidine-like effects on cardiac conduction, antidiuretic actions, and enzyme induction that can alter the effects of other drugs must be considered. Particularly common problems in the psychosomatic medicine setting are carbamazepine's interaction with the calcium channel blockers diltiazem and verapamil, two agents that may elevate carbamazepine levels into the toxic range (Stoudemire et al. 1993). Two different hematological reactions to carbamazepine may occur. One is a predictable and usually transient decline in both red and white blood cell counts when treatment is initiated; the other is aplastic anemia—a rare side effect that can occur at any time after initiation of therapy. The latter occurs in approximately 1 in 575,000 treated patients per year (Seetharam and Pellock 1991).

Hepatic side effects related to carbamazepine are usually limited to a benign, asymptomatic elevation of alanine aminotransferase or aspartate aminotransferase, usually less than twice the upper limit of normal values. This benign reaction is seen in no more than 5% of patients (Jeavons 1983). However, a rare, idiosyncratic, and life-threatening hepatotoxicity is reported to occur in fewer than 1 in 10,000 patients (Jeavons 1983), usually within the first month of therapy. Because carbamazepine is a potent inducer of cytochrome P450 (CYP) 3A4, it influences the metabolism of many drugs that rely on this enzyme. Thus, the blood levels of some drugs may decrease if carbamazepine is added to a patient's medication regimen. Carbamazepine induces its own metabolism, necessitating gradual increases in dosage over the first few weeks of treatment to maintain a steady blood level.

When valproate is prescribed for medically ill patients, the clinician should be alert to gastrointestinal side effects, hepatotoxicity, coagulation effects, and possible drug-drug interactions. In most patients, the most troublesome side effect of valproate is nausea, often accompanied by vomiting. Although hepatic toxicity is a concern when prescribing valproate, it is relatively rare. Hepatic necrosis, a major risk factor for children younger than 2 years, is an uncommon complication in adults, occurring in 1 in 10,000 patients (Eadie et al. 1988). Aside from this rare hepatic complication, a more common and benign hepatic effect of valproate is an increase in serum ammonia levels resulting from valproate's inhibition of urea synthesis. Although this elevation in serum ammonia usually causes no difficulties in most patients, it is potentially problematic for patients with preexisting liver disease, especially those prone to hepatic encephalopathy. Therefore, significant liver disease is a relative contraindication to valproate therapy. In contrast to carbamazepine, which induces CYP3A4, valproate inhibits CYP2C enzymes that metabolize drugs. For example, prolonged and elevated benzodiazepine levels can result in increased sedation and ataxia.

Gabapentin's adverse effects are usually mild and transient and include somnolence, dizziness, and ataxia. Gabapentin has dose-limited absorption, reducing the risk of overdose. Lamotrigine's side effects are dose related and involve CNS symptoms: dizziness, headache, diplopia, ataxia, and nausea (McDaniel and Sharma 2002). The most important side effect is an 11% rate of skin rash, with a risk of Stevens-Johnson syndrome (Gilman 1995). Most rashes are transient and resolve even if treatment with lamotrigine is continued.

Medical Psychotherapy

A manic patient frequently resists medications that will decrease euphoria. A strong therapeutic alliance with the patient can help with treatment adherence. The clinician should offer relief for symptoms that are most bothersome to the patient. Family therapy in the clinic and hospital settings can comfort the patient and family, particularly as they attempt to cope with both the stress of underlying medical illness and the manic syndrome.

References

American Psychiatric Association: Diagnostic and Statistical Manual of Mental Disorders, 4th Edition, Text Revision. Washington, DC, American Psychiatric Association, 2000

Cassem NH, Papakostas GI, Fava M, et al: Mood-disordered patients, in Massachusetts General Hospital Handbook of General Hospital Psychiatry, 5th Edition. Edited by Stern TL, Fricchione GL, Cassem NH, et al. St. Louis, MO, Mosby, 2004, pp 69–92

Cohen LM: Renal disease, in The American Psychiatric Publishing Textbook of Consultation-Liaison Psychiatry: Psychiatry in the Medically Ill, 2nd Edition. Edited by Wise MG, Rundell JR. Washington, DC, American Psychiatric Publishing, 2002, pp 557–562

Cohen LS, Sichel DA, Robertson LM, et al: Postpartum prophylaxis for women with bipolar disorder. Am J Psychiatry 152:1641–1645, 1995

Clayton PJ: Bipolar illness, in The Medical Basis of Psychiatry. Edited by Winokur G, Clayton PJ. Philadelphia, PA, WB Saunders, 1986, pp 39–59

Eadie MJ, Hooper WD, Dickinson RG: Valproate-associated hepatotoxicity and its biochemical mechanisms. Med Toxicol Adverse Drug Exp 3:85–106, 1988

Geddes JR, Burgess S, Hawton K, et al: Long-term lithium therapy for bipolar disorder: systematic review and meta-analysis of randomized controlled trials. Am J Psychiatry 161:217–222, 2004

Gilman J: Lamotrigine: an antiepileptic agent for the treatment of partial seizures. Ann Pharmacother 29:144–151, 1995

Goodwin FK, Jamison KR: Manic-Depressive Illness. New York, Oxford University Press, 1990

Hirschfeld RMA, Keck PE, Kramer M, et al: Rapid antimanic effect of risperidone monotherapy: a 3-week multicenter, double-blind, placebo-controlled trial. Am J Psychiatry 161:1057–1065, 2004

Jeavons PM: Hepatotoxicity in antiepileptic drugs, in Chronic Toxicity in Antiepileptic Drugs. Edited by Oxley J, Janz D, Meinardi H. New York, Raven, 1983, pp 1–46

Kessler RC, Rubinow DR, Holmes C, et al: The epidemiology of DSM-III-R bipolar disorder in a general population survey. Psychol Med 27:1079–1089, 1997

Llewellyn A, Stowe ZN, Strader JR: The use of lithium and management of women with bipolar disorder during pregnancy and lactation. J Clin Psychiatry 59 (suppl 6): 57–64, 1998

McDaniel JS, Sharma SM: Mania, in The American Psychiatric Publishing Textbook of Consultation-Liaison Psychiatry, 2nd Edition. Edited by Wise MG, Rundell JR. Washington, DC, American Psychiatric Publishing, 2002, pp 339–359

Post RM: Use of the anticonvulsant carbamazepine in primary and secondary affective illness: clinical and theoretical implications. Psychol Med 12:701–704, 1982

Post RM, Frye MA, Denicoff KD, et al: Beyond lithium in the treatment of bipolar illness. Neuropsychopharmacology 19:206–219, 1998

Sachs GS, Grossman F, Ghaemi SN, et al: Combination of a mood stabilizer with risperidone or haloperidol for treatment of acute mania: a double-blind, placebo-controlled comparison of efficacy and safety. Am J Psychiatry 159:1146–1154, 2002

Seetharam MN, Pellock JM: Risk-benefit assessment of carbamazepine in children. Drug Saf 6:148–158, 1991

Starkstein SE, Robinson RG: Neuropsychiatric aspects of cerebrovascular disorders, in The American Psychiatric Press Textbook of Neuropsychiatry. Edited by Yudofsky SC, Hales RE. Washington, DC, American Psychiatric Press, 1992, pp 449–472

Stoudemire A, Fogel BS, Gulley LR, et al: Psychopharmacology in the medical patient, in Psychiatric Care of the Medical Patient. Edited by Stoudemire A, Fogel BS. New York, Oxford University Press, 1993, pp 155–206

Weissman MM, Bland RC, Canino GJ, et al: Cross-national epidemiology of major depression and bipolar disorder. JAMA 276:293–299, 1996

Additional Readings

Bennett J, Goldman W, Suppes T: Gabapentin for treatment of bipolar and schizoaffective disorders. J Clin Psychopharmacol 17:141–142, 1997

Cassidy F, Forest K, Murry E, et al: A factor analysis of the signs and symptoms of mania. Arch Gen Psychiatry 55:27–32, 1998

DePaulo JR: Genetics of bipolar disorder: where do we stand? Am J Psychiatry 161:595–597, 2004

Grisaru N, Chudakov B, Yaroslavsky Y, et al: Transcranial magnetic stimulation in mania: a controlled study. Am J Psychiatry 155:1608–1610, 1998

Janicak PG, Levy NA: Rational copharmacy for acute mania. Psychiatr Ann 28:204–212, 1998

Krauthammer C, Klerman GL: Secondary mania: manic syndromes associated with antecedent physical illness or drugs. Arch Gen Psychiatry 35:1333–1339, 1978

Massand PS: Lamotrigine as prophylaxis against steroid-induced mania. J Clin Psychiatry 60:708–709, 1999

Solomon DA, Keitner GI, Ryan CE, et al: Lithium plus valproate as maintenance polypharmacy with bipolar disorder: a review. CNS Spectr 5:19–28, 2000

7

Anxiety and Insomnia

Anxiety and Anxiety Disorders

In medically ill patients, anxiety, panic, or insomnia may be a reaction to the stress of illness or hospitalization, a manifestation of a medical or psychiatric disorder, or an adverse effect of medication. Anxiety accounts for 10% of all visits to physicians (Colón and Popkin 1999). Anxiety symptoms are easily mistaken for cardiac arrhythmia, asthma, coronary disease, vertigo, cerebrovascular disease, or an endocrine disorder. Consequently, patients with anxiety disorders are frequently referred for expensive and unnecessary examinations, such as ambulatory electrocardiogram (ECG) monitoring, cardiac catheterization, and pheochromocytoma testing (Simon and Walker 1999). Most anxiety seen in the general hospital is not pathological. Mild anxiety syndromes (normal situational anxiety and adjustment disorder with anxiety) usually resolve with disappearance of the stressor. However, more severe anxiety, or even mild anxiety in patients with respiratory or cardiac compromise, can cause acute distress, interfere with the medical evaluation, interfere with treatment, or increase morbidity. Anxiety severity also correlates with health care use and length of hospital stay, even when accounting for illness severity (Colón and Popkin 2002; Saravay et al. 1991).

Epidemiology

Anxiety disorders are among the most common of all psychiatric disorders. Lifetime prevalence of anxiety disorders is 24.9%; 12-month prevalence is 17.2% (Colón and Popkin 2002). Women are at higher risk for having a current anxiety disorder than are men (about 2:1). Of patients with chronic medical conditions, 18% have a lifetime prevalence of an anxiety disorder, compared with 12% of patients without chronic medical conditions (Wells et al. 1988). Panic disorder is present in 3–10 times more patients with asthma than in the general population (Colón and Popkin 2002). When panic disorder is treated in these patients, hospitalization rates decline (Katon 1984). Hospitalized patients identified as highly anxious have longer hospital stays and higher hospitalization costs than do other hospitalized patients (Levenson et al. 1992).

Biology of Anxiety

Basic science and clinical research implicate noradrenergic, serotonergic, and γ-aminobutyric acid (GABA)–ergic systems, and possibly neuropeptides, in the genesis of normal and pathological anxiety. Patients with anxiety disorders appear to have unstable autonomic nervous systems, hypersensitive respiratory control mechanisms, and hypersensitive central nervous system (CNS) carbon dioxide (CO_2) chemoreceptors (Colón and Popkin 2002). Pharmacological challenge studies and functional CNS imaging suggest that key CNS structures important in producing normal and pathological anxiety include the locus coeruleus, amygdala, hippocampus, temporal lobes, and frontal lobes. Projections from the amygdala and hypothalamus modulate autonomic and endocrine responses associated with regulation of vigilance and anxiety; amygdala stimulation in humans induces anxiety and fear (Colón and Popkin 2002). Functional imaging studies have reported metabolic abnormalities in the hippocampus, parahippocampal areas, and inferior frontal cortex in patients with panic disorder (Bisaga et al. 1998; Nordahl et al. 1998).

Clinical Characteristics

Anxiety Disorder Due to a General Medical Condition and Substance-Induced Anxiety Disorder

Pathological anxiety that is an integral part of the pathophysiology of the medical illness is called "anxiety disorder due to a general medical condition." Secondary panic and obsessive-compulsive symptoms are also included in this diagnosis. Sometimes the diagnosis is only finalized after the fact, when the psychiatric consultant shows that removing the medical etiology was associated with remediation of the anxiety or panic symptoms. Even then, relations between organic and reactive aspects of an overall anxiety syndrome are complex; having a medical condition causally related to a secondary anxiety syndrome does not rule out reactive anxiety.

Substance-induced anxiety disorder is reserved for instances in which a clinical constellation of generalized anxiety, panic attacks, or obsessive-compulsive symptoms is linked to substance intoxication or withdrawal. The symptoms must emerge within a month of substance intoxication or withdrawal and are not better accounted for by another anxiety disorder. Medical conditions and substances associated with anxiety and panic are listed in Table 7–1.

Generalized Anxiety Disorder

Generalized anxiety disorder (GAD) is characterized by excessive anxiety plus apprehensive expectations about events or activities. A patient's incessant worry is difficult to control and commonly evokes restlessness, fatigue, irritability, muscle tension, and sleep dysfunction (American Psychiatric Association 2000). When encountered in psychosomatic medicine, GAD is often an established condition that is exacerbated or unmasked in the general hospital setting. Patients with GAD usually have other psychiatric disorders. Motor tension is a routine part of GAD and may include trembling and twitching. Age at onset is usually in the 20s or 30s.

Panic Disorder

Primary panic disorder patients have recurrent, unexpected panic attacks followed by worry, concern, and behavior changes related to the attacks. The attacks are not due to a general medical condition or the direct effects of a substance. Panic disorder is underrecognized, underdiagnosed, and undertreated in outpatient medical settings. Panic disorder was present in 33%–43% of the patients with chest pain whose cardiac catheterizations indicated normal coronary arteries (Colón and Popkin 2002).

Agoraphobia Without Panic Disorder

Patients with agoraphobia are not seen in medical-surgical settings for the simple reason that they rarely leave home unless there is a life-threatening emergency or unless the family or a community outreach program brings them to medical attention.

Table 7–1. Medical/toxic causes of anxiety and panic

Cardiovascular conditions	Metabolic conditions
Angina pectoris	Anemia
Cerebral insufficiency	Heavy metal toxicity
Congestive heart failure	Hyperthermia
Coronary insufficiency	Hyperkalemia
Dysrhythmia	Hypoglycemia
Hypovolemia	Hyponatremia
Intra-aortic balloon pump	Insulinoma
Myocardial infarction	Porphyria
Paroxysmal atrial tachycardia	Vitamin deficiency states
Syncope	Wilson's disease
Valvular disease, especially mitral valve prolapse	
	Drugs
	Alcohol and its withdrawal
Endocrine conditions	Aminophylline
Carcinoid syndrome	Amphetamine
Hyperadrenalism	Anticholinergics
Hyperparathyroidism	Antidepressants, especially fluoxetine and
Hyperthyroidism	bupropion
Hypocalcemia	Antihypertensives: reserpine, hydralazine
Hypoparathyroidism	Antituberculous agents
Hypothyroidism	β-Blockers (withdrawal)
Ovarian dysfunction	Caffeine
Pancreatic tumor	Calcium channel blockers
Pheochromocytoma	Cannabis
Pituitary disorders	Cocaine
Pseudohyperparathyroidism	Digitalis (toxicity)
	Dopamine
Immunological and collagen vascular conditions	Ephedrine
Anaphylaxis	Epinephrine
Polyarteritis nodosa	Estrogen
Rheumatoid arthritis	Hallucinogens
Systemic lupus erythematosus	Heavy metals
Temporal arteritis	Insulin
	Levodopa

Table 7–1. Medical/toxic causes of anxiety and panic *(continued)*

Drugs *(continued)*	Respiratory conditions
Lidocaine	Asthma
Methylphenidate	Chronic obstructive pulmonary disease
Monosodium glutamate (MSG)	Pneumonia
Neuroleptics (akathisia)	Pneumothorax
Nicotinic acid	Pulmonary edema
Nonsteroidal anti-inflammatory agents	Pulmonary embolus
Phenylephrine	Respirator dependence
Phenylpropanolamine	
Procaine	**Gastrointestinal conditions**
Procarbazine	Crohn's disease
Pseudoephedrine	Peptic ulcer disease
Salicylates	Ulcerative colitis
Sedative-hypnotics (and withdrawal)	
Steroids	**Neurological conditions**
Sympathomimetics	Encephalitic and postencephalitic disorders
Theophylline	Essential tremor
Thyroid preparations	Huntington's disease
Yohimbine	Multiple sclerosis
	Myasthenia gravis
	Neurosyphilis
	Postconcussional syndrome
	Restless legs syndrome
	Seizure disorder, especially temporal lobe epilepsy
	Stroke
	Subarachnoid hemorrhage
	Transient ischemic attacks
	Vascular headaches
	Vertigo (e.g., Meniere's disease)

Specific and Social Phobias

Specific phobias and social phobias are usually hidden by the patient and are seldom identified by the primary physician (Colón and Popkin 2002), unless the degree of impairment is pronounced or interferes with clinical care, such as when a claustrophobic patient cannot tolerate the magnetic resonance imaging procedure or when phobias involve blood, injection, or injury. Patients often delay seeking medical attention because of avoidance associated with specific phobias.

Obsessive-Compulsive Disorder

Ego-dystonic obsessions and irresistible compulsive behaviors can produce somatic manifestations. For example, patients can develop dermatoses from frequent hand washing. Obsessive-compulsive disorder is highly comorbid with major depressive disorder. Primary obsessive-compulsive disorder, when it appears or recurs during a hospitalization or an outpatient workup for a new medical problem, may be related to the stress, uncertainty, and loss of control experienced by patients. Secondary obsessive-compulsive syndromes occur in several neuropsychiatric conditions, including Gilles de la Tourette's syndrome, epilepsy, and after head injury.

Acute Stress Disorder and Posttraumatic Stress Disorder

Acute stress disorder involves exposure to a life-threatening or affectively overwhelming traumatic event that produces dissociative symptoms, reexperiencing of the trauma, avoidance of associated stimuli, increased arousal, and significant distress or social or occupational impairment (American Psychiatric Association 2000). Symptoms must last for more than 2 days but no more than 4 weeks and emerge within a month of the trauma. The symptoms are not substance induced or the result of metabolic aspects of a general medical condition, although a life-threatening medical condition can certainly be the stressor associated with the psychological symptoms. Acute stress disorder identifies patients at risk for posttraumatic stress disorder (PTSD) because 50% of those with acute stress disorder go on to develop PTSD.

A diagnosis of PTSD requires that a life-threatening trauma is "persistently reexperienced," that the duration of the symptoms is longer than 1 month, that emotional numbing and increased arousal are present, and that stimuli linked to the trauma are avoided (American Psychiatric Association 2000).

The experience of hospitalization or severe illness can trigger reexperiencing phenomena, nightmares, strong emotions, and autonomic arousal. A PTSD diagnosis should alert the clinician to the potential presence of comorbid psychiatric disorders, especially substance-related disorders, mood disorders, and panic disorder.

Adjustment Disorder With Anxiety

Adjustment disorder is a maladaptive response to an identifiable stressor. For many patients, the stressors are the medical illness, the clinic or hospital environment, and the treatment.

Differential Diagnosis

Medical or Psychiatric Etiology

When pathological anxiety is present, the symptoms may be due to 1) situational stress, 2) a primary psychiatric disorder, 3) long-standing character pathology, or 4) a medical or toxic etiology (see Table 7–1). Two important questions must be answered when attempting to differentiate among causes of pathological anxiety: 1) What past and family historical data are present? (Past or family history of a primary anxiety disorder increases the probability that current signs and symptoms are manifestations or recurrences of a primary anxiety disorder.) 2) Is there an identifiable potential medical or toxic cause for the anxiety? The differential diagnosis of anxiety disorders includes a wide range of physical illnesses and psychoactive substances (Table 7–1). Evaluation directed toward the body system most prominently affected by anxiety symptoms (e.g., gastrointestinal, respiratory) may provide the most diagnostic evidence for the etiology.

Psychiatric Differential Diagnosis

Anxiety disorders are sometimes mistaken for other psychiatric disorders, especially agitated depression. Anxiety disorders usually have an earlier age at onset and are less episodic than mood disorders. The mental status examination differentiates agitated delirium and psychotic disorders from anxiety disorders. The akathisia that occasionally occurs with neuroleptics can resemble anxiety. Substance-related disorders are an underdiagnosed cause of anxiety. Anxiety disorders frequently coexist with other psychiatric disorders, especially depression and substance-related disorders.

Treatment and Management

Anxiety Disorder Due to a General Medical Condition or Substance

When a remediable etiology for an anxiety syndrome is found, the clinician should reverse it, unless medically impossible or contraindicated. Unless anxiety symptoms are reversible or self-limited, pharmacological treatment should be considered. Symptoms are usually undertreated, and concerns about iatrogenic addiction are overstated.

Acute Anxiety and GAD

Benzodiazepines.   Benzodiazepines are effective anxiolytics. Few features make them potentially dangerous in the medically ill, especially for short-term use. However, tolerance, dependence, and accident proneness present limitations to long-term use of benzodiazepines. Table 7–2 summarizes clinical and pharmacodynamic information about the most commonly used benzodiazepines. Doses for elderly and medically ill patients are often lower than normally used.

Agents with longer half-lives (e.g., diazepam, clorazepate) can be administered less frequently and may be easier to taper after prolonged use than agents with shorter half-lives. However, they are more likely to accumulate in patients who have impaired hepatic function or who are taking multiple medications. Agents with shorter elimination half-lives reach steady state much more rapidly and are eliminated more quickly, making them reasonable options for the short-term management of anxiety. Lorazepam and oxazepam have no active metabolites and are better suited for patients with liver impairment or patients taking multiple medications. Among benzodiazepines, only lorazepam is reliably absorbed when administered intramuscularly.

The most common side effect of benzodiazepines is sedation. Dizziness, weakness, anterograde amnesia (correlated with decreasing duration of action), nausea, and impaired motor performance are also reported. After chronic use, tolerance can develop. Withdrawal syndromes occur when dosage is reduced too rapidly.

Buspirone.   The mechanism of action of buspirone, a nonbenzodiazepine antianxiety agent, is related to its actions on serotonin$_{1A}$ receptors. Buspirone has several advantages in the medically ill because it is not sedating and has

Table 7–2. Benzodiazepines

Generic name	Trade name	Onset	Duration of action	Usual therapeutic dosage range (mg/day)[a]	Approximately equivalent antianxiety dose (mg)	Approximately equivalent hypnotic dose (mg)
Alprazolam	Xanax	Intermediate	Short	2–8	0.5	1
Chlordiazepoxide	Librium	Intermediate	Long	15–150	10	25
Clonazepam	Klonopin	Intermediate	Short	1–3	1	1
Clorazepate	Tranxene	Rapid	Long	15–60	7.5	15
Diazepam	Valium	Rapid	Long	5–40	5	10
Estazolam	ProSom	Rapid	Intermediate	1–2	—	1
Flurazepam	Dalmane	Rapid to intermediate	Long	15–30	—	30
Lorazepam	Ativan	Intermediate	Intermediate	1–6	1	2
Midazolam	Versed	Rapid	Very short	0.1 mg/kg	2	2
Oxazepam	Serax	Intermediate to slow	Intermediate	30–120	15	30
Prazepam	Centrax	Slow	Long	20–60	10	20
Quazepam	Doral	Rapid	Long	7.5–15	—	15
Temazepam	Restoril	Intermediate to slow	Short	15–30	15	30
Triazolam	Halcion	Intermediate	Short	0.125–0.5	—	0.5
Zolpidem	Ambien	Rapid	Short	5–10	—	10

[a]Doses for elderly and medically ill patients are often lower.
Source.   Adapted from Fair et al. 2002. Used with permission.

no known abuse potential. Considerable evidence indicates that buspirone is as effective for GAD as are benzodiazepines. Buspirone may be a particularly desirable choice in treating chronic anxiety in patients with pulmonary conditions; it may be associated with an actual increase in respiratory drive (Garner and Eldridge 1989). Buspirone is not useful in the treatment of acute anxiety because its onset of therapeutic response requires 2 or more weeks; buspirone is also not effective as a primary treatment for panic disorder. Average total daily dose is 30 mg, but initial dosage is 5 mg twice daily, which can be increased by 5 mg/day every 3–4 days.

The adverse effects of buspirone include nausea, vomiting, headache, and dizziness. It can produce a serotonin syndrome when taken with monoamine oxidase inhibitors (MAOIs) or with other medications that increase serotonin activity (Fait et al. 2002). It also can displace less firmly protein-bound drugs such as digoxin.

Antidepressants.   Antidepressants, especially selective serotonin reuptake inhibitors (SSRIs) and serotonin-norepinephrine reuptake inhibitors (SNRIs), are effective in the treatment of GAD and other anxiety disorders (Gorman and Kent 1999). Venlafaxine's extended-release form, which is taken once daily, became the first antidepressant approved for the treatment of GAD. Most patients obtain some benefit within 2 weeks, with additional improvement seen over the next 6 weeks of treatment (Schatzberg 2003, pp. 80–81). Paroxetine and escitalopram also have been approved by the U.S. Food and Drug Administration (FDA) for treatment of GAD.

Neuroleptics.   Low-dose neuroleptics are particularly beneficial in the medical setting when fear, agitation, or delirium is present. For example, 0.5 mg of haloperidol two or three times per day can markedly reduce the extreme fear that patients sometimes experience when they are being weaned from a respirator. Neuroleptics such as haloperidol are sometimes combined with benzodiazepines such as lorazepam to treat delirium. The clinical synergism provides additional sedation and lowers the likelihood of extrapyramidal side effects (Menza et al. 1988). In addition, neuroleptics are particularly useful in treating secondary anxiety disorders and other secondary psychiatric disorders resulting from high-dose steroids. Patients who are medically ill and have severe, refractory anxiety or panic or those in whom sedation from benzodiazepine agents cannot be tolerated also may benefit from a cautious trial of neuroleptics.

The treating physician must observe the patient for acute dystonia, akathisia, and early signs of neuroleptic malignant syndrome.

β-Blockers.   Propranolol helps control some sympathetic nervous system symptoms of anxiety, such as palpitations and sweating. The psychological components of anxiety may remain. The adverse effects of β-blockers include bradycardia, hypotension, and fatigue.

Medical psychotherapy.   Supportive psychotherapy can help patients cope with the acute stressors during a hospitalization or series of clinic visits. Attention has focused on the potential efficacy of cognitive-behavioral therapy for anxiety disorders (Welkowitz et al. 1991). Cognitive psychotherapy involves active exploration, clarification, and testing of the patient's perceptions and beliefs. Common psychodynamic themes in anxious patients are loss, real and metaphorical physical threats, and lack of control. It is important in the hospitalized patient to address potential hospital environment factors that may be associated with anxiety (Table 7–3).

Table 7–3.   Hospital environment factors associated with anxiety

Financial burden

Intrusive medical procedures

Isolation

Loss of autonomy

Loss of privacy

Noise

Pain

Physical discomfort

Possibility of death

Sleep deprivation

Uncertainty regarding cause of illness

Uncertainty regarding prognosis

Source.   Adapted from Colón EA, Popkin MK: "Anxiety and Panic," in *The American Psychiatric Publishing Textbook of Consultation-Liaison Psychiatry: Psychiatry in the Medically Ill,* 2nd Edition. Edited by Wise MG, Rundell JR. Washington, DC, American Psychiatric Publishing, 2002, p. 405. Copyright 2002, American Psychiatric Publishing. Used with permission.

Behavioral management.   Behavior therapies provide an opportunity for reduction of acute anxiety, enhancement of the patient's sense of mastery, and clarification of measurable goals. Behavioral interventions commonly used in psychosomatic medicine include relaxation techniques, systematic desensitization, biofeedback, meditation, hypnosis, and establishing graded goals with simple reinforcement schedules.

Panic Disorder

Benzodiazepines.   Alprazolam and clonazepam are approved by the FDA for treatment of panic disorder; they may be most useful when rapid control of attacks is necessary. A significant limitation of alprazolam in treating panic is the potential for dependence, withdrawal, and rebound symptoms on discontinuation and between doses. Discontinuation of alprazolam should be *very* gradual. Clonazepam has a longer half-life than alprazolam (24–48 hours); it is quite sedating for many patients.

Antidepressants.   Most antidepressants exert antipanic effects (Ballenger 1991). Three SSRI antidepressants (paroxetine, fluoxetine, and sertraline) have received U.S. FDA-approved indications for panic disorder. After a 2-week single-blind, placebo lead-in, one group of 168 research patients receiving SSRIs experienced an 88% decrease in mean number of panic attacks per week, compared with a 53% decrease in the placebo-treated group (Pohl et al. 1998). SSRI doses used for panic are similar to those used for depression, but higher doses are frequently necessary for complete control of panic attacks, including the elimination of limited-symptom panic attacks. Tricyclic antidepressants, trazodone, nefazodone, and MAOIs are also efficacious. Bupropion is not effective in treating panic disorder. (Chapter 5, "Depression," in this volume contains information on normal antidepressant doses and potential adverse effects.)

Neuroleptics.   Neuroleptics are effective for rapid relief of acute panic attacks that endanger life or medical status. Parenteral haloperidol, 4–10 mg (or higher doses if needed), can help control attacks.

Other medications.   Propranolol blocks some peripheral manifestations of panic attacks. Clonidine is effective in decreasing symptoms in some patients.

Medical psychotherapy.   Explaining panic disorder to the patient as a part of supportive psychotherapy is helpful and reassuring. Behavioral, cognitive-behavioral, and relaxation therapies are effective primary or adjunctive treatments of panic disorder. Cognitive-behavioral approaches emphasize the combination of symptom control (especially breathing) and cognitive restructuring to give physical symptoms a noncatastrophic interpretation. Use of medication and psychotherapy together is particularly efficacious, especially for patients with severe panic disorder.

Specific and Social Phobias

The treatment of choice for specific phobia is graded exposure. In the hospitalized patient, exposure treatments do not have to be in vivo. Imagery-based exposure that uses a graded hierarchy of anxiety-producing stimuli is also effective (Hollander et al. 1988). Social phobia is amenable to treatment with SSRIs and SNRIs. Paroxetine, sertraline, and venlafaxine's extended-release version are approved by the FDA to treat social phobia and are superior to placebo, although overall, fewer than half of the patients taking SSRIs respond favorably (Stein et al. 1999).

Obsessive-Compulsive Disorder

Clomipramine is a potent serotonin reuptake blocker but is not well tolerated because of side effects. Two-thirds of the patients with obsessive-compulsive disorder can expect significant symptomatic improvement; some patients have almost complete remission (Hollander et al. 1988). SSRIs are also effective for obsessive-compulsive symptoms, and they lack anticholinergic and sedating side effects. Three SSRI antidepressants—paroxetine, sertraline, and fluoxetine—are approved by the FDA for treating obsessive-compulsive disorder. The most successful obsessive-compulsive disorder treatment is enhanced when medication is combined with behavioral treatments, such as graded exposure and response prevention techniques.

Acute Stress Disorder and PTSD

It is important to remember that traumatic events often result in hospitalization (e.g., motor vehicle accidents) and can occur in medical facilities (e.g., cardiac arrests). The development of significant anxiety and dissociative symptoms after exposure to an extreme stressor identifies an individual as at risk for acute stress disorder (ASD) and PTSD. The mainstay of ASD and PTSD treatment is group and individual psychotherapy. Increasingly, however, case reports and controlled trials have documented successful treatment of ASD and PTSD with SSRI antidepressant medications. Paroxetine and sertraline now have FDA approval to treat PTSD. Benzodiazepines also provide symptomatic relief for some PTSD patients, but caution is advised because of the high risk of comorbid substance-related disorders. Other psychiatric disorders that frequently accompany ASD and PTSD, such as major depression, are sometimes more treatment responsive than the actual ASD or PTSD symptoms.

Insomnia

Mild, transient sleep disturbance secondary to anxiety or physical discomfort is the most common form of insomnia seen in hospitalized or severely ill patients. The most common DSM-IV-TR (American Psychiatric Association 2000) insomnia subtype is sleep disorder due to a general medical condition, insomnia type. To make this diagnosis, a specific medical disorder must produce a significant, new sleep disturbance and/or related daytime distress (Weilburg and Winkelman 2002). Insomnias secondary to psychiatric disorders, primary sleep disorders (e.g., primary or idiopathic insomnia), sleep apnea, and narcolepsy are not included in this category.

Patients in hospitals or nursing homes may have disrupted sleep in any of three ways: decreased total sleep time, disrupted day/night or circadian cycles, and disrupted sleep architecture (Weilburg and Winkelman 2002). In particular, patients in the intensive care unit have periods of sleep that are brief and distributed fairly evenly throughout the 24-hour day rather than consolidated at night. Intensive care unit patients also tend to have frequent awakenings and to spend very little time in rapid eye movement (REM) and delta sleep. Insomnia has many individual toxic and medical causes. A vigorous evaluation of sleep complaints, sometimes including a full-scale sleep study, will yield a treatable psychiatric, neurological, or medical etiology in most cases.

Treatment

Reversal of Causes

The consulting psychiatrist must determine whether potentially reversible psychiatric or medical illnesses are present that could disrupt sleep, such as depression, delirium, mania, psychoactive substance dependence, anxiety disorders, pain, and psychosis. Several medications can interfere with sleep. The treatment of obstructive sleep apnea has evolved from tracheostomy to a variety of options that include weight loss, nasal continuous positive airway pressure, pharyngeal surgery, and medications. Myoclonic sleep disorders such as restless legs syndrome are difficult to treat. Dopaminergic agents, such as levodopa, pergolide, and bromocriptine, offer some benefit; reports indicate that pramipexole is particularly effective (Montplaisir et al. 1999).

Behavioral and Environmental Manipulations

Changing a patient's surroundings by recommending different lighting, altering the schedule of medications (especially those known to interfere with sleep), modifying vital sign requirements, and preventing daytime naps frequently can resolve or improve insomnia. Caffeine appears to increase insomnia in hospitalized patients, so simply removing coffee, tea, and cola from the diets of patients complaining of insomnia may be of practical utility (Weilburg and Winkelman 2002).

Sedative-Hypnotic Medications

Once remediable causes of insomnia are corrected and behavioral and environmental manipulations attempted, the consulting psychiatrist must decide if a patient could benefit from a hypnotic agent. Table 7–2 summarizes the most commonly used sedative-hypnotic medications in general hospital and outpatient settings.

Benzodiazepine hypnotic agents should be used at the lowest effective dose and only for a brief period. In general, drugs with a rapid onset of action, such as diazepam, triazolam, and zolpidem, help patients who have trouble falling asleep; medications with a somewhat delayed onset of action, such as clonazepam, temazepam, and quazepam, are recommended for patients who have sleep interruption (Weilburg and Winkelman 2002). Discontinuation of a benzodiazepine sedative-hypnotic, especially a shorter-acting agent used for more than a few nights, may lead to rebound insomnia. If this occurs, the clinician should reassure the patient that it is temporary and substitute an antihistamine (e.g., diphenhydramine 25–50 mg orally) for a few nights. Short-acting benzodiazepine sedative-hypnotics, such as triazolam, sometimes cause anterograde amnesia. For outpatients who have long-standing insomnia or who are taking activating medications (e.g., bupropion, fluoxetine), many clinicians have success with low-dose trazodone (25–100 mg nightly). The use of trazodone avoids problems with tolerance and anterograde amnesia, but some patients may report mild "hangover," orthostatic dizziness, or, very rarely, priapism.

References

American Psychiatric Association: Diagnostic and Statistical Manual of Mental Disorders, 4th Edition, Text Revision. Washington, DC, American Psychiatric Association, 2000

Ballenger JC: Long-term pharmacologic treatment of panic disorder. J Clin Psychiatry 52 (suppl):18–23, 1991

Bisaga A, Katz J, Antonini A, et al: Cerebral glucose metabolism in women with panic disorders. Am J Psychiatry 155:1178–1183, 1998

Colón EA, Popkin MK: Anxiety and panic, in The American Psychiatric Publishing Textbook of Consultation-Liaison Psychiatry: Psychiatry in the Medically Ill, 2nd Edition. Edited by Wise MG, Rundell JR. Washington, DC, American Psychiatric Publishing, 2002, pp 393–415

Fait ML, Wise MG, Jachna JS, et al: Psychopharmacology, in The American Psychiatric Publishing Textbook of Consultation-Liaison Psychiatry: Psychiatry in the Medically Ill, 2nd Edition. Edited by Wise MG, Rundell JR. Washington, DC, American Psychiatric Publishing, 2002, pp 939–987

Garner SJ, Eldridge FL: Buspirone, an anxiolytic drug that stimulates respiration. Am Rev Respir Dis 139:945–950, 1989

Gorman JM, Kent JM: SSRIs and SNRIs: broad spectrum of efficacy beyond major depression. J Clin Psychiatry 60 (suppl 4):33–38, 1999

Hollander E, Liebowitz MR, Gorman JM: Anxiety disorders, in The American Psychiatric Press Textbook of Psychiatry. Edited by Talbott JA, Hales RE, Yudofsky SC. Washington, DC, American Psychiatric Press, 1988, pp 443–491

Katon W: Panic disorder and somatization: review of 55 cases. Am J Med 77:101–106, 1984

Levenson JL, Hamer RM, Rossiter C: Psychopathology and pain in medical inpatients: predict resource use during hospitalization but not rehospitalization. J Psychosom Res 36:585–592, 1992

Menza MA, Murray GB, Holmes VF, et al: Controlled study of extrapyramidal reactions in the management of delirious, medically ill patients: intravenous haloperidol versus intravenous haloperidol plus benzodiazepines. Heart Lung 17:238–241, 1988

Montplaisir J, Nicolas A, Denesle R, et al: Restless legs syndrome improved by prami-pexole: a double-blind randomized trial. Neurology 52:938–943, 1999

Nordahl T, Stein M, Benkelfat C, et al: Regional cerebral metabolic asymmetries replicated in an independent group of patients with panic disorders. Biol Psychiatry 44:998–1006, 1998

Pohl RB, Wolkow RM, Clary CM: Sertraline in the treatment of panic disorder: a double-blind multicenter trial. Am J Psychiatry 155:1189–1195, 1998

Saravay SM, Steinberg MD, Weinschel B, et al: Psychological comorbidity and length of stay in the general hospital. Am J Psychiatry 148:324–329, 1991

Schatzberg A: Antidepressants, in Manual of Clinical Psychopharmacology, 4th Edition. Edited by Schatzberg AF, Cole JO, DeBattista C. Washington, DC, American Psychiatric Publishing, 2003, pp 37–157

Simon GE, Walker EA: The consultation psychiatrist in the primary care clinic, in Essentials of Consultation-Liaison Psychiatry. Edited by Rundell JR, Wise MG. Washington, DC, American Psychiatric Press, 1999, pp 513–520

Stein MB, Fyer AJ, Davidson JRT, et al: Fluvoxamine treatment of social phobia (social anxiety disorder): a double-blind, placebo-controlled study. Am J Psychiatry 156: 756–760, 1999

Weilburg JB, Winkelman JW: Sleep disorders, in The American Psychiatric Publishing Textbook of Consultation-Liaison Psychiatry: Psychiatry in the Medically Ill, 2nd Edition. Edited by Wise MG, Rundell JR. Washington, DC, American Psychiatric Publishing, 2002, pp 495–518

Welkowitz LA, Papp LA, Cloitre M, et al: Cognitive-behavior therapy for panic disorder delivered by psychopharmacologically oriented clinicians. J Nerv Ment Dis 179: 472–476, 1991

Wells KB, Golding JM, Burnham MA: Psychiatric disorder in a sample of the population with and without chronic medical conditions. Am J Psychiatry 145:976–981, 1988

Additional Readings

Ballenger JC: Treatment of panic disorder in the general medical setting. J Psychosom Res 44:5–15, 1998

Davidson J: Pharmacotherapy of social anxiety disorder. J Clin Psychiatry 59:47–51, 1998

Nierenberg AL, Adler EA: Trazodone for antidepressant-associated insomnia. Am J Psychiatry 151:1069–1072, 1994

Salzman C, Miyawake EK, le Bars P, et al: Neurobiologic basis of anxiety and its treatment. Harv Rev Psychiatry 1:197–206, 1993

Silber MH: Restless legs syndrome. Mayo Clin Proc 72:261–264, 1997

Smoller JW, Simon NM, Pollack MH, et al: Anxiety in patients with pulmonary disease: comorbidity and treatment. Semin Clin Neuropsychiatry 4:84–97, 1999

Wise MG, Rundell JR: Anxiety and neurological disorders. Semin Clin Neuropsychiatry 4:98–102, 1999

Zaubler TS, Katon W: Panic disorder in the general medical setting. J Psychosom Res 44:5–15, 1998

8

Somatoform and Related Disorders

Physicians have certain expectations for patients who have physical complaints; according to Lipowski (1988), "A patient should complain in reasonable proportion to demonstrative pathology, report physical distress in bodily terms and emotional distress in psychological terms, and accept a doctor's opinion and advice compliantly" (p. 1361). Between 60% and 80% of people in the general population experience somatic complaints during any given week; physicians cannot find an organic cause in 20%–84% of the patients who present with physical symptoms (Kellner 1985). When a physiological cause cannot be found for a symptom or when the physician thinks that a significant disparity exists between the patient's subjective complaints and objective findings, a psychiatric consultation is sometimes requested. A typical consult asks for psychiatric evaluation to rule in or rule out a "functional," "psychogenic," or "psychosomatic" symptom.

The amplification or magnification of somatic sensations varies widely among patients. This amplification process has both trait and state characteristics. Barsky et al. (1992) reported that amplification is influenced by the patient's cognition (information, beliefs, opinions, and attribution), context of the symptom (feedback from others and expectations), amount of attention to the symptom (when attention is increased, the symptom is amplified; when decreased, the symptom is diminished), and mood (anxiety and depression amplify symptoms). A large differential diagnosis must be considered in a patient who presents with physical symptoms (Table 8–1). Patients who amplify somatic symptoms (somatizers) are a heterogeneous group and defy simple categorization or explanation. Not all somatizers have a somatoform disorder. In this chapter, we review somatization and then review DSM-IV-TR (American Psychiatric Association 2000) somatoform disorders and three related conditions: psychological factors affecting medical condition, factitious disorders, and malingering.

Table 8–1.   Differential diagnosis of physical complaint(s)

General medical disorder

Medically unexplained symptom(s)

Somatic presentation of a psychiatric disorder:

    Mood disorder, especially major depressive disorder

    Anxiety disorder, especially generalized anxiety disorder and panic disorder

    Psychotic disorder, especially delusional disorder, somatic type

    Substance-related disorder

    Dissociative disorder

    Adjustment disorder

    Psychological factors affecting medical condition

    Dementia or other cognitive disorder

Somatoform disorders

    Somatization disorder

    Undifferentiated somatoform disorder

    Hypochondriasis

    Conversion disorder

    Body dysmorphic disorder

    Pain disorder

    Somatoform disorder not otherwise specified

Factitious disorder

Malingering

Somatization

Definitions and Theoretical Concepts

Somatization is the tendency to experience, communicate, and amplify psychological and interpersonal distress in the form of somatic distress and medically unexplained symptoms (Abbey 2002). Most patients fall into one of these four categories:

1. *Medically unexplained symptoms*—somatic symptoms are not explained after appropriate medical and psychiatric assessment. These patients are often described as the "worried well." A good example of such patients are the 70%–80% of all medical students who at some point in their medical education become convinced or fear that they have a disease (Ford 1983).

2. *Somatic presentation of psychiatric disorder*—patients with psychiatric disorders, especially mood and anxiety disorders, commonly present to primary care physicians with somatic symptoms as the most prominent part of the clinical picture. Many psychiatrists who do not work closely with primary care practitioners are unaware of this association. In addition, psychiatrists do not inquire about physical symptoms as part of evaluation or monitoring treatment, and patients are unlikely to spontaneously report physical symptoms to a psychiatrist. Therefore, psychiatrists cannot determine whether a patient is in full remission during treatment unless they monitor somatic symptoms along with other symptoms associated with the disorder (Pakel et al. 1995).

3. *Somatoform disorders*—patients present with physical symptoms that suggest a medical disorder; however, no medical disorder exists, or if one exists, it cannot fully explain the complaint(s). Despite medical evaluation and reassurance, the bodily preoccupation and worry about medical illness continue. For many of the patients with somatoform disorders, it is a "way of life" (Ford 1983).

4. *Factitious disorders or malingering*—patients intentionally produce or claim to have medical illness when they do not.

Illness Versus Disease

The distinction between *illness* and *disease* (Eisenberg 1977) is a useful concept for consultation psychiatrists to understand. Illness is the response of the individual and his or her family to symptoms. In contrast, disease is a patho-physiological process associated with documentable physical lesions or diagnosed by a physician. A patient can have a disease without an illness and an illness without a disease. Mismatches are common and are at the root of many management problems. For example, a patient with hypertension may not experience symptoms and thus not believe that he or she is ill; nonadherence to treatment soon follows. In contrast, the somatizing patient believes that he or she is ill despite the lack of evidence of a disease; or if evidence of disease is present, the patient's reaction is exaggerated.

Illness Behavior

Illness behavior refers to the manner in which individuals interpret their symptoms, take remedial action, and use sources of help (Mechanic 1986).

Abnormal Illness Behavior

Abnormal illness behavior is "an inappropriate or maladaptive mode of perceiving, evaluating or acting in relation to one's own health status" (Pilowsky 1987, p. 89). This behavior pattern persists despite the fact that a health care provider has offered an accurate explanation of the nature of the symptoms and an appropriate course of management.

Evaluation

Abbey (2002) recommends a comprehensive approach to evaluating patients who are identified by primary care physicians or specialists as potential somatizers. Although the patient may not have a somatoform or other psychiatric disorder, data gathering is similar to that of a typical psychiatric consultation. Table 8–2 summarizes the evaluation process for a potentially somatizing patient.

Epidemiology

Epidemiological and demographic characteristics are included in the discussions of each individual somatoform and related disorder later in this chapter. Fourteen common physical symptoms are responsible for almost half of all primary care visits; over a 1-year follow-up period, only 10%–15% of these symptoms are found to be caused by an organic illness (Katon and Walker 1998). Somatizing patients have higher average health costs than do other

Table 8–2. Psychiatric evaluation of a patient referred for somatization

Collaborate with referral sources: Understand clearly the reason for referral and what the patient was told about the consultation/evaluation.

Review the medical records: Review records before the consultation appointment.

Collaborate with family: Gain an accurate assessment of the patient's history, current and past functional capacity, and current or past psychosocial stressors.

Build an alliance with the patient: Address ambivalence about seeing a psychiatrist early, take the patient's symptoms seriously, and ask "how has this illness affected your life?"

Perform a mental status examination: Look for mental status examination findings suggestive of a psychiatric disorder. Pay particular attention to the range and depth of emotional response to issues raised during the examination, level of denial, meaning of symptoms and normal test results to the patient, and evidence of unwarranted hostility toward physicians.

Complete a physical examination: Perform an objective physical and laboratory examination of the patient (the referring physician already believes that the patient has no medical condition). Conduct relevant portions of a physical and neurological examination, which is likely to improve the alliance with the patient.

Use psychometric tests: Assess patients with the Minnesota Multiphasic Personality Inventory (MMPI), which is particularly useful for patients who may be malingering and/or who have severe characterological problems, and the Symptom Checklist–90 (SCL-90), which is brief and can be scored in the office.

Source. Adapted from Abbey SE: "Somatization and Somatoform Disorders," in *The American Psychiatric Publishing Textbook of Consultation-Liaison Psychiatry: Psychiatry in the Medically Ill,* 2nd Edition. Edited by Wise MG, Rundell JR. Washington, DC, American Psychiatric Publishing, 2002, pp. 361–392. Copyright 2002, American Psychiatric Publishing. Used with permission.

patients: total charges 9 times greater, hospital charges 6 times greater, and physician services 14 times greater. Somatizing patients spend up to 7 days per month sick in bed compared with the general population average of half a day (Smith et al. 1986).

Clinical Characteristics and Specific Management Strategies

The common feature shared by the somatoform disorders is the presence of physical symptoms that suggest a general medical condition but are not fully explained by a general medical condition, by the direct effects of a substance, or by another mental disorder. The physical symptoms are not intentional (i.e., malingering or factitious disorder) and cause significant disruption in social or occupational functioning (American Psychiatric Association 2000). DSM-IV-TR somatoform disorder diagnoses include somatization disorder, undifferentiated somatoform disorder, hypochondriasis, conversion disorder, body dysmorphic disorder (BDD), pain disorder, and somatoform disorder not otherwise specified. Epidemiology, clinical and associated features, clinical course and prognosis, and specific treatment and management strategies are discussed for each disorder.

Somatization Disorder (Briquet's Syndrome)

Epidemiology

The general population lifetime prevalence of somatization disorder is estimated at 0.1%–1.1%, depending on the criteria used (Karvonen et al. 2004; Regier et al. 1988). The prevalence in medical settings is higher—as high as 5% in some outpatient primary care clinics (deGruy et al. 1987). Somatization disorder is perhaps 10 times more common in women than in men. Symptom onset is usually in the teens, often with menarche. Of first-degree female relatives of women with somatization disorder, 20% have somatization disorder, and male relatives have a higher than expected rate of alcohol abuse and antisocial personality disorder (Golding et al. 1992).

Clinical Features

The typical patient with somatization disorder is a woman who describes herself as "always sickly." She began to experience medically unexplained symptoms in early adolescence and has, over the years, continued to have repeated unexplained physical complaints involving multiple organ systems. To make the diagnosis, DSM-IV-TR requires a history at some time of at least four pain symptoms, two gastrointestinal symptoms, one sexual symptom, and one pseudoneurological symptom, all unexplained medically.

Associated Features

As many as 75% of the patients with somatization disorder have comorbid Axis I diagnoses (Katon et al. 1991), most commonly major depressive disorder, dysthymic disorder, panic disorder, simple phobia, and substance abuse. As many as two-thirds of the patients with somatization disorder have symptoms that meet criteria for one or more personality disorders (see Rost et al. 1992), most frequently avoidant, paranoid, obsessive-compulsive, and histrionic.

Differential Diagnosis

Psychiatrists, even those who are inexperienced in psychosomatic medicine, can differentiate an undiagnosed medical illness, such as multiple sclerosis or systemic lupus, from somatization disorder. A detailed review of all past medical records is the key. Patients with somatization disorder have a life-long history of medically unexplained symptoms, typically beginning in their teens; along with this history are typically reports of numerous and recurrent conversion symptoms, a long list of medication "allergies" and unusual reactions, and a medical record that is best measured in pounds and not pages. A more complete discussion of the differential diagnosis of somatoform disorders is found in the section "Differential Diagnosis" later in this chapter (see also Table 8–1).

Clinical Course and Prognosis

The psychiatric consultant first must ensure that patients receive an appropriate diagnosis. Somatization disorder is a chronic but fluctuating disorder that rarely remits completely. The diagnosis of somatization disorder influences how physicians and the medical system respond to a patient. These patients are at risk for iatrogenic complications from numerous repetitive tests, procedures, and medications; the cost of the disorder is staggering.

Management

Appropriate management of somatization disorder is not easily implemented. It is a lifelong disorder, and most patients resist psychiatric consultation. The consultant must identify and treat comorbid psychiatric conditions. Table 8–3 contains a recommended management plan for patients with somatization disorder. To complicate management further, patients with somatization disorder also have primary and iatrogenically (often surgically) induced medical disorders, particularly as they grow older. When a patient with Briquet's syn-

Table 8–3. Management of somatization disorder

1. Establish one physician who can develop a doctor-patient relationship (usually a primary care physician, a physician with combined psychiatry–primary care training, or a medically oriented psychiatrist).

2. Treat comorbid mood or anxiety disorder, if present.

3. Maintain regular appointments. Even if the patient is doing well, continue regular appointments.

4. Gradually reduce the frequency of appointments. If physical symptoms recur in response to fewer appointments, reestablish more frequent appointments and try tapering appointments more slowly at a later date.

5. Perform regular physical examinations, and offer reassurance.

6. Do not pursue somatic complaints with further laboratory evaluations, referrals, or treatment unless objective evidence of disease is present.

7. Gradually shift the emphasis from listening to somatic complaints to talking about psychosocial stressors ("how is this illness affecting your life" often answers the question "how is your life affecting this illness?").

8. Work with the family or significant others to verify history and to monitor the patient's contacts with the health care system and medication intake.

9. Anticipate that the patient will receive prescription drugs or diagnostic procedures from other physicians; watch for drug misuse.

10. Protect the patient from iatrogenic problems, especially nonindicated surgical procedures.

drome also has a chronic medical illness, the primary physician is often reluctant to curtail medical evaluations. It is helpful in this situation to suggest to the primary physician that only complaints that have objective findings should be further evaluated and treated.

Undifferentiated Somatoform Disorder

Definition

Undifferentiated somatoform disorder is a residual diagnostic category for individuals whose symptoms do not meet criteria for somatization disorder or another somatoform disorder but who nevertheless have significant dysfunction caused by unexplained medical symptoms.

Epidemiology

No studies of undifferentiated somatoform disorder have been done, but studies of subsyndromal somatization disorder have attempted to identify a group of patients with sociodemographic and clinical characteristics similar to those of patients whose condition meets the full criteria for somatization disorder (Escobar et al. 1989). Further support for this diagnosis comes from the study of distressed high utilizers of medical care; this study documented significantly increased health care use by patients with functional somatic symptoms who had too few symptoms to meet DSM-IV (American Psychiatric Association 1994) criteria (Katon et al. 1991). In the general population, 4%–11% of the people have multiple medically unexplained symptoms consistent with a subsyndromal form of somatization disorder (Escobar et al. 1989).

Clinical Features

Undifferentiated somatoform disorder is diagnosed when the patient has one or more unexplained physical symptoms but does not meet the full criteria for somatization disorder. Most clinicians believe that the same principles of assessment and management for somatization disorder hold for patients with this diagnosis (see Tables 8–2 and 8–3).

Differential Diagnosis

As with somatization disorder, a detailed review of all past medical records is essential before rendering the diagnosis of undifferentiated somatoform disorder. When the history shows that the patient has the characteristics of somatization disorder but the disorder is early in the course or lacks the full criteria, this is a likely diagnosis. If one or just a few medically unexplained symptoms have occurred, especially if these symptoms occurred over a relatively short period of time, look for an alternative diagnosis. Remember, the absence of a general medical diagnosis (by itself) is never sufficient evidence for a psychiatric diagnosis. A more complete discussion of the differential diagnosis of somatoform disorders is found in the section "Differential Diagnosis" later in this chapter (see also Table 8–1).

Clinical Course and Prognosis

Individuals with undifferentiated somatoform disorder are probably a heterogeneous group. DSM-IV-TR notes that the "course of individual unexplained physical complaints is unpredictable. The eventual diagnosis of a general medical condition or another mental disorder is frequent" (American Psychiatric Association 2000, p. 491).

Management

See the earlier discussion of management in the "Somatization Disorder (Briquet's Syndrome)" section and Table 8–3.

Hypochondriasis

Definition

Hypochondriasis is the fear or the belief that one has a serious disease based on the misinterpretation of bodily symptoms. Anxiety and fear about the disease persist despite normal medical evaluations and reassurance (American Psychiatric Association 2000).

Epidemiology

The prevalence of hypochondriasis depends on the diagnostic criteria used (Barsky et al. 1986). A broad definition estimates that 50% of all patients seeing a physician have hypochondriacal symptoms or overlay (usually not a mental disorder); a narrow definition estimates a 1%–3% rate of hypochondriasis among various ethnic groups. Hypochondriasis is equally common in men and women (American Psychiatric Association 2000). The typical age at onset is in early adulthood.

Clinical Features

The core feature of hypochondriasis is fear of disease or conviction that one has a disease despite normal physical examination findings and physician reassurance. Bodily preoccupation (i.e., increased observation of and vigilance toward bodily sensations) is common. Patients with hypochondriasis believe that good health is a symptom-free state, and they are more likely than control patients to believe that symptoms mean disease (Barsky et al. 1992). Concern about the feared illness "often becomes a central feature of the individual's self-image, a topic of social discourse, and a response to life stresses" (American Psychiatric Association 2000, p. 504). Central clinical features of hypochondriasis are summed up by the four *D's*: 1) disease conviction, disease fear, disease preoccupation, and disability. According to DSM-IV-TR (American Psychiatric Association 2000), 6 months of symptoms are required before making the diagnosis.

Associated Features

Barsky et al. (1992) found that 88% of the hypochondriacal patients in a general medical outpatient clinic had one or more concurrent Axis I diagnoses; the most common were generalized anxiety disorder (71.4%), dysthymia (45.2%), major depression (42.9%), somatization disorder (21.4%), and panic disorder (16.7%). Patients with hypochondriasis are high utilizers of medical services and have the potential for iatrogenic complications from repeated investigations (Abbey 2002). Interestingly, research has shown that relatives of patients with hypochondriasis do not have a greater frequency of hypochondriasis than is found in the general population (Noyes et al. 1997).

Differential Diagnosis

Hypochondriasis in a general medical setting is most often secondary to a mood or anxiety disorder or to somatization disorder. A more complete discussion of the differential diagnosis of somatoform disorders is found in the section "Differential Diagnosis" later in this chapter (see also Table 8–1).

Clinical Course and Prognosis

Hypochondriasis is often a chronic condition; thus, one might argue that it is better understood as a personality style or an anxiety disorder (Barsky et al. 1992).

Treatment and Management

Hypochondriasis often remits or improves with resolution of underlying major life stressors, interpersonal situations, or mood and anxiety disorders. The clinician should reassure patients frequently—even though it does not change their behavior—and should protect them from iatrogenic harm, especially nonindicated surgical procedures. The family and significant others should be educated about the nature of hypochondriasis, which may help decrease anxiety and stress at home. In one study of pharmacological treatment of hypochondriasis, high-dose fluoxetine improved the conditions of 10 of 16 patients who did not have marked depressive features (Fallon et al. 1993), and a review of medication treatment suggested that the patients with "the obsessional cluster of somatoform disorders (hypochondriasis and body dysmorphic disorder)" respond well to selective serotonin reuptake inhibitors (Fallon 2004, p. 455). A recent randomized controlled trial of 6-session cognitive-behavioral therapy (CBT) compared with usual medical care showed clinically significant improvement at 6 and 12 months follow-up in the CBT-treated group (Barsky and Ahern 2004).

Conversion Disorder

Definition

Conversion disorder is a loss of or alteration in function that suggests a physical, usually neurological, disease, but one is not present. The initiation or exacerbation of the symptom is associated with a meaningful stressor.

Epidemiology

The prevalence of conversion disorder varies among studies. Toone (1990), in a review of several studies, estimated rates of 0.3% in the general population, 1%–3% in medical outpatient settings, and 1%–4.5% in inpatient neurological and medical settings. The prevalence in general medical practice has been estimated at 4%–9% (American Psychiatric Association 2000). Women outnumber men with the disorder by a ratio varying from 2:1 to 10:1 (Murphy 1990). Onset is typically in adolescence or early adulthood, although cases occur throughout the life cycle.

Clinical Features

Common presentations of conversion include motor symptoms (e.g., paralysis, disturbances in coordination or balance, localized weakness, akinesia, dyskinesia, aphonia, urinary retention, difficulty swallowing), sensory symptoms (e.g., blindness, double vision, anesthesia, paresthesia, deafness), and seizures or convulsions that may have voluntary motor or sensory components (Abbey 2002). When unilateral conversion symptoms appear in women, they are more likely to occur on the left side of the body. The reasons for this are unknown, but the same is true for somatoform pain and hypochondriasis symptoms (Toone 1990).

Persons with a conversion symptom frequently have a psychological "bind." For example, a teenager has perfectionistic parents who constantly pressure her to do numerous chores. When she does the chores, they always criticize her for inadequate performance. The teenager is in a "no-win" bind and must endure criticism whether or not the chores are done. She develops a "pain in the sacrum," which gives her an "out." She does not have to do the chores, avoids the usual criticism, and gets sympathetic attention. The association between her symptom and the fact that her parents are "pains in the butt" is an attractive hypothesis to the consulting psychiatrist but is not in conscious awareness for the teenager or her parents.

Conversion means that a conflict is converted by the unconscious to a physical symptom; this process is sometimes referred to as *primary gain.* The unconscious nature of conversion helps distinguish it from the consciously planned manipulative behaviors associated with malingering and factitious disorders. The consultation psychiatrist must exercise caution before diagnosing conversion. In follow-up studies, evidence of an actual disease process that retrospectively explained the "conversion" symptom was found in 12%–50% of cases (Ford and Folks 1985; Lazare 1981; Moene et al. 2000). Not all studies support this finding (Stone et al. 2003).

Associated Features

Protracted conversion reactions are sometimes associated with secondary physical changes (e.g., disuse atrophy). Patients frequently have a model for the symptom in a family member or close friend.

Differential Diagnosis

The pitfall in making a diagnosis of conversion disorder is the later appearance of a medical disorder that, in retrospect, explains the "conversion" symptom. For that reason, it is essential that positive evidence for conversion exists (e.g., conflicts or other stressor associated with initiation or exacerbation of symptom) prior to the diagnosis. Even then, you will occasional be wrong (see case example for pain disorder later in this chapter). A more complete discussion of the differential diagnosis of somatoform disorders is found in the section "Differential Diagnosis" later in this chapter (see also Table 8–1).

Clinical Course and Prognosis

Individual episodes of conversion usually are short, have a sudden onset, and resolve when the associated psychosocial stressor (bind) remits (American Psychiatric Association 2000; Murphy 1990). However, Stone et al. (2003) reported that 83% of the patients reported weakness and sensory symptoms at follow-up (range = 9- to 16-year follow-up).

Factors reported to predispose to conversion disorder are 1) prior physical disorders in the individual or a close contact who provides a model for the conversion symptoms and 2) severe social stressors, including bereavement, rape, incest, warfare, and other forms of psychosocial trauma (Toone 1990). A better prognosis is linked to 1) acute and recent onset, 2) traumatic or stressful life event at onset, 3) good premorbid health, and 4) absence of other major medical or psychiatric disorders (Lazare 1981).

Treatment and Management

A wide variety of successful treatments are reported. Spontaneous remission is common. The suggestion that the symptom will rapidly resolve and hypnosis sometimes are helpful and potentially curative; most conversion disorder patients are quite suggestible. When a clear relation between a conflict and a conversion symptom is identified, short-term focused or supportive therapy is indicated. Effective treatment focused on suggestion, combined with identifying and resolving unconscious psychological binds, will help the patient rapidly resolve the conversion symptom. Direct confrontation usually does not help and may worsen the symptom.

Most patients show a rapid response to treatment, but some do not (Stone et al. 2003). Multidisciplinary inpatient behavioral treatment was successful in 8 of 9 "acute" cases but failed in 27 of 28 "chronic" cases; whereas strategic-behavioral treatment (i.e., patient and patient's family were told that full recovery constituted proof of an organic etiology and that failure was proof of a psychiatric etiology) worked in 13 of 21 patients with chronic motor conversion disorder who had failed the initial behavioral therapy (Shapiro et al. 2004).

Pseudoseizures, tremor, and amnesia are least likely to have a rapid and good outcome (Toone 1990).

Body Dysmorphic Disorder

Definition

The hallmark of BDD is a preoccupation with an imagined defect in appearance (if a slight physical anomaly is present, the individual's concern with it is markedly excessive) that is accompanied by significant distress or impairment in social or occupational functioning (American Psychiatric Association 2000).

Epidemiology

Onset is typically in adolescence (Phillips et al. 1993), although the reported age at onset ranges from ages 6 to 33 years. Many years may pass before diagnosis because of the patient's reluctance to disclose symptoms (American Psychiatric Association 2000). With structured interviews, 3.2% of psychiatric patients met criteria for BDD (Zimmerman and Mattia 1998).

Clinical Features

The patient with BDD has an obsession or a preoccupation with an imagined physical body defect or flaw. The most common complaints involve facial appearance (e.g., wrinkles, nose, mouth), and less common complaints are about hair, breasts, genitalia, or other body parts. A minor flaw may exist, but the patient's concern is grossly excessive, and he or she may seek medical attention from a plastic surgeon or dermatologist. It is sometimes difficult to determine whether the patient's complaint is an overvalued idea or a somatic delusion (Hollander et al. 1992).

Associated Features

Most patients with BDD have at least one comorbid Axis I psychiatric disorder (Gunstad and Phillips 2003). In a study of 30 patients with BDD, the point prevalence of major depression was 50% and the lifetime prevalence was 60%, the point prevalence of bipolar disorder was 27% and the lifetime prevalence was 33%, the point prevalence of dysthymia was 7%, and the lifetime history of psychotic symptoms was 77% (Phillips et al. 1993). Psychosocial dysfunction is often profound, with social withdrawal and functioning below expected occupational capacity. Phillips et al. (1993) found that 97%

of patients with BDD avoid usual social and occupational activities; 30% were housebound, and 17% reported suicide attempts.

Differential Diagnosis

A few other disorders occur in the differential diagnosis of body dysmorphic disorder (e.g., major depression with and without psychotic features). If the somatic preoccupation is of delusional proportions, an additional diagnosis of delusion disorder, somatic type is made. A more complete discussion of the differential diagnosis of somatoform disorders is found in the section "Differential Diagnosis" later in this chapter (see also Table 8–1).

Clinical Course and Prognosis

BDD is usually chronic, with few symptom-free intervals, although the intensity of the symptoms often varies over time.

Treatment and Management

Surgical alteration of the perceived defect usually offers only temporary relief, if even that, and may create a real defect. Similarities are found between BDD and obsessive-compulsive disorder, so a trial of a serotonin reuptake blocker is warranted if symptoms persist (Abbey 2002; Fallon 2004). If the disorder is of psychotic proportion, pimozide is recommended (see section "Delusional Disorder, Somatic Type" later in this chapter). Successful pharmacotherapy for small series of patients with BDD also was reported with imipramine and doxepin (Brotman and Jenike 1984), clomipramine (Hollander et al. 1989), fluoxetine (Phillips et al. 1993, 2004), citalopram (Phillips and Najjar 2003), and tranylcypromine (Jenike 1984).

Pain Disorder

Definition

Pain disorder in DSM-IV-TR evolved from the previous concepts of somatoform pain disorder (DSM-III-R; American Psychiatric Association 1987) and psychogenic pain disorder (DSM-III; American Psychiatric Association 1980). In pain disorder, psychological factors are important in the onset, severity, exacerbation, or maintenance of the pain; if a medical disorder is also present, psychological factors exacerbate the pain.

Epidemiology

The prevalence of pain disorder is unknown.

Clinical Features

Chronic pain patients who were given the previous diagnoses of psychogenic or somatoform pain disorder were described as having "the disease of the *D's*": 1) disability, 2) disuse and degeneration of functional capacity secondary to pain behavior, 3) drug misuse, 4) doctor shopping, 5) dependency (emotional), 6) demoralization, 7) depression, and 8) dramatic accounts of illness (Brena and Chapman 1983). DSM-IV-TR lists three forms of this diagnosis: pain disorder associated with psychological factors, pain disorder associated with both psychological factors and a general medical condition, and pain disorder associated with a general medical condition.

Associated Features

Depression is diagnosed frequently in patients with chronic pain syndromes. Estimates range widely from 8% to 80%; most studies find that at least half of their chronic pain sample is depressed (Smith 1991).

Differential Diagnosis

A more complete discussion of the differential diagnosis of somatoform disorders is found in the section "Differential Diagnosis" later in this chapter (see also Table 8–1). Four pain symptoms are part of the diagnostic criteria for somatization disorder, so consider somatization disorder in your differential diagnosis. Also consider mood, anxiety, and psychotic disorders. As with conversion disorder, the most common pitfall in making a diagnosis of pain disorder is the later appearance of a medical disorder that, in retrospect, explains the pain. Therefore, look for positive evidence for somatoform pain disorder (e.g., conflicts or other stressor associated with initiation or exacerbation of the pain). Even then, the diagnosis may prove incorrect, as in the following case example:

> A 35-year-old man with a chief complaint of severe rectal pain was admitted to the neurology inpatient service. Medical examination and tests were WNL; psychiatric consultation was requested. During psychiatric examination, the

patient was very dramatic. He was constantly in motion, grimacing and complaining of rectal pain. He reported pain severity (scale from 1 [no pain] to 10 [worst pain you have every experienced] as "10." He had recently broken up with his fiancée. He also reported homosexual relationships in the past but spontaneously and emphatically stated that he was not homosexual. Past medical records showed few prior contacts with the medical system or physicians, except for two bouts with the flu and appendicitis. He denied anhedonia, weight loss, suicidal ideation, or decreased energy and past history of psychiatric disorders. He stated that his sleep and concentration were affected by the pain. On the basis of the lack of medical findings and the significant recent stressors (breakup with fiancée and conflicts over sexuality), a diagnosis of somatoform pain disorder was made. Four months later a tumor was discovered on his cauda equina.

Clinical Course and Prognosis

Iatrogenic complications are likely common and include dependence on narcotic analgesics and benzodiazepines, and unnecessary surgical interventions (Abbey 2002).

Treatment and Management

Management of pain syndromes is complex. The most effective treatments, especially when the pain is chronic and complicated by emotional issues and suffering, are provided by a multidisciplinary team that uses many modes of therapy. Serotonin-norepinephrine reuptake inhibitor types of antidepressants, which have analgesic and antidepressant actions (Arnold et al. 2004; Fishbain et al. 1998; Jones et al. 2005), and moclobemide (Pirildar et al. 2003) have been used. We discuss pain management in more detail in Chapter 12 ("Pain and Analgesics").

Somatoform Disorder Not Otherwise Specified

Somatoform disorder not otherwise specified is the diagnosis used for patients with somatoform symptoms that do not meet diagnostic criteria for any of the specific somatoform disorders. Examples include pseudocyesis and hypochondriacal and other unexplained physical symptoms lasting less than 6 months.

Psychological Factors Affecting Medical Condition

To diagnose psychological factors affecting medical condition, a temporal relation between a stressor and the initiation or exacerbation of a physical condition must exist. The physical condition is either tissue pathology (e.g., gastric ulcer) or a recognized physiological process (e.g., migraine headache). Common examples of physical conditions that can be exacerbated by psychological stress are tension or migraine headaches, hypertension, gastric and duodenal ulcers, asthma, and ulcerative colitis. The consultant must rule out a somatoform disorder during the patient's evaluation. A neutral way of uncovering stressors is to inquire, "How has this [*state the patient's somatic complaint in his or her own words*] affected your life?" The patient will frequently state what part of his or her life is most related to the symptom.

Factitious Disorders

Definition

Patients with factitious disorders intentionally feign or induce diseases or symptoms.

Epidemiology

Demographic analyses of factitious disorder patients suggest two general patterns. Patients with chronic factitious disorder (Munchausen syndrome) are usually middle-aged men, usually unmarried, and estranged from their families. Patients with more acute forms of factitious disorder are usually women, ages 20–40, who work in medical occupations such as nursing and medical technology (Ford and Feldman 2002). Gault and colleagues (1988) used an interesting mechanism for estimating factitious disorder frequency. They analyzed material submitted by patients as "kidney stones"; 3.5% of the "stones" were obviously nonphysiological and artifactual.

Clinical Features

Patients with factitious disorder are aware of their behaviors, although their underlying motivations are often unconscious. Factitious disorder may occur with predominantly physical symptoms, predominantly psychological symptoms, or combined physical and psychological symptoms. In chronic factitious disorder, or Munchausen syndrome, self-production of dramatic illnesses allows the patient to achieve the goal of multiple hospitalizations. In factitious disorder by proxy (Munchausen syndrome by proxy), signs and symptoms are created in another person, usually a child or an elderly relative (Ford and Feldman 2002). In factitious disorder by proxy, the perpetrators are the mothers in almost all reported cases. Several more and less common factitious behaviors are reported (Table 8–4).

Differential Diagnosis

The diagnosis of factitious disorder is difficult to make, unless direct evidence is found (e.g., a syringe and insulin found in the radio of a hospitalized patient with unexplained episodes of hypoglycemia). Indirect evidence, such as no medical diagnosis and a very dramatic presentation or a severe Axis II disorder, may cause frustrated medical staff to request psychiatric consultation because they suspect malingering (see case example under pain disorder). The psychiatric consultant must look past the staff's countertransference and look for positive evidence of a diagnosis. Some psychiatrists use "unlikely," "possible," "probable," or "definite" to indicate the likelihood of the diagnosis. A more complete discussion of the differential diagnosis of somatoform disorders is found in the section "Differential Diagnosis" later in this chapter (see also Table 8–1).

Clinical Course and Prognosis

Factitious disorders are associated with considerable morbidity and mortality. Few patients accept treatment, and even fewer are cured. If confronted, some patients may deny but stop behavior, very few may acknowledge behavior and enter treatment, and most will transfer their medical care elsewhere and continue factitious behavior (Wise and Ford 1999).

Treatment and Management

Recent changes in medical practice in the United States emphasize patients' rights and informed consent. As a result, many practices, such as clandestine searches of personal articles, are not acceptable and are probably illegal (Ford and Feldman 2002). Thus, when a patient is suspected of having a factitious disorder, it is prudent to take the steps outlined in Table 8–5.

Table 8–4. Some signs, symptoms, and diseases simulated or caused by factitious behavior

More common	Less common
Autoimmune diseases	Acquired immunodeficiency syndrome
Bleeding	Anaplastic anemia
Cancer	Cushing's disease
Chronic diarrhea	Diabetes mellitus
Epilepsy	Goodpasture's syndrome
Fever of unknown origin	Hemiplegia
Hematuria	Hypersomnia
Hypoglycemia	Hypertension
Intestinal bleeding	Hyperthyroidism
Iron deficiency anemia	Hypotension
Rashes	Myocardial infarction
Renal stones	Pheochromocytoma
Seizures	Pupillary dysfunction
	Reflex sympathetic dystrophy
	Septic arthritis
	Thrombocytopenia
	Torsion dystonia
	Uterine bleeding
	Ventricular tachycardia

Source. Adapted from Ford CV, Feldman MD: "Factitious Disorders and Malingering," in *The American Psychiatric Publishing Textbook of Consultation-Liaison Psychiatry: Psychiatry in the Medically Ill,* 2nd Edition. Edited by Wise MG, Rundell JR. Washington, DC, American Psychiatric Publishing, 2002, pp. 519–531. Copyright 2002, American Psychiatric Publishing. Used with permission.

Confrontation of the patient's behavior is best accomplished by having the primary physician and consulting psychiatrist approach the patient in a non-condemning but firm manner (Hollender and Hersh 1970). The patient is told that he or she is contributing to the illness and that this behavior must reflect a high degree of emotional distress and difficulty in directly communicating needs. The psychiatrist then offers therapeutic assistance. A small minority of patients will accept treatment, which preferably will begin in an inpatient psychiatric unit.

Table 8–5.   Steps to take when factitious disorders are suspected

1. Involve the hospital administration from the start.
2. Seek legal advice from the hospital's risk management department and/or the physician's own attorney.
3. Consult with the hospital's ethics committee early in the process.
4. Maintain confidentiality to the extent specified by law. The "blacklists" of Munchausen patients advocated and maintained by some institutions are not legally acceptable in the United States.

Source.   Adapted from Ford CV, Feldman MD: "Factitious Disorders and Malingering," in *The American Psychiatric Publishing Textbook of Consultation-Liaison Psychiatry: Psychiatry in the Medically Ill,* 2nd Edition. Edited by Wise MG, Rundell JR. Washington, DC, American Psychiatric Publishing, 2002, pp. 519–531. Copyright 2002, American Psychiatric Publishing. Used with permission.

Malingering

Definition

Malingering is grossly exaggerating, lying, or faking physical or psychological symptoms for the purpose of a concrete, recognizable gain (often called *secondary gain*). Individuals who have malingering are motivated by specific external incentives (Gorman 1982), including deferment from military service, avoidance of hazardous work assignments, receipt of financial rewards such as disability payments, escape from incarceration, or procurement of controlled substances (Ford and Feldman 2002).

Epidemiology

Malingering occurs when illness brings tangible gains. It is common in prisons, courtrooms, military settings, and settings where disability evaluations are performed. Even malingering by animal proxy is reported (LeBourgeois et al. 2002). This behavior adds considerably to the cost of insurance coverage (Gorman 1982).

Clinical Features

The following illustrates a case of malingering:

> A 24-year-old man en route to a trial for automobile theft complains of excruciating low back pain. Medical evaluation is equivocal for disc disease.

During his evaluation in the hospital, he requests and is given a pass to visit a "dying aunt." That night, he is observed dancing at a disco. The secondary gain for the individual was avoidance of prosecution.

Malingering is likely if more than one of the following factors is present: medicolegal presentation, marked disparity between the patient's claimed disability and objective findings, lack of cooperation with psychiatric or medical evaluation and treatment, and antisocial personality disorder. Psychological testing is often helpful in identifying malingering patients (Slick et al. 2004). The Minnesota Multiphasic Personality Inventory–2 (MMPI-2) is a useful test for patients who distort their presentations.

Differential Diagnosis

Malingering is difficult to prove, unless direct evidence is found (e.g., see case example in the clinical features section above). Some psychiatrists use "unlikely," "possible," "probable," or "definite" to indicate the likelihood of the diagnosis. A more complete discussion of the differential diagnosis of somatoform disorders is found in the section "Differential Diagnosis" later in this chapter (see also Table 8–1).

Treatment and Management

Malingering is a legal rather than a medical or psychiatric issue. With this fact in mind, the clinician must be circumspect in his or her approach to the patient. Every note should be written with the expectation that it will likely become a courtroom exhibit (Ford and Feldman 2002). The patient suspected of malingering usually is not confronted with a direct accusation. Direct confrontation can produce more sophisticated malingering (Youngblood et al. 1999). Instead, subtle communication indicates that the physician is "onto the game" (Kramer et al. 1979).

Differential Diagnosis

Other Somatoform and Related Disorders

Patients may have more than one somatoform or related disorder simultaneously (Table 8–1). These disorders are distinguished from one another by the diagnostic criteria and clinical characteristics described earlier in this chapter.

Medical Disorder

The consultant's first task is to rule out a medical disorder. Do *not* assume that the referring physician has eliminated this possibility. The patient's personality or exaggerated and inappropriate behavior may have decreased the primary physician's index of suspicion for medical diagnoses and shortened the preconsultation workup. In addition, these patients are sometimes medically complex. Therefore, the psychiatrist must thoroughly review current and past charts (an often time-consuming but worthwhile task) and perform physical, neurological, and mental status examinations.

Secondary Psychiatric Disorders

Patients with dementia, delirium, or other cognitive disorders may present with increased physical complaints, particularly when anxious. For example,

> A 69-year-old woman presents to the emergency department with hyperventilation, shaking, crying, and obvious anxiety. She is given a diagnosis of an "anxiety neurosis" by the emergency department physician, and psychiatric consultation is requested. Her mental status examination shows significant cognitive impairment (i.e., a Mini-Mental State Exam score of 9 out of 30). Symptoms started acutely when she could not understand how to operate an answering machine at her husband's business.

This is an example of a catastrophic reaction in a person with dementia.

Adjustment Disorder

If the symptom (e.g., fatigue, headache, backache) occurs acutely as a reaction to significant acute stress, it is often self-limited and can be diagnosed as an adjustment disorder (unspecified type). Identification of the stressor and its significance to the individual is the first and most important step to planning treatment. Short-term supportive, cognitive, focused insight-oriented, and group therapy are all potentially effective treatments.

Anxiety Disorders

A high correlation exists between anxiety, anxiety disorders, and the development of somatic symptoms (Simon and VonKorff 1991), sometimes called *secondary hypochondriasis*. Patients with an anxiety disorder, especially panic disorder, are hyperaware of body sensations and usually have increased sympathetic arousal. Those with panic disorder or generalized anxiety disorder frequently have numerous somatic symptoms (see also Chapter 7, "Anxiety and Insomnia," in this volume).

Depressive Disorder

Depressed patients typically have numerous somatic symptoms, including neurovegetative signs of depression such as sleep disturbance, decreased energy, anorexia, decreased libido, and other associated physical complaints (e.g., headache, tinnitus, dizziness, fatigue). Anxiety is a common feature of depression. Hypochondriacal preoccupation during depressive episodes increases with age (Cassem and Barsky 1991).

Substance-Related Disorders

Alcohol abuse and dependence, alcohol withdrawal, and the medical sequelae of chronic alcohol use are seen commonly by psychiatrists in the general hospital. Patients who abuse other drugs also have physical symptoms associated with active use or withdrawal. These patients will commonly report physical symptoms (e.g., sleep disturbance, palpitations, gooseflesh, tremor, irritability, dysthymia, gastrointestinal complaints).

Psychotic Disorder

Patients who are actively psychotic are easily recognized because the somatic symptoms reported are usually bizarre. The psychiatric consultant plays an important role in such cases. The consultant must ensure that physical symptoms are not ignored simply because the patient has a chronic psychotic disorder. On the other hand, the consultant must discourage unnecessary pursuit of bizarre physical symptoms that are secondary to psychosis. For example, a patient reported a "terrible buzzing sound in my head." Examination by an otolaryngologist showed no abnormalities. On further questioning, the patient stated that the buzzing was a result of a Central Intelligence Agency photon transmitter aimed at his head.

Delusional Disorder, Somatic Type

Delusional disorder, somatic type, is also called *monosymptomatic hypochondriasis* or *monosymptomatic hypochondriacal psychosis*. The three most common delusions are delusions of infestation (e.g., parasites, insects, worms, or foreign bodies on or under the skin), olfactory delusions (e.g., a foul odor from skin, mouth, rectum, or vagina), and dysmorphophobia (i.e., the belief that one's body is ugly or misshapen) (Munro and Chmara 1982). Pimozide (a neuroleptic) is the drug of choice for delusional disorder, somatic type. This medication should be begun at 2 mg in the morning and increased in 2-mg increments every 3 days. Doses rarely need to exceed 12 mg/day, and an 80% or higher rate of improvement is reported (Bhatia et al. 2000).

Additional Treatment and Management Considerations

Approach to the Patient

Specific management strategies for individual somatoform and related disorders were detailed in the specific discussions about those disorders earlier in this chapter. The key to the clinical management of the somatizing patient is to adopt "care" rather than "cure" as a goal. "Management" is a much more realistic goal than "treatment." Abbey (2002) suggested the following fundamental principles of managing patients with somatoform disorders:

- *Emphasize explanation.* To engage in treatment, patients require a sense that their primary physician and the consulting psychiatrist are taking them seriously, appreciate the magnitude of their distress, and have a rationale for the proposed management plan.
- *Arrange for regular follow-up.* Regular follow-up results in decreased use of other health care services. The best choice for most patients is management by their primary care practitioner in consultation with a psychiatrist.
- *Treat mood or anxiety disorders.* Mood and anxiety disorders have significant morbidity and interfere with participation in rehabilitation and psychotherapy. These disorders may fuel the somatization process or heighten somatic amplification.
- *Minimize polypharmacy.* Polypharmacy can cause iatrogenic complications. Unnecessary medications should be tapered and withdrawn. This process is often long and complicated, so it is important to take a staged approach with small, realistic, achievable steps.

- *Provide specific therapy when indicated.* A variety of specific therapies are suggested for the somatoform disorders. They are discussed elsewhere in this chapter.

- *Change social dynamics.* Many patients' lives revolve around their symptoms and the health care system. When possible, important members of the patient's social support system should be persuaded to consistently reward non-illness-related behaviors.

- *Recognize and control negative reactions and countertransference.* Somatizing patients evoke powerful negative emotional responses in physicians. These reactions result in less than optimal clinical care. The range of emotions experienced by physicians may include guilt for failing to help, fear that the patient will make a complaint (or sue), and anger at the patient.

Physical Reactivation and Physical Therapy

"Physical reactivation via a gradually escalating program of exercise (e.g., walking, swimming) often improves the quality of life in patients with a variety of somatoform disorders" (Abbey 2002, p. 384). Although it is often difficult to engage patients with somatoform disorders in exercise, once they become more active, they often find it pleasurable and report feelings of accomplishment, reduced stress, and greater confidence in their body. Physical therapy is helpful for patients with conversion disorder and may be the only treatment required.

Relaxation Therapies, Meditation, and Hypnotherapy

Various forms of relaxation therapies, biofeedback, meditation, and hypnotherapy are used in patients with somatoform disorders. Relaxation therapies aim to modulate somatic sensations and give patients a sense of self-empowerment.

Cognitive Therapy

Cognitive therapy is effective for some patients with somatization (Kronke and Swindle 2000) and hypochondriasis (Barsky and Ahern 2004; Hiller et al. 2002) and can reduce health care use (Hiller et al. 2003). It is used in both individual and group formats. A cognitive model directs attention to factors maintaining preoccupation with worries about health, including attentional factors, avoidant behaviors, beliefs, and misinterpretation of symptoms, signs, and medical communications (Salkovskis 1989). Cognitive therapy is a particularly valuable adjunct for pain disorders. It helps the patient identify and replace inappropriate negative beliefs or attributions with more appropriate ideas or coping strategies (Benjamin 1989). For chronic pain syndromes, cognitive therapy is reported to produce a greater reduction in pain complaints than do other forms of treatment (Benjamin 1989).

Group Psychotherapy

Group therapy is particularly useful in the management of somatoform disorders. With the gratification of social and affiliative needs via the group, the need to somatize to establish or maintain relationships may be reduced (Ford 1984). Confrontation by fellow group members regarding primary or secondary gain is usually much better tolerated than that by an individual's therapist (Abbey 2002). Anger at physicians and family and dependency needs are better tolerated in the group setting, which tends to diffuse intense affects. Group therapy is also useful in increasing interpersonal skills and in enhancing more direct forms of communication (Ford 1984).

References

Abbey SE: Somatization and somatoform disorders, in The American Psychiatric Publishing Textbook of Consultation-Liaison Psychiatry: Psychiatry in the Medically Ill, 2nd Edition. Edited by Wise MG, Rundell JR. Washington, DC, American Psychiatric Publishing, 2002, pp 361–392

American Psychiatric Association: Diagnostic and Statistical Manual of Mental Disorders, 3rd Edition. Washington, DC, American Psychiatric Association, 1980

American Psychiatric Association: Diagnostic and Statistical Manual of Mental Disorders, 3rd Edition, Revised. Washington, DC, American Psychiatric Association, 1987

American Psychiatric Association: Diagnostic and Statistical Manual of Mental Disorders, 4th Edition. Washington, DC, American Psychiatric Association, 1994

American Psychiatric Association: Diagnostic and Statistical Manual of Mental Disorders, 4th Edition, Text Revision. Washington, DC, American Psychiatric Association, 2000

Arnold LM, Lu Y, Crofford LJ, et al: A double-blind, multicenter trial comparing duloxetine with placebo in the treatment of fibromyalgia patients with or without major depressive disorder. Arthritis Rheum 50:2974–2984, 2004

Barsky AJ, Ahern DK: Cognitive behavior therapy for hypochondriasis: a randomized controlled trial. JAMA 291:1464–1470, 2004

Barsky AJ, Wyshak G, Klerman GL: Medical and psychiatric determinants of outpatient medical utilization. Med Care 24:548–560, 1986

Barsky AJ, Wyshade G, Klerman GL: Psychiatric comorbidity in DSM-III-R hypochondriasis. Arch Gen Psychiatry 49:101–108, 1992

Benjamin S: Psychological treatment of chronic pain: a selective review. J Psychosom Res 33:121–131, 1989

Bhatia MS, Jagawat T, Choudhary S: Delusional parasitosis: a clinical profile. Int J Psychiatry Med 30:83–91, 2000

Brena SF, Chapman SL (eds): Management of Patients With Chronic Pain. New York, Spectrum, 1983

Brotman AW, Jenike MA: Monosymptomatic hypochondriasis treated with tricyclic antidepressants. Am J Psychiatry 141:1608–1609, 1984

Cassem NH, Barsky AJ: Functional somatic symptoms and somatoform disorders, in Massachusetts General Hospital Handbook of General Hospital Psychiatry, 3rd Edition. Edited by Cassem NH. St Louis, MO, Mosby-Year Book, 1991, pp 131–157

deGruy F, Columbia L, Dickinson P: Somatization disorder in a family practice. J Fam Pract 25:45–51, 1987

Eisenberg L: Disease and illness: distinctions between professional and popular ideas of sickness. Cult Med Psychiatry 1:9–23, 1977

Escobar JI, Manu P, Matthews D, et al: Medically unexplained physical symptoms, somatization disorder and abridged somatization: studies with the Diagnostic Interview Schedule. Psychiatr Dev 7:235–245, 1989

Fallon BA: Pharmacotherapy of somatoform disorders. J Psychosom Res 56:455–460, 2004

Fallon BA, Liebowitz MR, Salman E, et al: Fluoxetine for hypochondriacal patients without major depression. J Clin Psychopharmacol 13:438–441, 1993

Fishbain DA, Cutler RB, Rosomoff HL, et al: Do antidepressants have an analgesic effect in psychogenic pain and somatoform pain disorder? A meta-analysis. Psychosom Med 60:503–509, 1998

Ford CV: The Somatizing Disorders: Illness as a Way of Life. New York, Elsevier, 1983

Ford CV: Somatizing disorders, in Helping Patients and Their Families Cope With Medical Problems. Edited by Roback HB. Washington, DC, Jossey-Bass, 1984, pp 39–59

Ford CV, Feldman MD: Factitious disorders and malingering, in The American Psychiatric Publishing Textbook of Consultation-Liaison Psychiatry: Psychiatry in the Medically Ill, 2nd Edition. Edited by Wise MG, Rundell JR. Washington, DC, American Psychiatric Publishing, 2002, pp 519–531

Ford CV, Folks DG: Conversion disorders: an overview. Psychosomatics 26:371–383, 1985

Gault MH, Campbell NR, Aksu AE: Spurious stones. Nephron 48:274–279, 1988

Golding JM, Rost K, Kashner TM, et al: Family psychiatric history of patients with somatization disorder. Psychiatr Med 10:33–47, 1992

Gorman WF: Defining malingering. J Forensic Sci 27:401–407, 1982

Gunstad J, Phillips KA: Axis I comorbidity in body dysmorphic disorder. Compr Psychiatry 44:270–276, 2003

Hiller W, Leibbrand R, Rief W, et al: Predictors of course and outcome in hypochondriasis after cognitive-behavioral treatment. Psychother Psychosom 71:318–325, 2002

Hiller W, Fichter MM, Rief W: A controlled treatment study of somatoform disorders including analysis of healthcare utilization and cost-effectiveness. J Psychosom Res 54:369–380, 2003

Hollander E, Liebowitz MR, Winchel R, et al: Treatment of body dysmorphic disorder with serotonin reuptake blockers. Am J Psychiatry 146:768–770, 1989

Hollander E, Neville D, Frenkel M, et al: Body dysmorphic disorder: diagnostic issues and related disorders. Psychosomatics 33:156–165, 1992

Hollender MH, Hersh SP: Impossible consultation made possible. Arch Gen Psychiatry 23:343–345, 1970

Jenike MA: A case report of successful treatment of dysmorphophobia with tranylcypromine. Am J Psychiatry 141:1463–1464, 1984

Jones CK, Peters SC, Shannon HE: Efficacy of duloxetine, a potent and balanced serotonergic and noradrenergic reuptake inhibitor, in inflammatory and acute pain models in rodents. J Pharmacol Exp Ther 312:726–732. 2005

Karvonen JT, Veijola J, Jokelainen J, et al: Somatization disorder in young adult population. Gen Hosp Psychiatry 26:9–12, 2004

Katon WJ, Walker EA: Medically unexplained symptoms in primary care. J Clin Psychiatry 59 (suppl 20):15–21, 1998

Katon W, Lin E, Von Korff M, et al: Somatization: a spectrum of severity. Am J Psychiatry 148:34–40, 1991

Kellner R: Functional somatic symptoms and hypochondriasis. Arch Gen Psychiatry 42:821–833, 1985

Kramer KK, LaPiana FG, Appleton B: Ocular malingering and hysteria: diagnosis and management. Surv Ophthalmol 24:89–96, 1979

Kronke K, Swindle R: Cognitive-behavioral therapy for somatization and symptom syndromes: a critical review of controlled clinical trials. Psychother Psychosom 69:205–215, 2000

Lazare A: Current concepts in psychiatry: conversion symptoms. N Engl J Med 305:745–748, 1981

LeBourgeois HW 3rd, Foreman TA, Thompson JW Jr: Novel cases: malingering by animal proxy. J Am Acad Psychiatry Law 31:520–524, 2002

Lipowski ZJ: Somatization: the concept and its clinical application. Am J Psychiatry 145:1358–1368, 1988

Mechanic D: The concept of illness behaviour: culture, situation and personal predisposition. Psychol Med 16:1–7, 1986

Moene FC, Landberg EH, Hoogduin KA, et al: Organic syndromes diagnosed as conversion disorder: identification and frequency in a study of 85 patients. J Psychosom Res 49:7–12, 2000

Munro A, Chmara J: Monosymptomatic hypochondriacal psychosis: a diagnostic checklist based on 50 cases of the disorder. Can J Psychiatry 27:374–376, 1982

Murphy MR: Classification of the somatoform disorders, in Somatization: Physical Symptoms and Psychological Illness. Edited by Bass C. Oxford, England, Blackwell Scientific, 1990, pp 10–39

Noyes R, Holt CS, Happel RL, et al: A family study of hypochondriasis. J Nerv Ment Dis 185:223–232, 1997

Pakel ES, Ramana R, Cooper Z, et al: Residual symptoms after partial remission: an important outcome in depression. Psychol Med 25:1171–1180, 1995

Phillips KA, Najjar F: An open-label study of citalopram in body dysmorphic disorder. J Clin Psychiatry 64:715–720, 2003

Phillips KA, Rasmussen SA: Change in psychosocial functioning and quality of life of patients with body dysmorphic disorder treated with fluoxetine: a placebo-controlled study. Psychosomatics 45:438–444, 2004

Phillips KA, McElroy SL, Keck PE, et al: Body dysmorphic disorder: 30 cases of imagined ugliness. Am J Psychiatry 150:302–308, 1993

Pilowsky I: Abnormal illness behavior. Psychiatr Med 5:85–91, 1987

Pirildar S, Sezgin U, Elbi H, et al: A preliminary open-label study of moclobemide treatment of pain disorder. Psychopharmacol Bull 37:127–134, 2003

Regier DA, Boyd JH, Burke JD, et al: One-month prevalence of mental disorders in the United States based on five Epidemiologic Catchment Area sites. Arch Gen Psychiatry 45:977–986, 1988

Rost KM, Akins RN, Brown FW, et al: The comorbidity of DSM-III-R personality disorders in somatization disorder. Gen Hosp Psychiatry 14:322–326, 1992

Salkovskis PM: Somatic problems, in Cognitive Behaviour Therapy for Psychiatric Problems. Edited by Hawton K, Salkovskis PM, Kirk J, et al. Oxford, England, Oxford University Press, 1989, pp 235–276

Shapiro AP, Teasell RW: Behavioural interventions in the rehabilitation of acute v. chronic non-organic (conversion/factitious) motor disorders. Br J Psychiatry 185:140–146, 2004

Simon GE, VonKorff M: Somatization and psychiatric disorder in the NIMH Epidemiologic Catchment Area study. Am J Psychiatry 148:1494–1500, 1991

Slick DJ, Tan JE, Strauss EH, et al: Detecting malingering: a survey of experts' practices. Arch Clin Neuropsychol 19:465–473, 2004

Smith GR: Somatization Disorder in Medical Settings. Washington, DC, American Psychiatric Press, 1991

Smith GR, Monson RA, Ray DC: Psychiatric consultation in somatization disorder: a randomized controlled study. N Engl J Med 314:1407–1413, 1986

Stone J, Sharpe M, Rothwell PM, et al: The 12-year prognosis of unilateral functional weakness and sensory disturbance. J Neurol Neurosurg Psychiatry 74:591–596, 2003

Toone BK: Disorders of hysterical conversion, in Somatization: Physical Symptoms and Psychological Illness. Edited by Bass C. Oxford, England, Blackwell Scientific, 1990, pp 207–234

Wise MG, Ford CV: Factitious disorders. Prim Care 26:315–326, 1999

Youngblood JR, Lees-Haley PR, Binder LM: Comment: Warning malingerers produces more sophisticated malingering. Arch Clin Neuropsychol 14:511–515, 1999

Zimmerman M, Mattia JI: Body dysmorphic disorder in psychiatric outpatients: recognition, prevalence, comorbidity, demographics, and clinical correlates. Compr Psychiatry 39:265–270, 1998

Additional Readings

Cloninger CR, Martin RL, Guze SB, et al: A prospective follow-up and family study of somatization in men and women. Am J Psychiatry 143:873–878, 1986

Derogatis LR, Lipman RS, Rickels K, et al: The Hopkins Symptom Check List (HSCL): a self-report symptom inventory. Behav Sci 19:1–15, 1974

Eisendrath SJ: Factitious physical disorders: treatment without confrontation. Psychosomatics 30:383–387, 1989

Ewald H, Rogne T, Ewald K, et al: Somatization in patients newly admitted to a neurological department. Acta Psychiatr Scand 89:174–179, 1994

Folks DG, Houck CA: Somatoform disorders, factitious disorders, and malingering, in Psychiatric Care of the Medical Patient. Edited by Stoudemire A, Fogel BS. New York, Oxford University Press, 1993, pp 267–287

Goldberg D, Gask L, O'Dowd T: The treatment of somatization: teaching techniques of reattribution. J Psychosom Res 33:689–695, 1989

Hahn SR, Thompson KS, Wills TA, et al: The difficult doctor-patient relationship: somatization, personality and psychopathology. J Clin Epidemiol 47:647–657, 1994

Lipowski ZJ: Somatization and depression. Psychosomatics 31:13–21, 1990

9

Substance-Related Disorders

Between 25% and 50% of general hospital patients have current alcohol abuse or dependence (Curtis et al. 1989; Gerke et al. 1997). Unfortunately, clinicians underrecognize substance-related disorders. Although psychiatrists positively identify alcohol abuse two-thirds of the time, other physicians recognize and diagnose the disorder only 10% of the time (Moore et al. 1989). Only 22% of the people who develop substance use disorders ever receive any addiction treatment during their lifetime; of these, about half receive treatment from specialty mental health or addiction professionals, and the other half receive treatment from general medical providers (Regier et al. 1993).

Consultation-liaison psychiatrists are in unique positions to identify and intervene in medically ill patients with substance-related disorders. A window of opportunity appears in patients while they are sick; they are often more open to treatment recommendations. Effective treatment or referral of patients who abuse substances requires close collaboration between the consultant and the referring physician. Both must communicate to the patient the medical, psychological, and social consequences of continued alcohol or drug use. Often, the health care team has strong feelings toward the substance-abusing patient. These feelings may need to be addressed in the context of the overall consultation.

DSM-IV-TR Substance-Related Disorders

Substance-related disorders are divided into *substance use disorders and substance-induced disorders*. Substance use disorders include alcohol and drug abuse and dependence. Substance-induced disorders include intoxication, withdrawal, delirium, dementia, amnestic, psychotic, mood, sexual dysfunction, anxiety, and sleep disorders. Table 9–1 summarizes DSM-IV-TR (American Psychiatric Association 2000) criteria for substance dependence and abuse. The loss of control over substance use has both a neurobiological and a behavioral basis that progresses over time as a result of substance-induced changes in the brain. For example, abused substances activate the mesolimbic dopamine system, which reinforces both natural and pharmacological rewards. All substances of abuse act on this system to increase synaptic levels of dopamine (Self 2004). Dopamine release leads to neuronal plasticity, which may underlie incentive learning that contributes to craving in human addictions.

Alcohol-Related Disorders

Alcohol is the most frequently abused substance. Sixty-seven percent of Americans drink, and 14% of men and 4% of women are heavy drinkers (Liskow and Goodwin 1986). Twenty-seven percent of the men and 26% of the women admitted to the hospital are heavy drinkers (Seppa and Makela 1993). Lifetime prevalence for alcohol dependence or abuse is 13%–14%; 1-year prevalence is 6%–7% for adults (American Psychiatric Association 2000). Alcohol-related problems usually begin between ages 16 and 30. Alcoholism runs in families. Children of alcoholic parents have alcoholism four to five times more often than do children of nonalcoholic parents. That this ratio holds even if the children are adopted away is evidence that the familial association is largely hereditary.

An estimated 200,000 deaths per year are alcohol-related (U.S. Department of Health and Human Services 1990). An estimated 25% of general hospital inpatients and 20% of medical outpatients have alcohol-related disorders (Yates 2002). Alcoholism contributes to several medical illnesses. The alcohol-attributable fractions of contribution to developing medical illnesses and events are highest for liver cirrhosis, esophageal cancer, fire injuries, motor vehicle accidents, and suicides (Yates 1999).

Table 9–1.   DSM-IV-TR criteria for substance dependence and abuse

Criteria for Substance Dependence

A maladaptive pattern of substance use, leading to clinically significant impairment or distress, as manifested by three (or more) of the following, occurring at any time in the same 12-month period:

(1) tolerance, as defined by either of the following:

    (a) a need for markedly increased amounts of the substance to achieve intoxication or desired effect

    (b) markedly diminished effect with continued use of the same amount of the substance

(2) withdrawal, as manifested by either of the following:

    (a) the characteristic withdrawal syndrome for the substance (refer to Criteria A and B of the criteria sets for Withdrawal from the specific substances)

    (b) the same (or a closely related) substance is taken to relieve or avoid withdrawal symptoms

(3) the substance is often taken in larger amounts or over a longer period than was intended

(4) there is a persistent desire or unsuccessful efforts to cut down or control substance use

(5) a great deal of time is spent in activities necessary to obtain the substance (e.g., visiting multiple doctors or driving long distances), use the substance (e.g., chain-smoking), or recover from its effects

(6) important social, occupational, or recreational activities are given up or reduced because of substance use

(7) the substance use is continued despite knowledge of having a persistent or recurrent physical or psychological problem that is likely to have been caused or exacerbated by the substance (e.g., current cocaine use despite recognition of cocaine-induced depression, or continued drinking despite recognition that an ulcer was made worse by alcohol consumption)

Specify if:

With Physiological Dependence: evidence of tolerance or withdrawal (i.e., either Item 1 or 2 is present)

Without Physiological Dependence: no evidence of tolerance or withdrawal (i.e., neither Item 1 nor 2 is present)

Course specifiers (see text for definitions):

Early Full Remission, Early Partial Remission, Sustained Full Remission, Sustained Partial Remission, On Agonist Therapy, In a Controlled Environment

Table 9–1.   DSM-IV-TR criteria for substance dependence and abuse *(continued)*

Criteria for Substance Abuse

A.   A maladaptive pattern of substance use leading to clinically significant impairment or distress, as manifested by one (or more) of the following, occurring within a 12-month period:

   (1)   recurrent substance use resulting in a failure to fulfill major role obligations at work, school, or home (e.g., repeated absences or poor work performance related to substance use; substance-related absences, suspensions, or expulsions from school; neglect of children or household)

   (2)   recurrent substance use in situations in which it is physically hazardous (e.g., driving an automobile or operating a machine when impaired by substance use)

   (3)   recurrent substance-related legal problems (e.g., arrests for substance-related disorderly conduct)

   (4)   continued substance use despite having persistent or recurrent social or interpersonal problems caused or exacerbated by the effects of the substance (e.g., arguments with spouse about consequences of intoxication, physical fights)

B.   The symptoms have never met the criteria for Substance Dependence for this class of substance.

Source.   Reprinted from American Psychiatric Association: *Diagnostic and Statistical Manual of Mental Disorders,* 4th Edition, Text Revision. Washington, DC, American Psychiatric Association, 2000. Used with permission.

Alcohol Abuse and Dependence

Screening and Laboratory Tests

Several brief diagnostic screens are available to assist with diagnosis of alcohol abuse and dependence (Soderstrom et al. 1997). One of these diagnostic aids, the CAGE questionnaire, continues to be particularly useful decades after its initial use (Table 9–2) (Ewing 1984). The clinician also should look for chronic anxiety or dysphoria, job loss, financial problems, legal problems, and absenteeism.

Several laboratory tests are highly suggestive, although not diagnostic, of alcohol abuse. Serum γ-glutamyltransferase is increased in more than half of problem drinkers and in 80% of alcoholic patients with liver dysfunction

Table 9–2. CAGE screen for diagnosis of alcoholism

Have you ever

C	Thought you should CUT back on your drinking?
A	Felt ANNOYED by people criticizing your drinking?
G	Felt GUILTY or bad about your drinking?
E	Had a morning EYE-OPENER to relieve hangover or nerves?

Note. 2–3 positive responses=high index of suspicion; four positive responses= pathognomonic.
Source. Reprinted from Ewing JA: "Detecting Alcoholism: The CAGE Questionnaire." *Journal of the American Medical Association* 25:1905–1907, 1984. Copyright 1984, American Medical Association. Used with permission.

(Trell et al. 1984). Aspartate aminotransferase levels are increased in 46% of alcoholic patients. Also common are increased uric acid, increased mean corpuscular volume, decreased white blood cell counts, increased triglycerides, increased alanine aminotransferase, and increased γ-glutamyltranspeptidase). Because alcohol abuse progressively damages many different organs, many laboratory test results become abnormal. A very high blood alcohol level (>200 mg/dL) found on routine clinical examination in a nonintoxicated patient is pathognomonic.

Medical Complications

Medical complications of chronic alcohol abuse include dementia, anemia, pancreatitis, esophageal disorders, cirrhosis, gastritis, insomnia, impotence, peripheral neuropathy, myopathy, cardiomyopathy, and Wernicke-Korsakoff syndrome. Physical examination may identify bruises, rib tenderness due to old or new fractures, spider angiomata, abdominal tenderness, muscle wasting, peripheral neuropathy, abducens nerve deficit, nystagmus, ataxia, and hypertension. Head imaging may show cerebral atrophy and/or subdural hematomas.

Management

It is foolish to recommend drinking in moderation to a medically ill alcoholic patient. After the patient is medically stabilized, the clinician should encourage the patient and family to become involved in community resources, especially Alcoholics Anonymous (AA). Of the patients who seriously commit to AA, 70% improve. Inpatient alcohol rehabilitation, day programs, or intensive outpatient alcohol rehabilitation also should be considered. In patients who have regular follow-up, a history of abstinence that culminates with impulsive drinking, and no hepatic impairment, the clinician should consider disulfiram. The clinician must inform the patient taking disulfiram that many over-the-counter and pharmacological agents contain alcohol. Naltrexone reduces the risk of relapse to heavy drinking (Garbutt et al. 1999). The usual dosage is 50 mg/day. Adverse effects include headache, nausea, and dysphoria.

Alcohol Intoxication

The body metabolizes alcohol at a rate of 100 mg/kg/hour. It takes approximately 1.5 hours to metabolize one shot of whiskey. Unless the person is alcohol-tolerant, blood levels of 30–50 mg/dL will cause mild euphoria; at 100 mg/dL, significant ataxia is present. Disorientation and stupor can occur at 200 mg/dL, and coma and death may occur at 400 mg/dL. Table 9–3 summarizes the salient features of alcohol intoxication and its management.

Management

The behavior associated with intoxication is managed by decreasing external stimuli, interrupting alcohol ingestion, and protecting individuals from harming themselves or others until the toxic effects of alcohol disappear. Unless medically contraindicated, food and/or coffee should be offered. The clinician should obtain a blood alcohol level and screen for other drug use. If the patient is severely agitated, the pharmacological treatments listed in Table 9–3 should be used.

Alcohol Overdose

Unfortunately, the lethal level of alcohol does not increase as tolerance develops (Mebane 1987). The LD_{50} (a lethal dose in 50% of patients) of alcohol is 500 mg/dL. Signs of life-threatening alcohol overdose are nonresponsiveness, slow and shallow breathing, and cardiac dysrhythmia.

Management

The clinician should immediately intubate the patient if he or she has respiratory compromise, hydrate the patient, monitor the patient's cardiac status, and provide other indicated emergency supportive measures. Hemodialysis is an option in potentially life-threatening alcohol overdoses.

Table 9–3.   Substance intoxication and its management

Substance	Signs and symptoms	Management
Alcohol	Alcohol smell, disinhibition, mood lability, impaired judgment, ataxia, dysarthria, nystagmus	If severely agitated, have security present, prevent more ingestion, provide a quiet room, reduce stimuli, offer food and/or coffee, use restraints if needed, sedate with lorazepam (1–2 mg iv/im every hour prn) or haloperidol (1–5 mg iv every half-hour until calm). Administer thiamine (100 mg/day im for 5 days) and folate (1 mg po four times a day).
Sedatives, hypnotics, or anxiolytics	Disinhibition, mood lability, dysarthria, ataxia, hyporeflexia, nystagmus, impaired attention	Observe for respiratory depression. Move to ICU if patient becomes stuporous, hypoxic, or unresponsive. If agitated, give haloperidol (1–5 mg iv/im) or lorazepam (1–2 mg iv/im) if there is no respiratory depression.
Opiates	Apathy, dysphoria or euphoria, psychomotor retardation, drowsiness, dysarthria, pinpoint pupils. If severe, respiratory depression, stupor, coma. Nystagmus is rare.	Observe for respiratory depression, pulmonary edema, seizures. Give naloxone (0.4 mg iv every 3–5 minutes) until symptoms clear; may have to repeat frequently.
Amphetamines and cocaine	Euphoria, heightened self-esteem, grandiosity, suspiciousness, perspiration, miosis, hypertension, tachycardia, nausea, anxiety, restlessness. More severe intoxication leads to hypervigilance, delusions (especially paranoid), hallucinations, psychomotor agitation, delirium, arrhythmias, and convulsions.	Obtain ECG and watch for dysrhythmias. Try to "talk the patient down." Watch for violent and suicidal behavior. Acidify the urine with vitamin C. Give lorazepam (1–3 mg hourly iv/im) to manage agitation and haloperidol (1–5 mg iv/po) for psychotic symptoms.

Note.   iv=intravenously; im=intramuscularly; prn=as needed; po=orally; ECG=electrocardiogram; ICU=intensive care unit.

Alcohol-Induced Psychotic Disorder

Diagnosis of alcohol-induced psychotic disorder is based on a history of recent heavy alcohol use and the absence of schizophrenia or mania. Auditory hallucinations are more prominent than other withdrawal symptoms, last at least 1 week, and occur while the patient has a clear sensorium.

Management

When patients develop alcohol-induced psychotic disorder during detoxification, a potent antipsychotic such as haloperidol, 2–5 mg orally twice a day, is typically needed to control agitation and hallucinations. After symptoms cease, neuroleptics should be discontinued.

Uncomplicated Alcohol Withdrawal

Within 6–48 hours after cessation of or reduction in prolonged alcohol use, withdrawal symptoms may appear (i.e., coarse tremor, nausea, weakness, autonomic hyperactivity, anxiety, irritability, mild transient illusions or hallucinations, insomnia, numbness, and/or paresthesias) (Table 9–4). The tremors typically peak 24–48 hours after the last drink and subside after 5–7 days of abstinence. Vital signs should be monitored during the abstinence syndrome, which is prevented by treatment with benzodiazepines.

Management

The choice of an inpatient or an outpatient setting to manage withdrawal depends on the severity of symptoms, stage of withdrawal, medical and psychiatric complications, presence of polysubstance abuse, patient cooperation, ability to follow instructions, social support systems, patient history, and, increasingly, insurance or managed care reimbursement policies. For outpatient alcohol withdrawal (Franklin et al. 2002), 50 mg of chlordiazepoxide is prescribed orally four times a day for four doses, followed by 25 mg orally for eight doses. Thiamine, 100 mg/day, should be given orally for 5 days. A standard, structured inpatient detoxification regimen is chlordiazepoxide, 50 mg orally every 6 hours for four doses, then 25 mg every 6 hours for eight doses (Franklin et al. 2002). Diazepam is recommended in patients with cross-addiction to other depressants or with a history of seizures. Lorazepam offers advantages in patients with liver disease, although care must be exercised in tapering it; it does not self-taper. Thiamine, 100 mg/day, and folic

Table 9–4. Substance withdrawal syndromes and their management

Substance	Signs and symptoms	Management
Alcohol	Coarse tremor, nausea, weakness, autonomic hyperactivity, anxiety, irritability, mild transient illusions or hallucinations, insomnia, numbness, paresthesias. *DTs:* disorientation, agitation, visual or tactile hallucinations, further autonomic hyperactivity, tremor, ataxia, fever, dilated pupils.	Monitor vital signs. Give thiamine (100 mg/day im for 5 days) and folic acid (1 mg daily for 5 days). Watch for fluid and electrolyte imbalances. Give chlordiazepoxide 50 mg every 6 hours for four doses, then 25 mg every 6 hours for eight doses; or oxazepam (15–45 mg every 4–6 hours); taper over 5–7 days. For psychotic symptoms or agitation, use haloperidol po, im, or iv. Watch for seizures.
Sedatives, hypnotics, or anxiolytics	Nausea, tremor, hyperreflexia, hyperphagia, tachycardia, dilated pupils, diaphoresis, irritability, insomnia, restlessness, anxiety. Seizures and delirium can occur in severe cases. Can be life-threatening.	Taper agent 10% daily. Alternatively, especially if the agent is short-acting (i.e., lorazepam, alprazolam), convert average daily dose to diazepam (or clonazepam). Give that dose for 2 days, then taper by 10% per day, adjusting as necessary for breakthrough withdrawal signs, if any.
Opiates	Rarely life-threatening but uncomfortable: dilated pupils, piloerection, rhinorrhea, fever, yawning, hypertension, tachycardia, cramps, drug craving, insomnia, restlessness, irritability, seizures.	Methadone 20 mg twice daily, supplemented by 5-mg doses up to four times daily for breakthrough signs. Taper total daily dose by 5 mg/day; slower taper in medically ill patients (10%/day).
Amphetamines and cocaine	Depression, irritability, fatigue, anxiety, insomnia or hypersomnia, drug craving, psychomotor agitation, hyperphagia.	Watch for suicidal and drug-seeking behavior. Give desipramine in antidepressant doses for depression and lorazepam (1–2 mg every 2–5 hours po, im, or iv) for severe anxiety or agitation.

Note.   im=intramuscularly; iv=intravenously; po=orally; DTs=delirium tremens.

acid, 1 mg/day for 5 days, should be given to correct nutritional deficiencies. If the patient has very poor nutrition, thiamine should be given intramuscularly or intravenously for 3 days. Fluid and electrolyte imbalances, hypoglycemia, fever, and hypomagnesemia must be monitored and treated.

Alcohol Withdrawal Seizures

Withdrawal seizures typically occur 7–38 hours after last alcohol use, with peak frequency at about 24 hours (Adams and Victor 1981). Hypomagnesemia, respiratory alkalosis, hypoglycemia, increased intracellular sodium, and up-regulation of N-methyl-D-aspartate (NMDA) receptors all potentially contribute to alcohol withdrawal seizures. One-third of patients who have withdrawal seizures go on to develop alcohol withdrawal delirium (delirium tremens [DTs]).

Management

Benzodiazepines are the treatment of choice for alcohol withdrawal seizures, but intramuscular administration should be avoided because of variable absorption (lorazepam is an exception). Diazepam, 2–10 mg intravenously, is a good choice if immediate seizure control is needed. For underlying seizure disorders, phenytoin maintenance is necessary. The most effective way to prevent alcohol withdrawal seizures is to detoxify the patient adequately with appropriate doses of benzodiazepines. Patients who have histories of alcohol withdrawal seizures should receive intramuscular magnesium sulfate, 1 g/2 mL four times daily for 2 days.

Alcohol Withdrawal Delirium (Delirium Tremens)

DTs begin 2–7 days after cessation of drinking. The risk for DTs is highest when the patient has a long history (>10 years) of heavy drinking and a major medical illness, especially liver disease, infection, trauma, poor nutrition, and metabolic disorders. Clinical signs and symptoms of DTs are disorientation, agitation, visual or tactile hallucinations, autonomic hyperactivity, tremor, ataxia, fever, and dilated pupils. Alcohol withdrawal delirium is life-threatening. Up to 40% of patients die if untreated. Fortunately, the mortality rate in hospitalized patients is less than 5% (Yost 1996). When patients die during DTs, the cause of death is usually heart failure, infection, or traumatic injury.

Management

The management of alcohol withdrawal delirium is the same as that for uncomplicated alcohol withdrawal, except more medications are required. The clinician should administer thiamine, reverse fluid and electrolyte imbalances, and correct hypoglycemia, if present. The addition of high-potency neuroleptics, such as haloperidol, is sometimes necessary if benzodiazepines do not adequately control confusion, delusions, hallucinations, or agitation.

Alcohol-Induced Persisting Amnestic Disorder (Wernicke-Korsakoff Syndrome)

Alcohol-induced persisting amnestic disorder (Wernicke-Korsakoff syndrome) begins with an abrupt onset of truncal ataxia, ophthalmoplegia (usually third nerve palsy), and delirium (Wernicke's encephalopathy). Ataxia may precede the mental status change. The clinician should not wait for all three signs; the presence of two suggests the disorder. The etiology of the disorder is thiamine deficiency. Long- and short-term memory impairment (Korsakoff's syndrome) usually develops if Wernicke's encephalopathy is unrecognized and goes untreated. The symptoms and signs are caused by lesions in the medial dorsal nucleus of the thalamus, the hippocampus, and the mammillary bodies. In Korsakoff's syndrome, memory losses are profound, but other cognitive functions are relatively spared.

Management

Patients should be given thiamine, 100 mg/hour intramuscularly or intravenously, with titration upward until ophthalmoplegia has resolved. Then thiamine, 100 mg/day parenterally, is continued for at least 7 days to treat alcohol-induced persisting amnestic disorder. Ocular findings improve first, followed by motor improvement, and, finally, mental status abnormalities resolve. Many patients are left with residual ataxia or confusion.

Sedative-, Hypnotic-, or Anxiolytic-Related Disorders

Abuse of sedative-hypnotics and benzodiazepines is rare in the inpatient setting; it is more common among chronically medically ill outpatients. All sedative-hypnotics and benzodiazepines induce tolerance to some degree. Unfortunately, even though the dose necessary for intoxication increases, the lethal dose does not. Whereas the opiate-dependent patient may double the dose and still not experience respiratory depression, barbiturate-addicted patients can develop potentially fatal respiratory depression with a dose only 20%–25% higher than the usual daily dose. Benzodiazepines have a much higher LD_{50} than barbiturates.

Sedative, Hypnotic, or Anxiolytic Abuse and Dependence

Diagnosis

Barbiturate and benzodiazepine abuse and dependence may develop secondary to street abuse or medical use. Table 9–1 summarizes DSM-IV-TR criteria for abuse and dependence diagnoses. An effective diagnostic aid is a positive "shopping bag sign"; the clinician asks the patient's family to bring in all the patient's medications. Benzodiazepines are frequently present in the bag.

Management

For sedative-hypnotic dependence in medical patients, simplification of medication regimens may be all that is required. If the patient has a positive "shopping bag sign," his or her medication needs should be reassessed and unnecessary medications thrown away. After medically supervised tapering and "dry out," any concurrent psychiatric disorders should be treated. The clinician should watch for drug-seeking behavior among patients and on the patient's behalf by friends and family members.

Sedative, Hypnotic, or Anxiolytic Intoxication

The most common features of intoxication are disinhibition, mood lability, dysarthria, ataxia, hyporeflexia, nystagmus, and impaired attention (see Table 9–3). The symptoms and signs are similar to those of alcohol intoxication. Accidental, iatrogenic, or suicidal overdose may cause respiratory depression. There is cross-reactivity between alcohol, benzodiazepines, and sedative-hypnotics.

Management

Because barbiturate withdrawal is life-threatening, close observation of anyone with barbiturate intoxication is necessary. The patient should be moved to the intensive care unit if stupor, hypoxia, or unresponsiveness occurs. When agitation threatens medical status, low doses of lorazepam (1–2 mg) intravenously or intramuscularly should be administered, and the patient should be observed for respiratory compromise. An alternative is haloperidol, 1–5 mg orally, intramuscularly, or intravenously. In life-threatening overdose situations, the clinician should consider hemodialysis. Benzodiazepine antagonists, such as flumazenil, can reverse coma in some individuals with hepatic coma or benzodiazepine overdose.

Sedative, Hypnotic, or Anxiolytic Withdrawal

The features of sedative, hypnotic, or anxiolytic withdrawal are similar to those of alcohol withdrawal; the time of onset and duration of sedative-hypnotic withdrawal vary with the half-life of the drugs (see Chapter 7, "Anxiety and Insomnia," in this volume). The most common withdrawal features are hyperreflexia, nausea, tremulousness, tachycardia, dilated pupils, diaphoresis, irritability, insomnia, restlessness, and anxiety (see Table 9–4). Seizures and delirium occur in severe cases. Like alcohol withdrawal, sedative-hypnotic withdrawal is potentially life-threatening. Withdrawal is sometimes missed in hospitalized patients because of a low index of suspicion or because symptoms can occur 7–10 days after admission. Changes in mental status in a hospitalized elderly patient taking many medications should alert the clinician to the possibility of sedative-hypnotic withdrawal, especially if accompanied by fever, autonomic hyperactivity, seizures, insomnia, or tremor.

Management

Because of potential medical complications during detoxification, especially among high-dose abusers, inpatient treatment is preferred. The clinician can construct a withdrawal regimen with the same medication the patient is taking. If, however, the drug's half-life is too short to permit comfortable tapering, as is sometimes the case with lorazepam or alprazolam, longer-acting agents should be used. For benzodiazepine detoxification, the patient's average daily dose should be converted into an equivalent diazepam dosage and administered for 2 days. The diazepam dosage then should be decreased 10% per day thereafter, adjusting for breakthrough withdrawal signs if they appear (Franklin et al. 2002).

Sedative-, Hypnotic-, or Anxiolytic-Induced Persisting Amnestic Disorder

Long- and short-term memory impairment may occur after prolonged and heavy use of a sedative-hypnotic agent. The clinical findings are equivalent to those of Korsakoff's syndrome.

Management

The sedative-, hypnotic-, or anxiolytic-induced amnestic disorder usually gradually reverses. The clinician should attend to nutritional needs.

Opioid (Narcotic)–Related Disorders

Narcotics are used to relieve pain, cough, diarrhea, agitation, and severe anxiety in the intensive care unit. Unfortunately, tolerance begins within days, so narcotics' potential effectiveness in long-term treatment is limited. Psychiatrists are frequently consulted to examine patients in pain who do not respond to an "adequate" narcotic regimen or to evaluate a patient's "overuse" of narcotics. In the course of such consultations, underuse rather than abuse of narcotic analgesics is often found.

It is sometimes difficult to determine whether a patient has crossed the line between "appropriate" and "excessive" use of narcotics. At least 19% of patients who have chronic pain syndromes use opiates chronically, and 27% of them meet three or more abuse criteria (Chabal et al. 1997). A careful examination includes psychiatric history, family psychiatric history, personality style, pattern of medical resources use, and physical and laboratory examination. More than 90% of opiate-addicted patients have at least one other diagnosable psychiatric disorder—most commonly, depression, alcoholism, or antisocial personality disorder (Khantzian and Treece 1985).

Psychiatric effects such as euphoria, paranoia, psychomotor agitation, and sedation can occur because an opiate receptor site is occupied. There are several subtypes of opioid receptors (i.e., mu, delta, kappa, iota, and epsilon). Opiates that occupy different receptor types have little cross-tolerance. The mu receptor mediates analgesia, euphoria, sedation, meiosis, and respiratory depression (Kosten et al. 1990) and has selective affinity for heroin, meperidine, hydromorphone, and methadone. The mu receptor is also sensitive to the opioid antagonist naloxone. Neuroadaptive changes at receptor sites are hypothesized to produce dependence and tolerance, especially tolerance to respiratory depression (Franklin et al. 2002). Once neuroadaptation occurs, removal of the opioid from receptors produces withdrawal symptoms.

Opioid Abuse and Dependence

Diagnosis and Symptoms

The DSM-IV-TR criteria for substance dependence and abuse are presented in Table 9–1. Table 9–3 and 9–4 summarize signs of clinical toxicity and withdrawal to watch for.

Management

After medical stabilization and drug detoxification, the patient should be referred for treatment. Both inpatient and outpatient treatment programs are available. In general, success and retention rates of methadone programs exceed those of programs that require abstinence.

Opioid Intoxication

Cardinal features of opioid intoxication include apathy, dysphoria or euphoria, psychomotor retardation, drowsiness, dysarthria, impaired attention, and pinpoint pupils; with more severe toxic states, respiratory depression, stupor, or coma can occur (see Table 9–3). Pupils are pinpoint unless respiratory depression or meperidine caused dilation. Clinicians should suspect an opiate overdose in any patient who presents in a coma, especially when associated with respiratory depression, pupillary constriction, and/or the presence of needle marks.

Management

The clinician should observe patients for respiratory depression, pulmonary edema, and seizures. In a comatose patient suspected of opiate overdose, 0.4 mg of naloxone should be given immediately and repeated every 3–5 minutes until symptoms clear significantly. Naloxone is administered repeatedly because of its short duration of action relative to the opiate.

Opioid Withdrawal

Narcotic or opioid withdrawal is uncomfortable but not life-threatening; opiate overdose, alcohol withdrawal, barbiturate overdose, and barbiturate withdrawal are potentially life-threatening. The course and presentation of symptoms for opioid withdrawal vary with the half-life of the agent and hepatic status. Classic features include pupillary dilation, yawning, piloerection, rhinorrhea, nausea, fever, hypertension, tachycardia, cramps, drug craving, insomnia, restlessness, irritability, and seizures (see Table 9–4). Untreated symptoms can last 2–3 weeks.

Management

Methadone is an excellent treatment for withdrawal because of its long half-life (24–36 hours). In opioid-dependent patients hospitalized on a general medical unit, methadone is started at 30–40 mg/day in divided doses. According to signs of breakthrough withdrawal, 5 mg may be added two to four times a day. The amount given the first day is divided into two doses on the second day and then tapered by 5 mg/day. Methadone is tapered more slowly in medically ill patients. Clinicians must observe patients closely for oversedation or undertreatment. An average daily maintenance dose is 60–80 mg; 80–120 mg is occasionally needed.

Because of meperidine's short duration of action, use of methadone for detoxification is sometimes too difficult; slow tapering of meperidine itself is often necessary. Clonidine also can be used for opioid withdrawal, alone or in combination with naltrexone.

Amphetamine-Related Disorders

Amphetamines block the reuptake of dopamine, serotonin, and norepinephrine and profoundly affect dopamine storage release. Amphetamines are especially abused by night workers, students, dieters, persons who work long hours, and persons who are chronically dysphoric. Legitimate medical uses of amphetamines include treatment of depression, attention-deficit/hyperactivity disorder, and narcolepsy; doses range from 5 to 25 mg/day. On the street, daily doses reach 100 mg or more. Higher doses can cause psychosis or delirium. Repeated use leads to postintoxication depression, which can perpetuate further abuse.

Amphetamine Abuse and Dependence

Diagnosis

Table 9–1 summarizes the DSM-IV-TR criteria for substance dependence and abuse. The clinician should obtain a toxicology screen because polydrug abuse is common. Poor nutrition may lead to anemia.

Management

The patient must discontinue amphetamine use. If postamphetamine depression occurs, the clinician should consider antidepressants and psychiatric hospitalization. Individuals who abuse amphetamines daily or intravenously require inpatient hospitalization to treat aggression, psychosis, depression, and suicidal ideation during withdrawal.

Amphetamine Intoxication

Symptoms and signs of mild amphetamine intoxication include euphoria, heightened self-esteem, grandiosity, suspiciousness, miosis, tachycardia, nausea, perspiration, hypertension, and anxiety (see Table 9–3). More severe intoxication leads to hypervigilance, paranoia, psychomotor agitation, delirium, arrhythmias, and convulsions.

Management

Amphetamine-intoxicated patients should be "talked down." The clinician should watch for hypertension, hyperpyrexia, seizures, violence, and suicidal ideation. Urine should be tested for concurrent drug use. Benzodiazepines, such as lorazepam (1–3 mg hourly), should be used to treat severe anxiety or agitation and to help prevent seizures in patients with a seizure history. In an amphetamine overdose, the urine should be acidified with vitamin C to speed elimination. Paranoid or delusional symptoms are treated with antipsychotic medications, such as haloperidol.

Amphetamine Intoxication Delirium

An agitated confusional state may develop within 24 hours of amphetamine use. Hallucinations, delusions, and signs of autonomic hyperactivity are frequently present.

Management

Haloperidol, 2–10 mg every half-hour, should be administered as needed for agitation and psychosis. The clinician must watch for violence and hyperpyrexia, obtain a toxicology screen to rule out other drug use, and acidify the urine to enhance excretion.

Amphetamine-Induced Psychotic Disorder, With Delusions

Amphetamines can induce paranoia that can last several days in a patient with a clear sensorium. Amphetamine psychosis resembles acute paranoid schizophrenia.

Management

Haloperidol, 2–10 mg every half-hour, should be administered. The clinician should obtain a toxicology screen to rule out other drug use and acidify the urine to enhance excretion.

Amphetamine Withdrawal

When amphetamines are abruptly discontinued, several treatable postintoxication findings can occur, including depression (especially if the patient is at risk for depression already), irritability, anxiety, fatigue, insomnia or hypersomnia, psychomotor agitation, and hyperphagia (see Table 9–4).

Management

The drug should not be restarted; postintoxication symptoms are usually self-limited or treatable. Benzodiazepines (lorazepam or diazepam) should be given as needed for severe anxiety or agitation. Neuroleptics are occasionally required if agitation is accompanied by psychosis or delirium. The clinician must observe the patient carefully for postwithdrawal depression. If depression appears, the patient may need antidepressant medications or a transfer to the psychiatry unit.

Cocaine-Related Disorders

Cocaine blocks the reuptake of neuronal dopamine, serotonin, and norepinephrine. Cocaine has a fairly specific activating effect on mesocortical and mesolimbic dopaminergic pathways. Dopamine is an important neurotransmitter in limbic pleasure centers, including those related to food and sexual activity. A patient's inability to control cocaine intake is probably related to the highly rewarding properties of the drug. With repeated cocaine use, tolerance develops secondary to decreased reuptake inhibition and altered receptor sensitivity. Cocaine also causes cortical kindling (Halikas et al. 1991). *Kindling* is the process by which brief bursts of central nervous system stimulation at regular intervals and constant intensity result in lasting changes in brain excitability. Limbic areas of the brain are uniquely sensitive to kindling and its neuropsychiatric consequences.

Cocaine Abuse and Dependence

Diagnosis

Table 9–1 summarizes the DSM-IV-TR diagnostic criteria for substance dependence and abuse. The chronic cocaine user may have severe financial problems because of the large amounts of the drug needed (often several times hourly) to stave off the cocaine "crash."

Management

When a patient who abuses cocaine is admitted to the hospital, the staff should watch for drug-seeking behavior, depression, suicidal behavior, and insomnia. A toxicology screen can help make the diagnosis and rule out potential contributions by other drugs of abuse. Periodic toxicology screens are often needed. After the patient is medically stabilized, he or she should be referred for treatment. Inpatient drug rehabilitation is indicated when outpatient treatment has failed, when the patient is unmotivated, when concurrent psychiatric illness is present, or when a complicating psychosocial situation exists.

Cocaine Intoxication

Features of cocaine intoxication vary but may include euphoria, grandiosity, hypervigilance, increased libido, psychomotor agitation, tachycardia, miosis, hypertension, perspiration, nausea, delirium, and hallucinations (see Table 9–3). Sudden death has been reported with acute cocaine intoxication; death usually is the result of cardiac arrest or ventricular fibrillation. Cocaine binges can last a few hours to several days. Tolerance to the euphoric effects develops rapidly during the course of a binge.

Management

Agitation and anxiety associated with cocaine intoxication are treated with diazepam or lorazepam. Reassurance and the constant presence of family or friends are frequently enough to help the patient get through the acute phase. The clinician should observe the patient for suicidality, arrhythmias, and psychotic symptoms. Because cocaine is rapidly metabolized, symptoms of acute intoxication usually clear within hours. Life-threatening levels decline quickly, so airway support and cardiac monitoring are required for only a few hours. Prolonged cocaine use is usually followed by a severe dysphoric syndrome ("crash"), which, if persistent, may require antidepressant medication or a transfer to the psychiatry ward.

Cocaine Intoxication Delirium

An agitated confusional state may appear within 24 hours of cocaine use.

Management

The clinician should obtain a toxicology screen immediately. Cocaine intoxication delirium usually disappears rapidly as the serum level decreases. Violence is common, so restraints should be ready (both physical and chemical—lorazepam or haloperidol, 1–4 mg intravenously, intramuscularly, or orally as needed). The patient must be watched for seizures.

Cocaine-Induced Psychotic Disorder, With Delusions

Paranoid delusions can appear shortly after cocaine use. Unlike the confusional state, psychosis is often prolonged, lasting weeks or months in an occasional patient.

Management

Cocaine delusional disorder requires neuroleptics (haloperidol, 1–5 mg intravenously, intramuscularly, or orally, every 6 hours). Psychiatric hospitalization is often required. The clinician should obtain a toxicology screen and watch for seizures.

Cocaine Withdrawal

Although abrupt discontinuation of cocaine is medically safe, postintoxication sequelae can occur after prolonged use. For most patients, the worst dysphoria and craving occur in the first day of abstinence. However, profound dysphoria may last 2 weeks or longer. It is typically accompanied by strong drug craving and insomnia (see Table 9–4). After several weeks of improvement, a second period of craving and depression may occur, which resolves slowly over weeks to months (Gawin and Kleber 1986). Episodic craving, often triggered in response to environmental stimuli, can continue indefinitely.

Management

Persistent depression that meets criteria for major depressive episode should be treated pharmacologically. Gawin et al. (1989) conducted a double-blind, random-assignment, 6-week comparison of desipramine and placebo in outpatient cocaine abusers. Cocaine craving and use were significantly reduced in the group given desipramine (40% relapse to cocaine use after 6 weeks, compared with 80% relapse among placebo recipients). The consultant should make the patient and hospital staff aware of the phases of abstinence and watch for suicidal and drug-seeking behavior.

References

Adams RD, Victor M: Principles of Neurology. New York, McGraw-Hill, 1981

American Psychiatric Association: Diagnostic and Statistical Manual of Mental Disorders, 4th Edition, Text Revision. Washington, DC, American Psychiatric Association, 2000

Chabal C, Erjavec MK, Jacobson L, et al: Prescription opiate abuse in chronic pain patients: clinical criteria, incidence and predictors. Clin J Pain 13:150–155, 1997

Curtis JR, Geller G, Stokes EG, et al: Characteristics, diagnosis, and treatment of alcoholism in elderly patients. J Am Geriatr Soc 37:310–316, 1989

Ewing J: Detecting alcoholism: the CAGE questionnaire. JAMA 25:1905–1907, 1984

Franklin JE Jr, Leamon MH, Frances RJ: Substance-related disorders, in The American Psychiatric Publishing Textbook of Consultation-Liaison Psychiatry: Psychiatry in the Medically Ill, 2nd Edition. Edited by Wise MG, Rundell JR. Washington, DC, American Psychiatric Publishing, 2002, pp 417–453

Garbutt JC, West SL, Carey TS, et al: Pharmacological treatment of alcohol dependence: a review of the evidence. JAMA 281:1318–1325, 1999

Gawin FH, Kleber HD: Abstinence symptomatology and psychiatric diagnosis in cocaine abusers. Arch Gen Psychiatry 43:107–113, 1986

Gawin FH, Kleber H, Buck R, et al: Desipramine facilitation of initial cocaine abstinence. Arch Gen Psychiatry 46:117–121, 1989

Gerke P, Hapke U, Rumpf HJ, et al: Alcohol-related diseases in general hospital patients. Alcohol Alcohol 32:179–184, 1997

Halikas JA, Crosby RD, Carlson GA, et al: Cocaine reduction in unmotivated crack users using carbamazepine versus placebo in a short term, double-blind crossover design. Clin Pharmacol Ther 50:81–95, 1991

Khantzian IF, Treece C: DSM-III psychiatric diagnoses of narcotic addicts. Arch Gen Psychiatry 42:1067–1071, 1985

Kosten TR, Gawin FH, Morgan C: Evidence for altered desipramine disposition in methadone-maintained patients treated for cocaine abuse. Am J Drug Alcohol Abuse 16:329–336, 1990

Liskow B, Goodwin DW: Alcoholism, in The Medical Basis of Psychiatry. Edited by Winokur G, Clayton PJ. Philadelphia, PA, WB Saunders, 1986, pp 190–211

Mebane AH: Drug abuse issues in critically ill patients, in Problems in Critical Care. Edited by Wise MG. Philadelphia, PA, JB Lippincott, 1987, pp 623–685

Moore RD, Bone LR, Geller G, et al: Prevalence, detection and treatment of alcoholism in hospitalized patients. JAMA 261:403–407, 1989

Regier DA, Narrow WE, Rae DS, et al: The de facto US mental and addictive disorders service system: Epidemiologic Catchment Area prospective 1-year prevalence rates of disorders and services. Arch Gen Psychiatry 50:85–94, 1993

Self D: Drug dependence and addiction: neural substrates. Am J Psychiatry 161:223, 2004

Seppa K, Makela R: Heavy drinking in hospital patients. Addiction 88:1377–1382, 1993

Soderstrom CA, Smith GS, Kufera JA, et al: The accuracy of the CAGE, the Brief Michigan Alcoholism Screening Test, and the Alcohol Use Disorder Identification Test in screening trauma center patients for alcoholism. J Trauma 43:962–969, 1997

Trell E, Kristenson H, Fex G: Alcohol-related problems in middle-aged men with elevated serum gamma-glutamyltransferase: a preventive medical investigation. J Stud Alcohol 45:301–309, 1984

U.S. Department of Health and Human Services: The Health Consequences of Alcohol Use: A Report of the Surgeon General (DHHS Publ No CDC-88-8406). Washington, DC, U.S. Dept of Health and Human Services, 1990

Yates WR: Epidemiology of psychiatric disorders in the medically ill, in Psychiatric Treatment of the Medically Ill. Edited by Robinson RG, Yates WR. New York, Marcel Dekker, 1999, pp 41–64

Yates WR: Epidemiology of psychiatric disorders in medically ill patients, in The American Psychiatric Publishing Textbook of Consultation-Liaison Psychiatry: Psychiatry in the Medically Ill, 2nd Edition. Edited by Wise MG, Rundell JR. Washington, DC, American Psychiatric Publishing, 2002, pp 237–256

Yost DA: Alcohol withdrawal syndrome. Am Fam Physician 54:657–664, 1996

Additional Readings

Allen JP, Litten RZ, Fertig JB, et al: Carbohydrate-deficient transferrin: an aid to early recognition of alcohol relapse. Am J Addict 10 (suppl):24–28, 2001

Brouette T, Anton R: Clinical review of inhalants. Am J Addict 10:79–94, 2001

Burgess C, O'Donohoe A, Gill M: Agony and ecstasy: a review of MDMA effects and toxicity. Eur Psychiatry 15:287–294, 2000

Center for Substance Abuse Treatment: CSAT TIPs (Web page). Available at: http://www.treatment.org/Externals/tips.html. Accessed January 5, 2001

Daley DC, Salloum IM, Zuckoff A, et al: Increasing treatment adherence among outpatients with depression and cocaine dependence: results of a pilot study. Am J Psychiatry 155:1611–1613, 1998

Gastfriend DR, Renner JA, Hackett TP: Alcoholic patients—acute and chronic, in Massachusetts General Hospital Handbook of General Hospital Psychiatry, 5th Edition. Edited by Stern TL, Fricchione GL, Cassem NH, et al. St. Louis, MO, Mosby, 2004, pp 203–216

McClellan AT, Lewis DC, O'Brien CP, et al: Drug dependence, a chronic medical illness: implications for treatment, insurance, and outcomes evaluation. JAMA 284:1689–1695, 2000

Palmistierna T: A model for predicting alcohol withdrawal delirium. Psychiatr Serv 52:820–823, 2001

Renner JA, Gastfriend DR: Drug-addicted patients, in Massachusetts General Hospital Handbook of General Hospital Psychiatry, 5th Edition. Edited by Stern TL, Fricchione GL, Cassem NH, et al. St. Louis, MO, Mosby, 2004, pp 217–229

10

Important
Pharmacological Issues

Amedically ill patient almost always receives medications. The patient's well-being is already threatened by the medical illness, and the patient's health should not be further compromised by medication-related adverse events. Therefore, it is essential that the psychiatrist performing consultations in medically ill patients understand the pharmacological issues discussed in this chapter. (For a more detailed discussion of psychopharmacology in the medically ill, see Fait et al. 2002.)

Diagnosis or, sometimes, specific symptoms provide a consultant with the rationale for the use of medications. After a diagnosis is made, baseline symptoms are documented, and target symptoms are identified, the clinician has the basis for evaluating the patient's response to medication and side effects. A symptom rating scale helps to quantify a patient's response. If a response does not occur, document changes in the patient's symptoms and symptom severity, as well as potential side effects.

Adherence to Pharmacological Treatment

Forming an alliance with the patient during consultation and follow-up is fundamental to achieving the best possible outcome but is often difficult. The patient has beliefs about "psychiatric" medications that must be explored and clarified. Most patients are also affected by feelings of failure about needing a "chemical crutch," fear of addiction, magical hopes for cure, and transference feelings toward the physician.

Patients benefit from education about the medication. An integral part of this process includes a realistic discussion of potential adverse reactions, how to take the medication properly, expected time until response, and what to do if a dose is missed. Lin et al. (2003) found that such discussions improved the patient's attitude toward medication, increased confidence that side effects can be managed, and improved adherence. A discussion that includes the patient as a partner facilitates formation of the doctor-patient alliance. The consultant should always obtain and document informed consent. Clinicians can use these principles to improve patient care and adherence (see Table 10–1).

Drug Actions

Drug Absorption

Absorption rates differ among administration routes, although absorption from different forms of oral medications (capsule, pill, liquid) is generally similar (Fait et al. 2002). Parenteral administration generally results in more rapid effects, although the erratic absorption of some medications given intramuscularly, such as diazepam, makes their clinical benefits less predictable. Gastric absorption increases when the stomach is empty, and emptying into the jejunum is more rapid. Aluminum or magnesium antacids can impair absorption and clinical efficacy of psychotropic medications. Cholestyramine, an exchange resin used to decrease cholesterol, can significantly impair absorption of several drugs (e.g., doxepin), even when the medications are ingested many hours apart (Geeze and Wise 1988). Intestinal absorption of most drugs is not altered in the elderly (Turnheim 2003).

Table 10–1. Medication principles in the psychosomatic medicine setting

Review all medications the patient is taking, including herbal and over-the-counter medications.

Keep the medication regimen simple. Whenever possible, use only one medication to treat a symptom or disorder.

Educate the patient about the medication. A therapeutic alliance is your best guarantee of adherence.

Monitor target symptoms and side effects closely when starting a medication.

Remember that discontinuing a medication is often a valuable intervention, especially when an elderly patient is taking multiple medications.

Avoid prescribing medications on an as-needed basis, particularly in patients with pain, withdrawal syndromes, and delirium.

When as-needed medication dosing is required, monitor frequency of use to determine a standing dosage.

Change one medication at a time, and use the minimum dose necessary to obtain the desired response.

Treat prophylactically if a clear rationale exists (e.g., can give benztropine to avoid a dystonic reaction from neuroleptics in an anxious young man with first-break psychosis).

Use a medication that was previously effective for the patient or a family member who had the same disorder.

If treatment fails, reexamine your diagnosis. Always reconsider the possibility of occult substance abuse.

Note that serum drug levels are not a certification of efficacy or toxicity.

Be aware that generic drugs are cost-effective, but bioavailability can vary.

Recognize that social and characterological issues strongly influence treatment acceptance and adherence.

Remember that each patient is unique.

Source. Adapted from Fait ML, Wise MG, Jachna JS, et al.: "Psychopharmacology," in *The American Psychiatric Publishing Textbook of Consultation-Liaison Psychiatry: Psychiatry in the Medically Ill,* 2nd Edition. Edited by Wise MG, Rundell JR. Washington, DC, American Psychiatric Publishing, 2002, pp. 939–987. Copyright 2002, American Psychiatric Publishing. Used with permission.

Drug Distribution

With the exception of lithium, psychotropic medications are lipophilic and drawn to fatty tissues. Thus, psychotropic medications generally have large volumes of distribution. With aging, the water content of the body decreases and the fat content rises, so the distribution volume of hydrophilic compounds is reduced in the elderly, whereas that of lipophilic drugs is increased. In addition, most psychiatric medications are bound to plasma proteins, such as albumin and glycoprotein. When medication is bound to proteins, it is not available for biological activity, such as occupying receptors in the brain (Fait et al. 2002). Protein binding also complicates removal of toxic levels of medications (e.g., by dialysis). With aging and chronic medical illness, albumin levels decrease, and the proportion of unbound (free) drug generally increases. Some medications compete with psychotropic medications for protein binding. For example, warfarin is greater than 90% plasma protein bound. If the patient taking warfarin is then prescribed chloral hydrate for insomnia, a metabolite of chloral hydrate (trichloroacetic acid) may displace warfarin from plasma proteins (Csernansky and Whiteford 1987). This can increase the amount of active anticoagulant severalfold and place the patient at risk for complications, including death.

Drug Receptors

Receptors are the site of action for medications in the central nervous system (CNS) and elsewhere. A medication's receptor activity can be modified in several ways: 1) competitive inhibition, 2) alteration of the receptor, or 3) activation of multiple receptor sites by several drugs. The latter activation may produce side, additive, or opposite effects.

Competitive Inhibition

A patient who develops a severe hypotensive reaction to chlorpromazine is given epinephrine. The epinephrine, which normally stimulates both α-adrenergic and β-adrenergic receptors, cannot stimulate the α-adrenergic receptor because it is blocked by chlorpromazine. As a result, epinephrine's unopposed β-adrenergic stimulation further lowers blood pressure. Competitive inhibition can also produce a desired response, such as the administration of naloxone hydrochloride to reverse the effects of an opioid overdose.

Alteration of the Receptor

Alteration of the receptor by a neuromodulator may influence drug efficacy. Thyroid medication (particularly triiodothyronine) or lithium in some patients appears to increase the effectiveness of antidepressant medication. In addition, continued stimulation of a receptor by an agonist generally results in downregulation, such that subsequent exposure to the same agonist has a diminished effect.

Activation of Multiple Receptor Sites

Activation of multiple receptor sites by one or several medications can produce unwanted side effects, additive effects (e.g., CNS depression), unpredictable effects, or opposite effects. The effect of multiple drugs on receptors is often integrated through second messenger pathways (Gilman et al. 1990).

Drug Metabolism

Absorbed drugs first pass through the liver before entering the systemic circulation ("first-pass effect"). Liver enzymes act on these drugs; the metabolites produced are inactive or active psychopharmacological compounds. Once in the liver, a medication, whether on a first or a subsequent pass, is exposed to two main groups of metabolizing enzymes. The oxidative process occurs via the monooxygenase or cytochrome P450 (CYP) enzyme system. Conjugation is usually the second catabolic enzymatic process; the medication or its metabolites are coupled with other compounds to form more easily excreted (i.e., more hydrophilic) compounds. The metabolism rate, especially the oxidative process, is affected by many factors and disease states, which are discussed later in this chapter.

Cytochrome P450 System

The hepatic CYP enzyme system (vesicles containing the enzymes have a great deal of red pigment, whose wavelength happens to be 450 nm) evolved to eliminate toxic substances from the body. The P450 system did not evolve to metabolize medications; it just happens to do so. This helps explain why different ethnic groups and individuals metabolize the same medication at different rates (i.e., have widely different blood levels after an identical dose).

Four CYP enzymes are especially important in the oxidative metabolism of medications: CYP1A2, CYP2C (2C9/2C19), CYP2D6, and CYP3A3/4.

These enzymes are subject to inhibition, genetic variation, and, in some cases, induction. Table 10–2 lists some of the more common interactions among these enzymes and medications. Medications are often metabolized by a particular enzyme, can compete for metabolism with other substrates, or can inhibit an enzyme without being metabolized by it. Hepatic enzyme inhibition slows metabolism (i.e., increases the half-life and AUC [area under the curve]) and increases the concentration and potential toxicity of psychotropic and other drugs affected. In general, paroxetine is greater than fluoxetine, which is greater than sertraline, at inhibiting the 2D6 isoenzyme, whereas fluvoxamine strongly inhibits 1A2 activity. Among the selective serotonin reuptake inhibitors (SSRIs), citalopram appears to have no significant effects on the CYP system. Hepatic enzyme induction can decrease the efficacy of a medication because it increases metabolism (i.e., decreases the half-life and AUC).

Some consultation psychiatrists advocate the use of sertraline or citalopram for most psychosomatic medicine patients; however, dual-action (serotonin-norepinephrine reuptake inhibitors [SNRIs]) and noradrenergic antidepressants may be particularly important in treating chronic pain and painful physical symptoms (Greco et al. 2004; Jones et al. 2005; Max et al. 1992). The former medications are associated with fewer drug–drug interactions attributable to hepatic enzyme inhibition; drug interactions are important in the hospital setting, where the average inpatient takes eight medications (Adson et al. 1998).

Drug Elimination

A medication and its metabolites are usually excreted by the kidneys, as well as into the bile or feces. Small amounts are also lost through sweat, saliva, or tears. Drug excretion via the kidneys declines with age; therefore, elderly patients should be treated as having renal insufficiency (Turnheim 2003). Water-soluble drugs (e.g., lithium) are readily excreted by the kidneys. Biological or elimination half-life measures the amount of time needed to excrete half of the medication from the body. This is usually expressed as plasma half-life, which is how long it takes to remove half of the medication from plasma. Frequency of drug administration is estimated by the length of its half-life. A steady-state drug level is generally achieved after four to five half-lives of a drug; at this point, more stable serum medication levels are obtained. Plasma half-life does not necessarily reflect biological activity in the brain.

Table 10–2.   Cytochrome P450 (CYP)–drug interactions[a]

	Substrates	Inhibitors	Inducers
CYP1A2			
Psychotropic	Caffeine Clozapine Duloxetine Haloperidol Olanzapine Propranolol Tertiary TCAs (amitriptyline, imipramine)	Fluvoxamine	Cigarettes Caffeine Modafinil (?)
Nonpsychotropic	Phenacetin Theophylline Verapamil Warfarin	Ciprofloxacin Grapefruit juice Tacrine	Cabbage Charbroiled food Omeprazole Rifampin
CYP2C (2C9/2C19)			
Psychotropic	Barbiturates Diazepam Propranolol Tertiary TCAs	Fluoxetine Fluvoxamine Modafinil (?) Serraline (?)	St. John's wort
Nonpsychotropic	NSAIDs Phenytoin Tolbutamide Warfarin		Phenobarbital Phenytoin

Table 10–2. Cytochrome P450 (CYP)–drug interactions[a] *(continued)*

	Substrates	Inhibitors	Inducers
CYP2D6			
Psychotropic	Clozapine	Duloxetine	Not induced
	Duloxetine	Fluoxetine	
	Haloperidol[b]	Fluphenazine	
	Olanzapine	Fluvoxamine	
	Paroxetine	Methylphenidate[d]	
	Phenothiazines[c]	Norfluoxetine	
	Risperidone	Paroxetine	
	Secondary TCAs (nortriptyline,	Phenothiazines[c]	
	desipramine)	Sertraline	
	Venlafaxine	TCAs	
Nonpsychotropic	β-Blockers	Cimetidine	
	Codeine → morphine	Quinidine[e]	
	Type 1C antiarrhythmics (flecainide,		
	propafenone)		
CYP3A3/4			
Psychotropic	Alprazolam	Fluoxetine	Carbamazepine
	Carbamazepine	Fluvoxamine	Modafinil
	Clozapine	Nefazodone	St. John's wort
	Midazolam	Norfluoxetine	
	Nefazodone	Sertraline	
	Pimozide		

Table 10–2. Cytochrome P450 (CYP)–drug interactions[a] *(continued)*

	Substrates	Inhibitors	Inducers
CYP3A3/4 *(continued)*			
Psychotropic *(continued)*	Quetiapine	Cimetidine	Dexamethasone
	Serraline	Cyclosporine	Phenobarbital
	Tertiary TCAs	Diltiazem	Phenytoin
	Triazolam	Erythromycin[c]	Primidone
	Venlafaxine	Fluconazole	Rifabutin
	Ziprasidone	Grapefruit juice	Rifampin
		Itraconazole[c]	
		Ketoconazole[c]	
Nonpsychotropic	Anticancer drugs	Miconazole	
	Astemizole	Protease inhibitors	
	Calcium channel blockers		
	Cisapride		
	Cyclosporine		
	Erythromycin		
	Lidocaine		
	Quinidine		
	Steroids		

Note. Tricyclic antidepressants (TCAs) are metabolized by CYP2D6, CYP3A, CYP2C, and CYP1A2. (?) = incomplete or inconsistent data; NSAIDs = nonsteroidal anti-inflammatory drugs.
[a]Includes both in vivo and in vitro data. [b]Complex interaction. [c]Phenothiazines include chlorpromazine, prochlorperazine, perphenazine, trifluoperazine, fluphenazine, thioridazine, and mesoridazine. [d]Methylphenidate likely has CYP effects, but particular isoenzymes have not been identified. [e]Extraordinarily powerful inhibitors of CYP enzymes, sometimes referred to as "killers."
Source. Data compiled by M.G. Wise, J.R. Rundell, and L. Ereshefsky.

Lithium Clearance

Administration of a medication that inhibits the synthesis of renal prostaglandins, such as nonsteroidal anti-inflammatory drugs, can impair renal clearance of lithium. Thus, lithium clearance is decreased by indomethacin, ibuprofen, diclofenac, piroxicam, and phenylbutazone. Renal disease also can impair lithium clearance.

Renal Failure

The adjustment of psychotropic medications in patients with renal failure is not too cumbersome because almost all psychotropics and their active metabolites are eliminated by hepatic metabolism (Bennett et al. 1999). Lithium is the exception. The lithium dose should be decreased to 50%–75% of normal for a glomerular filtration rate (GFR) of 10–50 mL/min and 25%–50% of normal for a GFR less than 10 mL/min. Most antidepressants do not require dosage adjustment as GFR declines. The dosage of the longer-acting benzodiazepines, such as diazepam, chlordiazepoxide, and flurazepam, may need to be lowered by up to 50% in patients with a GFR of less than 10 mL/min. Avoid the use of chloral hydrate, nomifensine, and ethchlorvynol in patients with renal failure.

Drug Interactions

Drugs Being Taken by the Patient

Recognizing drug interactions is a crucial part of consultation work (Tables 10–2 and 10–3). Table 10–3 lists the most important clinical interactions involving psychotropic medications (Malone et al. 2004). The effect of one drug on another can be *pharmacokinetic* (i.e., affecting the absorption, distribution, biotransformation, and excretion of the other drug) or *pharmacodynamic* (i.e., changing the effect of the drug at its point of action) (Fait et al. 2002).

The clinician should obtain a complete medication list, including medications recently discontinued, over-the-counter medications used, and herbal or other alternative drug preparations used, from the patient or from the patient's chart if he or she is hospitalized. The clinician should also ask a family member to bring in all medications from the patient's house; he or she must

Table 10–3.   Clinically important psychotropic drug–drug interactions

Drug or drug class	Precipitant drug or drug class	Interaction
Benzodiazepines (alprazolam, triazolam)	Azole antifungal agents (fluconazole, itraconazole, ketoconazole)	CYP3A4 inhibition
Carbamazepine	Propoxyphene	CYP3A4 inhibition
Dextromethorphan	MAOIs (isocarboxazid, phenelzine, selegiline, tranylcypromine)	Serotonin syndrome
MAOIs (isocarboxazid, phenelzine, selegiline, tranylcypromine)	Anorexiants (amphetamine, benzphetamine, dexfenfluramine, dextroamphetamine, diethylpropion, fenfluramine, mazindol, methamphetamine, phendimetrazine, phentermine, phenylpropanolamine, sibutramine)	Serotonin syndrome
	Sympathomimetics (dopamine, ephedrine, isometheptene mucate, mephentermine, metaraminol, phenylephrine, pseudoephedrine)	Serotonin syndrome
Meperidine	MAOIs (isocarboxazid, phenelzine, selegiline, tranylcypromine)	Serotonin syndrome
Pimozide	Macrolide antibiotics (clarithromycin, dirithromycin, erythromycin, troleandomycin)	CYP3A4 inhibition
	Azole antifungal agents (fluconazole, itraconazole, ketoconazole)	CYP3A4 inhibition

Table 10–3. Clinically important psychotropic drug–drug interactions *(continued)*

Drug or drug class	Precipitant drug or drug class	Interaction
SSRIs, SNRIs (citalopram, duloxetine, fluoxetine, fluvoxamine, nefazodone, paroxetine, sertraline, venlafaxine)[a]	MAOIs (isocarboxazid, phenelzine, selegiline, tranylcypromine)	Serotonin syndrome
Theophyllines	Fluvoxamine	CYP1A2 inhibition
Warfarin	Barbiturates (amobarbital, butabarbital, butalbital, mephobarbital, phenobarbital, secobarbital)	CYP2C9 induction

Note. CYP = cytochrome P450; MAOIs = monoamine oxidase inhibitors; SNRIs = serotonin-norepinephrine reuptake inhibitors; SSRIs = selective serotonin reuptake inhibitors.
Source. Adapted from Malone et al. 2004.

watch for the "shopping bag sign," in which the family member brings in massive quantities of current and expired medications that require a large bag or box. The most important clinically significant drug interactions are summarized in Table 10–3. Psychiatrists may find it helpful to have this list with them when performing psychiatric consultations.

Monoamine Oxidase Inhibitors and Diet

Tyramine in the diet can interact with a monoamine oxidase inhibitor (MAOI) to cause a hypertensive crisis. If the patient ingests food containing significant amounts of tyramine, the catecholamine produced can cause severe hypertension. Reasonable dietary restraint is the best prevention.

Neuroleptic Malignant Syndrome

Clinical Characteristics

Neuroleptic malignant syndrome (NMS) is a rare, potentially fatal idiosyncratic reaction to rapid alteration in CNS dopamine activity. NMS is typically caused by medications that block dopamine, such as neuroleptics, metoclopramide, and (rarely) clozapine. In 89% of cases, NMS symptoms start within the first 10 days of neuroleptic treatment or dosage increase. The full syndrome usually develops within 48 hours of initial onset (Shalev and Munitz 1986). The clinical characteristics of NMS are listed in Table 10–4. The core symptoms of NMS—fever, skeletal muscle rigidity, autonomic instability, and altered mental state—are present in most cases.

It is of interest that atypical antipsychotics, although they have low rates of extrapyramidal side effects (EPS) in general, produce EPS in 95% or more of the patients with NMS (Ananth et al. 2004). Laboratory abnormalities in NMS are elevated creatine kinase in 92% of patients, leukocytosis in 70% of patients, myoglobinemia in 75% of patients, and reduced serum iron levels in 96% of patients during an episode of NMS (Rosebush and Steward 1989). Laboratory values also may reflect dehydration and elevated liver enzymes. Brain scan and computed tomography rarely have abnormal results, and the cerebrospinal fluid may (in 2 of 54 patients; Addonizio et al. 1987) show elevated protein levels. Electroencephalograms commonly show nonspecific slowing (21 of 45 patients; Addonizio et al. 1987).

Table 10–4.   Clinical characteristics of neuroleptic malignant syndrome and their frequency

	Kurlan et al. 1984	Levenson 1985	Rosebush/ Steward 1989
Core features (%)			
Fever	100	98	100
Rigidity	92	89	96
Autonomic instability			
Tachycardia	79	89	100
Diaphoresis	60	67	100
Labile blood pressure	54	74	100
Altered mental state			
Stupor	27		
Coma	27		
Associated features (%)			
Tremor	56	45	92
Akinesia	38		
Dystonia	33		
Sialorrhea	31		
Tachypnea	25		29

Epidemiology

Various authors have estimated the incidence of NMS in psychiatric inpatients receiving neuroleptics to be 0.02%–3.23% (Pelonero et al. 1998). If milder variants of NMS are included, the frequency among some populations may be as high as 12.2% (Levinson and Simpson 1986). The prevalence of NMS is unknown. NMS has an estimated mortality rate of 1%–20%, depending on the population being studied (Caroff 1980); atypical antipsychotics are associated with lower mortality rates (Ananth et al. 2004). NMS occurs at all ages, with a range from 3 to 78 years (Shalev and Munitz 1986). However, Caroff (1980) summarized 60 NMS cases and noted that nearly 80% were in patients younger than 40. He also noted that young adult men predominated (male-to-female ratio of 2:1). Addonizio et al. (1987), in a review of 115 NMS patients, reported that 63% were male and 37% were female.

The mean age was higher (40 years). Ananth et al. (2004) identified 68 cases of NMS associated with atypical antipsychotics. Again, males greatly outnumbered females (47 to 21).

Risk Factors

The three most significant risk factors for NMS (Table 10–5) are a rapid decrease in CNS dopamine activity, which can be achieved by rapid neuroleptization with intramuscular haloperidol or withdrawal of levodopa therapy (Serrano-Duenas 2003); extreme neuroleptic sensitivity in patients with Lewy body dementia (Baskys 2004); and rechallenge with a neuroleptic within 2 weeks after NMS. Addonizio and Susman (1991) reported 68 instances of post-NMS patients who safely restarted neuroleptics (28 received thioridazine) and 41 who experienced a recurrence. High-potency neuroleptics, such as haloperidol, may be associated with a higher risk for NMS. Shalev and Munitz's (1986) review of 202 patients with NMS found that haloperidol was involved in 49.5% of cases. This association likely reflects haloperidol's popularity; however, it more likely indicates that rapid increases in neuroleptic dosage that occur with haloperidol are an important risk factor (Addonizio and Susman 1991; Keck et al. 1987; Shalev and Munitz 1986). Patients who have dementia with Lewy bodies, debatably the second most common cause of dementia after Alzheimer's disease, have extensive destruction of their dopaminergic and anticholinergic pathways; therefore, these patients are very sensitive to extrapyramidal symptoms and fatal complications of neuroleptics (Baskys 2004). Other risk factors associated with the development of NMS are listed in Table 10–5.

Occurrence in Medically Ill Patients

Except for neuroleptic use in patients with Lewy body dementia and withdrawal of medications in patients with Parkinson's disease (Ueda et al. 2001), no clear association exists between a particular medical illness and NMS. Because dehydration and exhaustion occur in a wide variety of medical diseases, medical disease may increase the risk for NMS. Shalev et al. (1989) found that patients with organic brain disease who develop NMS have a higher mortality rate than do patients with NMS who have a normal CNS (i.e., 39% vs. 19% for the overall group). Patients with NMS develop secondary medical problems, including pneumonia, pulmonary emboli, and renal failure

Table 10–5.   Risk factors for neuroleptic malignant syndrome (NMS)

Rapid decrease in central nervous system dopamine activity (essential)

Prior episode of NMS within the last few weeks

Neuroleptic use in patient with Lewy body dementia

Treatment with haloperidol (lower mortality)

Intramuscular administration of neuroleptic

Dehydration

Use of lithium

Diagnosis of mood disorder

Male (especially young male)

Brain disorder (increases mortality)

Concurrent medical illness

(secondary to rhabdomyolysis), that are potentially lethal. "Lead-pipe" muscle rigidity leads to muscle contractures, rhabdomyolysis, and myoglobinemia and potentially to acute myoglobinuric renal failure. Chest wall rigidity may decrease pulmonary function. Other medical complications resulting from NMS include dehydration, malnutrition, infections, deep venous thrombosis, exacerbation of preexisting coronary disease, and myocardial infarction.

Differential Diagnosis

EPS Accompanied by Fever

EPS accompanied by fever are very likely to be misdiagnosed as NMS. In an examination of 67 patients with NMS, Levinson and Simpson (1986) found that 41% of the patients had a medical illness to explain the fever, 23% probably had complicating medical factors, and only 36% of the patients had no medical factors (i.e., had NMS). The lesson seems clear—when a febrile patient who is taking a neuroleptic is examined, the clinician should have a high index of suspicion that the fever is caused by a medical illness.

Neuroleptic-Induced Catatonia

A patient with neuroleptic-induced catatonia presents with a combination of catatonia and parkinsonian signs. As Gelenberg and Mandel (1977) noted in eight patients, "All [patients] developed posturing, waxy flexibility, negativism, regressive behavior, incontinence of urine, and slowness of response. Parkinsonian features noted in all patients included stiffness, bradykinesia, and lack of associated movements" (p. 949). Significant temperature elevation and autonomic instability were not seen in these patients.

Catatonia

Signs and symptoms of catatonia *predate* neuroleptic treatment, and significant temperature elevation and autonomic instability are absent. Catatonia is treated by *increasing* neuroleptic medication or administering electroconvulsive therapy.

Heatstroke

Heatstroke is a potential complication of neuroleptic agents. Therefore, a neuroleptic-treated patient during hot, humid weather is at risk for heatstroke. Symptoms are fever, tachycardia, hyperventilation, and mental confusion, which may rapidly progress to coma. Sweating is usually not present; vomiting and nausea occur in most patients. The clinician can differentiate heatstroke from NMS by a history of heat exposure, absence of sweating, and flaccid muscle tone.

Malignant Hyperthermia

Malignant hyperthermia is caused by a genetic abnormality. Vulnerable individuals, after exposure to inhalation anesthesia (e.g., halothane), skeletal muscle relaxants (e.g., succinylcholine hydrochloride), certain chemicals (e.g., carbon tetrachloride), or even stress, may develop profound muscular rigidity and fever. In malignant hyperthermia, a defect in cellular calcium transport causes muscle contraction and heat generation. Several differences are found between malignant hyperthermia and NMS. Malignant hyperthermia occurs after exposure to anesthetics, and NMS occurs after a rapid decrease in CNS dopamine (exposure to neuroleptics or withdrawal of dopaminergic therapy). Malignant hyperthermia occurs within minutes to hours, and NMS occurs in hours to days. Both respond well to dantrolene, but *only* patients with NMS show muscular relaxation with curare or diazepam.

Anticholinergic Delirium or Coma

Anticholinergic delirium or coma can result from treatment with a variety of anticholinergic medications. Signs of toxicity include blurred vision; ileus; urinary retention; tachycardia; dry, flushed skin without sweating; mild temperature elevation; disorientation; and hallucinations. Anticholinergic delirium, but not NMS, is briefly relieved by 1–2 mg of intravenous physostigmine infused over 2–3 minutes and repeated in 20–30 minutes if needed (cardiac and vital sign monitoring is recommended, and seizures are possible). In anticholinergic toxicity, muscle rigidity is lacking.

Serotonin Syndrome

Characteristics of serotonin syndrome are similar to those of NMS, although differences in etiology, presentation, and treatment are seen. Serotonin syndrome results from excessive serotonin activity in the CNS. NMS is an idiosyncratic reaction, but serotonin syndrome is not. Serotonin syndrome is dose related, and any patient, given sufficient serotonergic activity, will develop serotonin syndrome. Therefore, the risk factors for serotonin syndrome are pharmacologically related, although constitutional factors may alter the threshold. Serotonin syndrome is most closely associated with MAOIs (MAOI overdose, combination of two MAOIs, MAOI plus meperidine, MAOI plus L-tryptophan, and MAOI plus an SSRI). Serotonin syndrome very rarely occurs secondary to a single antidepressant, even in overdose (except an MAOI). Serotonin syndrome typically develops from a combination of medications (see Table 10–3), each medication augmenting serotonergic activity by a different mechanism.

Table 10–6 lists the clinical characteristics of serotonin syndrome. Early warning signs for serotonin syndrome include myoclonus, clonus, hyperreflexia, shivering, and restlessness. The generalized rigidity ("lead-pipe" rigidity) present in NMS is typically absent in serotonin syndrome, although an individual with serotonin syndrome can experience muscle tension (e.g., clenched jaws, bruxism).

The management of serotonin syndrome is similar to that of NMS, in that all offending agents are discontinued and supportive care is provided. Pharmacological treatment is based on nonspecific blockade of excessive postsynaptic serotonergic activity. Medications used for treatment include cyproheptadine 0.5 mg/kg/day maximum; methysergide 4–8 mg; or propranolol (insufficient experience to recommend a specific dose).

Table 10–6. Clinical characteristics of serotonin syndrome and their frequency

Feature	Frequency (%)
Altered mental state	
Confusion	42
Hypomania	21
Restlessness	45
Myoclonus	34
Hyperreflexia	29
Diaphoresis	26
Shivering	26
Tremor	26
Diarrhea	16
Incoordination	13

Source. Adapted from Sternbach 1991.

Treatment and Management

Death does not occur from the same mechanism that triggers NMS but is caused by medical complications. Treatment consists of neuroleptic discontinuation, supportive care, and pharmacological therapies such as dantrolene and bromocriptine. When supportive measures (respiratory therapy, external cooling, hydration, physical therapy, nutritional measures) alone are used, the mean time until clinical improvement is 6.8 days. The addition of dantrolene or bromocriptine reduces recovery time to 1.2 and 1.0 days, respectively. Pharmacological treatment with dantrolene is initially given intravenously, 2–3 mg/kg over 10–15 minutes (daily total=0.8–10 mg/kg/day intravenously), or is given orally, 50–700 mg/day in four divided doses. Bromocriptine is given orally, 2.5–10 mg three times a day. Several treatments are not recommended for NMS: electroconvulsive therapy (except for lethal catatonia), benzodiazepines, anticholinergics, and nitroprusside.

Pregnancy

Psychotropic drug use during pregnancy is a common and an important issue. Risks associated with drug therapy during pregnancy include teratogenic effects, direct neonatal toxicity, perinatal effects, and potential long-term neurobehavioral sequelae (Fait et al. 2002). The patient and the clinician must weigh these risks against the consequences of treatment without medication(s). Table 10–7 presents general guidelines for psychotropic medication use during pregnancy and breast-feeding.

Antipsychotics

In a meta-analysis, Altshuler et al. (1996) reported a higher than normal rate of fetal malformation after first-trimester exposure to low-potency neuroleptic agents. Exposure to other neuroleptic agents showed no clear pattern of teratogenicity (Arana and Rosenbaum 2000). Perinatal effects of neuroleptic agents include EPS, such as tremors, hypertonicity, and dyskinesias (Auerbach et al. 1992). Although it is best to avoid antipsychotics during pregnancy, failure to treat psychosis in a pregnant woman typically poses a greater risk to the fetus than does the risk of exposure to an antipsychotic drug. Also, remember that electroconvulsive therapy is the treatment of choice for a pregnant woman who has psychotic depression (Wise et al. 1984).

Antidepressants

Tricyclic antidepressants are relatively safe during pregnancy (Altschuler et al. 1996), although withdrawal syndromes (i.e., jitteriness, irritability, and seizures) are described in newborns when exposure occurs close to the time of delivery. Fluoxetine is not associated with major congenital malformations. However, minor malformations were reported, as well as more admissions to special care nurseries, when women took fluoxetine during the later stages of pregnancy (Chambers et al. 1996); this study had methodological problems (Cohen and Rosenbaum 1997). Other SSRIs, such as fluvoxamine, paroxetine, and sertraline, were not associated with increased risk of major malformations or higher rates of miscarriage, stillbirth, or prematurity (Kulin et al. 1998). Data regarding the safety of the MAOIs and newer antidepressants in pregnancy are lacking, so these drugs should be avoided in pregnant women, whenever possible.

Mood Stabilizers and Antianxiety Agents

Lithium may cause cardiovascular defects, particularly when taken during the first trimester; this risk is significantly lower than previously believed (Cohen

Table 10–7. Guidelines for medication use during pregnancy or breast-feeding

1. Perform a risk-benefit analysis.

2. Document the mother's problems in daily living and her ability to care for the fetus/infant, target symptoms, and the rationale for medication use.

3. Record all drug exposures (prescribed, over-the-counter, herbal, and illicit) during pregnancy and during postpartum period, if the patient is breast-feeding. Ask about and document alcohol consumption during pregnancy.

4. Obtain informed consent. Discuss with the mother the risks and unknown aspects of taking psychotropic medication while pregnant or breast-feeding, to include the remote possibility of long-term effects on the child. Document this discussion, and have the patient sign the informed consent, especially if the patient insists on taking medications despite recommendations to the contrary (e.g., patient has a severe, chronic psychotic illness that responds only to clozapine and insists on breast-feeding despite recommendations against breast-feeding while taking clozapine). If the patient's capacity to make an informed decision is influenced by the illness, have the spouse participate in the decision-making process and have him also sign the informed consent.

5. Use a medication that has worked in the past, unless contraindicated.

6. Choose medication that has some data rather than a novel compound with no data.

7. Attempt monotherapy. Data on combination pharmacotherapy do not exist. Do not forget that electroconvulsive therapy is the treatment of choice when a woman has a psychotic depression.

8. While the patient is breast-feeding, try to avoid prescribing medications that require invasive monitoring (e.g., clozapine).

9. Use the minimum effective dose.

10. Urge the mother who is breast-feeding to take doses so that the medication level in breast milk is minimized at the time the infant nurses (i.e., take medication immediately after the infant nurses, or take dose immediately prior to infant's long afternoon nap).

Source. Adapted from recommendations found in Llewellyn and Stowe 1998.

et al. 1994). When lithium is used during the first trimester, fetal echocardiography and ultrasonography are recommended. Carbamazepine and valproic acid are known to cause fetal neural tube defects (Lammer et al. 1987; Rosa 1991); these medications should be avoided, especially during the first trimester. At one time, diazepam was thought to increase the incidence of fetal oral clefts (Saxen 1975), but no increased risk was found in large cohort and case-controlled studies (Rosenberg et al. 1983).

Breast-Feeding

Breast-feeding has many advantages and few drawbacks for the newborn and the mother. As a result, most women breast-feed during puerperium (Llewellyn and Stowe 1998). Unfortunately, for some of these women, the postpartum period is complicated by depression, mania, or psychosis, and treatment with psychotropic medications becomes necessary. Is it safe for the infant to breast-feed while the mother is taking a psychotropic medication? Information available to answer this question is limited and is mainly found in case reports. In addition, medication's passage into breast milk and then into the infant is quite complicated. Independent variables include the mother (e.g., metabolism, volume of distribution, amount of medication taken, and timing of dose), the breast milk (e.g., breast-feeding schedule in relation to time of ingestion, pH, composition), and the infant (e.g., absorption, metabolism, volume of distribution, excretion) (Llewellyn and Stowe 1998). The American Academy of Pediatrics's Committee on Drugs (1994) has categorized medications according to their risk to the breast-feeding infant (see Table 10–8). However, clinical judgment still must prevail because some of these recommendations must be qualified. For example, valproate is considered compatible with breast-feeding; however, others recommend against its use because of the potential risk of hepatotoxicity in children (Chaudron and Jefferson 2000). Carbamazepine is considered compatible with breast-feeding; however, poor feeding and hepatic dysfunction have been reported (Chaudron and Jefferson 2000). Lithium is contraindicated with breast-feeding; however, information is insufficient to support such a strong recommendation (Chaudron and Jefferson 2000).

References

Addonizio G, Susman VL: Neuroleptic Malignant Syndrome: A Clinical Approach. St. Louis, MO, Mosby-Year Book, 1991

Addonizio G, Susman VL, Roth SD: Neuroleptic malignant syndrome: review and analysis of 115 cases. Biol Psychiatry 22:1004–1020, 1987

Table 10–8.   Medications and breast-feeding

Drug/Medication	Classification	Reason (if listed)
Mood stabilizers		
Carbamazepine	Compatible with breast-feeding	
Lithium	Contraindicated	Infant's levels one-third to one-half of mother's level
Valproic acid	Compatible with breast-feeding	
Anxiolytics		
Diazepam	Unknown but may be of concern	
Lorazepam	Unknown but may be of concern	
Midazolam	Unknown but may be of concern	
Prazepam[a]	Unknown but may be of concern	
Quazepam	Unknown but may be of concern	
Temazepam	Unknown but may be of concern	
Antipsychotics		
Chlorpromazine	Unknown but may be of concern	Drowsiness and lethargy in infants
Haloperidol	Unknown but may be of concern	
Perphenazine	Unknown but may be of concern	

Table 10–8. Medications and breast-feeding *(continued)*

Drug/Medication	Classification	Reason (if listed)
Antidepressants		
Amitriptyline	Unknown but may be of concern	
Amoxapine	Unknown but may be of concern	
Desipramine	Unknown but may be of concern	
Doxepin	Unknown but may be of concern	
Fluoxetine	Unknown but may be of concern	
Fluvoxamine	Unknown but may be of concern	
Imipramine	Unknown but may be of concern	
Trazodone	Unknown but may be of concern	
Hypnotics		
Chloral hydrate	Compatible with breast-feeding	
Zolpidem	Compatible with breast-feeding	

[a] Accumulates in breast milk.
Source. Adapted from American Academy of Pediatrics, Committee on Drugs 1994.

Adson DE, Crow SJ, Meller WH, et al: Potential drug-drug interactions on a tertiary care hospital consultation-liaison psychiatry service. Psychosomatics 39:360–365, 1998

Altshuler LL, Cohen LS, Szuba MP, et al: Pharmacological management of psychiatric illness in pregnancy: dilemmas and guidelines. Am J Psychiatry 153:592–606, 1996

American Academy of Pediatrics, Committee on Drugs: The transfer of drugs and other chemicals into human milk. Pediatrics 93:137–150, 1994

Ananth J, Parameswaran S, Gunatilake S, et al: Neuroleptic malignant syndrome and atypical antipsychotic drugs. J Clin Psychiatry 65:464–470, 2004

Arana GW, Rosenbaum JF: Handbook of Psychiatric Drug Therapy, 4th Edition. Philadelphia, PA, Lippincott Williams & Wilkins, 2000, pp 37–38

Auerbach JG, Hans SL, Marcus J, et al: Maternal psychotropic medication and neonatal behavior. Neurotoxicol Teratol 14:399–406, 1992

Baskys A: Lewy body dementia: the litmus test for neuroleptic sensitivity and extrapyramidal symptoms. J Clin Psychiatry 65 (suppl 11):16–22, 2004

Bennett WM, Aronoff GR, Golper TA, et al: Drug Prescribing in Renal Failure, 4th Edition. Philadelphia, PA, American College of Physicians, 1999

Caroff SN: The neuroleptic malignant syndrome. J Clin Psychiatry 41:79–83, 1980

Chambers C, Johnson K, Dick L, et al: Birth outcomes in pregnant women taking fluoxetine. N Engl J Med 335:1010–1015, 1996

Chaudron LH, Jefferson JW: Mood stabilizers during breastfeeding: a review. J Clin Psychiatry 61:79–90, 2000

Cohen LS, Rosenbaum JR: Fluoxetine in pregnancy (letter). N Engl J Med 336:872, 1997

Cohen LS, Friedman JM, Jefferson JW, et al: A reevaluation of risk of in utero exposure to lithium [published erratum appears in JAMA 271:1485, 1994]. JAMA 271:146–150, 1994

Csernansky JG, Whiteford HA: Clinically significant psychoactive drug interactions, in Psychiatry Update: The American Psychiatric Association Annual Review, Vol 6. Edited by Hales RE, Frances AJ. Washington, DC, American Psychiatric Press, 1987, pp 802–815

Fait ML, Wise MG, Jachna JS, et al: Psychopharmacology, in The American Psychiatric Publishing Textbook of Consultation-Liaison Psychiatry: Psychiatry in the Medically Ill, 2nd Edition. Edited by Wise MG, Rundell JR. Washington, DC, American Psychiatric Publishing, 2002, pp 939–987

Geeze D, Wise MG: Doxepin-cholestyramine interaction. Psychosomatics 29:233–236, 1988

Gelenberg AL, Mandel MR: Catatonic reactions to high-potency neuroleptic drugs. Arch Gen Psychiatry 34:947–950, 1977

Gilman AG, Rall TW, Neis AS, et al: Goodman and Gilman's The Pharmacological Basis of Therapeutics, 8th Edition. New York, Pergamon, 1990

Greco T, Eckert G, Kroenke K: The outcome of physical symptoms with treatment of depression. J Gen Intern Med 19:813–818, 2004

Jones CK, Peters SC, Shannon HE: Efficacy of duloxetine, a potent and balanced serotonergic and noradrenergic reuptake inhibitor, in inflammatory and acute pain models in rodents. J Pharmacol Exp Ther 312:726–732, 2005

Keck PE, Pope HG, McElroy SL: Frequency and presentation of neuroleptic syndrome: a prospective study. Am J Psychiatry 144:1344–1346, 1987

Kulin NA, Pastuszak A, Sage SR, et al: Pregnancy outcome following maternal use of the new selective serotonin reuptake inhibitors. JAMA 279:609–610, 1998

Kurlan R, Hamill R, Shoulson I: Neuroleptic malignant syndrome. Clin Neuropharmacol 7:109–120, 1984

Lammer EJ, Sever LE, Oakley GP Jr: Teratogen update: valproic acid. Teratology 35:465–473, 1987

Levenson JL: Neuroleptic malignant syndrome. Am J Psychiatry 142:1137–1145, 1985

Levinson DF, Simpson GM: Neuroleptic induced extrapyramidal symptoms with fever—heterogeneity of the neuroleptic malignant syndrome. Arch Gen Psychiatry 43:839–848, 1986

Lin EH, VonKorff M, Ludman EJ, et al: Enhancing adherence to prevent depression relapse in primary care. Gen Hosp Psychiatry 25:303–310, 2003

Llewellyn A, Stowe ZN: Psychotropic medications in lactation. J Clin Psychiatry 59 (suppl 2):41–52, 1998

Malone DC, Abarca J, Hansten PD, et al: Identification of serious drug-drug interactions: results of the Partnership to Prevent Drug-Drug Interactions. J Am Pharm Assoc (Wash DC) 44:142–151, 2004

Max MB, Lynch SA, Muir J: Effects of desipramine, amitriptyline, and fluoxetine on pain in diabetic neuropathy. N Engl J Med 326:1250–1256, 1992

Pelonero AL, Levenson JL, Pandurangi AK: Neuroleptic malignant syndrome: a review. Psychiatr Serv 49:1163–1172, 1998

Rosa FW: Spina bifida in infants of women treated with carbamazepine during pregnancy. N Engl J Med 324:674–677, 1991

Rosebush PI, Steward T: A prospective analysis of 24 episodes of neuroleptic malignant syndrome. Am J Psychiatry 146:717–725, 1989

Rosenberg L, Mitchell AA, Parsells JL, et al: Lack of relation of oral clefts to diazepam use during pregnancy. N Engl J Med 309:1282–1285, 1983

Saxen I. Associations between oral clefts and drugs taken during pregnancy. Int J Epidemiol 4:37–44, 1975

Serrano-Duenas M: Neuroleptic malignant syndrome-like, or—dopaminergic malignant syndrome—due to levodopa therapy withdrawal: clinical features in 11 patients. Parkinsonism Relat Disord 9:175–178, 2003

Shalev A, Munitz H: The neuroleptic malignant syndrome: agent and host interaction. Acta Psychiatr Scand 73:337–347, 1986

Shalev A, Hermesh H, Munitz H: Mortality from neuroleptic malignant syndrome. J Clin Psychiatry 50:18–25, 1989

Sternbach H: The serotonin syndrome. Am J Psychiatry 148:705–713, 1991

Turnheim K: When drug therapy gets old: pharmacokinetics and pharmacodynamics in the elderly. Exp Gerontol 38:843–853, 2003

Ueda M, Hamamoto M, Nagayama H: Biochemical alterations during medication withdrawal in Parkinson's disease with and without neuroleptic malignant–like syndrome. J Neurol Neurosurg Psychiatry 71:111–113, 2001

Wise MG, Ward SC, Townsend-Parchman W, et al: Case report of ECT during a high risk pregnancy. Am J Psychiatry 141:99–101, 1984

Additional Readings

Roose SP, Glassman AH: Antidepressant choice in the patient with cardiac disease: lessons from the Cardiac Arrhythmia Suppression Trial (CAST) studies. J Clin Psychiatry 55:83–100, 1994

Rosebush PI, Mazurek MF: Serum iron and neuroleptic malignant syndrome. Lancet 338:149–151, 1991

Stotland NL: Obstetrics and gynecology, in The American Psychiatric Publishing Textbook of Consultation-Liaison Psychiatry: Psychiatry in the Medically Ill, 2nd Edition. Edited by Wise MG, Rundell JR. Washington, DC, American Psychiatric Publishing, 2002, pp 701–716

11

Violence and Aggression

Emergency Consultation

Aside from a suicide attempt, few events focus the attention of medical staff and other patients faster than violence or the threat of violence in a hospital. When this situation arises, a "stat" psychiatric consultation is often requested. The psychiatrist usually is faced with one of three situations: 1) a patient is actively violent and combative; 2) a patient is threatening violence; or 3) violence has already occurred, and the patient may or may not now appear acutely violent.

When first contacted about an acute or emergency psychiatric consultation for a potentially violent or violent patient (usually by telephone), the consultant should ask the referring physician or staff whether the individual is armed with a gun, knife, or other potentially lethal weapon. He or she should inquire about medical and mental state. If the family is available, the staff or referring physician should gather information about the patient's history of violence and recent mental state. This information can be collected while the psychiatrist is en route to the location. When the psychiatrist arrives, a sufficient number of personnel should be ready to restrain the individual if necessary. The organization and instruction of the restraint team are important. When the instruction is properly given, injury to the patient, the members of the restraint team, and the psychiatrist is less likely (see Table 11–1).

Table 11–1. Procedure for physical restraint

1. If the patient is armed, call security or police.

2. If the patient is unarmed, get sufficient help. At least five adults are required.

3. Assign each individual a specific extremity or the head (e.g., "You secure the right arm"). Personnel should wait for the team leader's command for restraint to proceed.

4. Ensure that a nurse has a sedative injection prepared and ready to administer.

5. Ensure that leather restraints are readily available. If the patient is already hospitalized and has intravenous and other lines attached, soft restraints are recommended.

6. Ensure that properly trained personnel who know how to quickly apply the restraints are available.

7. Do not remove the restraints unless adequate force is available to reapply restraints or until it is certain that the patient or staff is not at risk.

8. Evaluate the patient for medical or toxic explanations for the violent episode.

9. Monitor the patient closely for changes in medical status (especially vital signs and circulatory function distal to the restraints) and mental status and the need for medication.

10. Document carefully the reasons for the restraint and the lack of alternatives; ensure that all medical facility operating instructions are adhered to.

The Combative, Actively Violent Patient

The combative, actively violent patient needs restraint and sedation. If the patient is armed, restraint is best performed by police or security personnel. Neuroleptic medications (e.g., haloperidol) are frequently used to calm the acutely aggressive patient. The initial dose is 1–2 mg intravenously (if an intravenous line is still in place) or intramuscularly. The dose should be increased by 1 mg every half-hour until aggression is controlled. Young, strong patients often require higher doses (e.g., 5 mg). Interestingly, women who are psychotic and require psychiatric hospitalization are more likely to be both verbally and physically assaultive than men are (Krakowski and Czobor 2004). Neuroleptics are not appropriate long-term management medications (unless the violence is related to a psychotic disorder) and may cause potentially complicating adverse effects, such as dystonias, akathisia, and extrapyramidal signs. Lorazepam is also frequently used in the acute violent setting because it is short acting and can be administered by several routes. Lorazepam, 1–2 mg, should be administered orally or intramuscularly every hour until control is achieved. If lorazepam is given intravenously, to avoid respiratory depression and laryngospasm, the clinician should push slowly and not exceed 2 mg/minute (Hales et al. 2002).

A Patient Who Is Threatening Violence

An individual who is threatening violence requires immediate intervention. A clinician should not knowingly place him- or herself in harm's way. However, if the person indicates during an evaluation that he or she is armed, the clinician should ask the individual why he or she needs a weapon. The psychiatrist can then formulate an appropriate request for the person to relinquish the weapon. If he or she refuses, the psychiatrist is advised not to continue the interview and to call police and/or security personnel to disarm the person.

The psychiatrist should use a calm, reassuring voice to tell the patient that he or she will help him or her maintain control. The psychiatrist must avoid angry confrontation and determine the reason for the aggressiveness. Is the patient paranoid, confused, and/or filled with rage? Common psychiatric etiologies are delirium, mania, psychosis, drug or alcohol intoxication, and drug or alcohol withdrawal. Persons with primitive character pathology often become enraged and act out impulsively.

Most patients will respond to an emphatic inquiry, and, in this way, the situation can be defused. Sedation should be offered, but if the patient's behavior escalates and becomes violent, the restraint team should be signaled to restrain the patient and administer sedation. The patient's family is often helpful, particularly if the patient is delirious and paranoid. If a hospitalized patient believes that the hospital staff is about to kill him or her, calm reassurance from loved ones is helpful. In some situations, family involvement is not indicated. If the individual has a character disorder or is angry with the family, the family's involvement may escalate the person's anger rather than calm it.

A Patient Who Has Already Committed Violence

If violence has already occurred and the patient is now calm, the clinician should immediately try to answer the following:

1. Does the person still have the urge and the means to be violent?
2. What was the reason(s) for the violence, and is that stimulus still present?
3. What is the patient's current mental status, and what was the mental status before and at the time of the violence?
4. What is the environment (physical and social) in which the violence occurred?
5. Is a potentially contributory psychiatric disorder present?

Physiological Basis for Violence and Aggression

Multiple neurotransmitters mediate aggression. Serotonin, dopamine, acetylcholine, and γ-aminobutyric acid all play important roles (Hales et al. 2002). Neurotransmitters probably interact with one another to influence aggression. Norepinephrine tracks originate in the locus coeruleus in the lateral tegmental system and terminate in the forebrain. Frontal and temporal lobes of the forebrain, when damaged, are associated with rage and violent behavior. β_1-Adrenergic receptors are also located in the limbic forebrain and are implicated in mediating aggressive behavior (Alexander et al. 1979).

Differential Diagnosis of Violence and Aggression

Many medical and psychiatric disorders are associated with violence and aggression. Neurological conditions such as dementia, epilepsy, stroke, and degenerative conditions (e.g., Parkinson's disease, multiple sclerosis) predispose patients to aggression. Violent behavior is common among psychiatric patients with intermittent explosive disorder, conduct disorder, oppositional defiant disorder, antisocial personality disorder, and borderline personality disorder. It is somewhat less common among patients with psychotic disorders and bipolar disorder, manic. Several psychoactive substances can precipitate or lower the threshold for aggression: alcohol, amphetamines, antianxiety medications, anticholinergic drugs, cocaine, hypnotics, and steroids (Hales et al. 2002).

Treatment and Prevention of Chronic Aggression

Pharmacological Treatment

Pharmacological treatment is sometimes necessary to help manage chronic aggression. When selecting a medication, consultation-liaison psychiatrists must search for the underlying cause of the chronic aggression. Unless unique and specific indications for other pharmacological agents are present, many clinicians consider β-blockers (e.g., propranolol, nadolol, pindolol) as the first-line treatment of chronic aggression (Greendyke et al. 1986; Hales et al. 2002; Ratey et al. 1992; Yudofsky et al. 1987). Table 11–2 summarizes medications used for chronic aggression, underlying conditions that might lead a clinician to use that medication, and dosage ranges.

Nonpharmacological Treatment

Patients with aggressive syndromes almost always require a multimodal management approach that includes behavioral, psychoeducational, and family approaches. Behavioral treatments are highly effective for patients with aggression related to central nervous system dysfunction. Behavioral strategies include token economy, aggression replacement strategies, and decelerative techniques (Corrigan and Jakus 1994; Corrigan et al. 1993). Patients and their families must learn to identify behaviors (e.g., yelling, cursing, and threatening) that are warning signs that aggression or violence is likely to occur (Hales et al. 2002). Patients and families can then apply alternative behaviors such as sitting quietly or engaging in pleasurable activities. Family therapy may assist families in coping with and more effectively managing aggressive household members.

The Overt Agitation Severity Scale (Kopecky et al. 1998; Yudofsky et al. 1997) includes 47 characteristics of agitation that are organized into 12 functionally related units. Domains of observation on this scale include verbal aggression, physical aggression against self, physical aggression against objects, physical aggression against other people, and interventions. The scale can be scored, providing a quantitative way to follow up a patient's level of violence. Consultation psychiatrists may wish to obtain copies of this scale to keep for consultations with aggressive and agitated patients.

Table 11–2. Pharmacological management of chronic aggression

Medication	Indication	Dosage range
β-Blockers		
Propranolol	Chronic or recurrent aggression	Start at 20 mg tid, increase by 60 mg/day every 3–5 days. Target is symptom control or 12 mg/kg/day.
Antianxiety medications		
Buspirone	Traumatic brain injury	10–20 mg tid
Clonazepam	Aggression associated with anxiety or tics	0.5–3.0 mg tid
Lorazepam	Acute aggression or agitation	Initially give 1–2 mg (po or im); repeat hourly until agitation is controlled. Maintain at maximum of 2 mg every 4 hours. When no longer agitated for 48 hours, decrease at 10% per day.
Anticonvulsants		
Carbamazepine	Aggressive behavior associated with brain disorders	400–1,200 mg/day. Watch for bone marrow suppression and hepatotoxicity.
Valproic acid	Aggressive behavior associated with brain disorders	1,000–1,500 mg/day. Watch for hepatotoxicity.
Lithium	Aggressive behavior associated with mania	300–1,800 mg/day. Watch for neurotoxicity and confusion.

Table 11–2. Pharmacological management of chronic aggression *(continued)*

Medication	Indication	Dosage range
Antidepressants		
SSRIs	Impulsive aggressivity, mental retardation, CNS lesions, depression with lability	Begin at relatively low doses (e.g., 10 mg fluoxetine, 25 mg sertraline, 10 mg paroxetine). If antiaggression effects not achieved over several weeks, the dosage may be slowly increased at 1- to 2-week intervals toward higher levels (up to 80 mg/day fluoxetine, 200 mg/day sertraline, 60 mg/day paroxetine).
Trazodone	Aggressive behavior associated with depression and insomnia	50–300 mg/day. Watch for oversedation.
Neuroleptics	Psychotic symptoms	Depends on medication.

Note. tid = three times a day; po = orally; im = intramuscularly; CNS = central nervous system; SSRIs = selective serotonin reuptake inhibitors.
Source. Adapted from Hales RE, Silver JM, Yudofsky SC, et al.: "Aggression and Agitation," in *The American Psychiatric Publishing Textbook of Consultation-Liaison Psychiatry: Psychiatry in the Medically Ill*, 2nd Edition. Edited by Wise MG, Rundell JR. Washington, DC, American Psychiatric Publishing, 2002, pp. 149–166. Copyright 2002, American Psychiatric Publishing. Used with permission.

References

Alexander RW, Davis JN, Lejkowitz RJ: Direct identification and characterization of beta-adrenergic receptors in rat brain. Nature 258:437–440, 1979

Corrigan PW, Jakus MR: Behavioral treatment, in Neuropsychiatry of Traumatic Brain Injury. Edited by Silver JM, Yudofsky SC, Hales RE. Washington, DC, American Psychiatric Press, 1994, pp 733–769

Corrigan PW, Yudofsky SC, Silver JM: Pharmacological and behavioral treatments for aggressive psychiatric inpatients. Hosp Community Psychiatry 44:125–133, 1993

Greendyke RM, Kanter DR, Schuster DB, et al: Propranolol treatment of assaultive patients with organic brain disease: a double-blind crossover, placebo-controlled study. J Nerv Ment Dis 174:290–294, 1986

Hales RE, Silver JM, Yudofsky SC, et al: Aggression and agitation, in The American Psychiatric Publishing Textbook of Consultation-Liaison Psychiatry: Psychiatry in the Medically Ill, 2nd Edition. Edited by Wise MG, Rundell JR. Washington, DC, American Psychiatric Publishing, 2002, pp 149–166

Kopecky HJ, Kopecky CR, Yudofsky SC: Reliability and validity of the Overt Agitation Severity Scale in adult psychiatric inpatients. Psychiatr Q 39:301–323, 1998

Krakowski M, Czobor P: Gender differences in violent behaviors: relationship to clinical symptoms and psychosocial factors. Am J Psychiatry 161:459–465, 2004

Ratey JJ, Sorgi P, O'Driscoll GA, et al: Nadolol to treat aggression and psychiatric symptomatology in chronic psychiatric inpatients: a double-blind, placebo-controlled study. J Clin Psychiatry 53:41–46, 1992

Yudofsky SC, Silver JM, Schneider SE: Pharmacologic treatment of aggression. Psychiatr Ann 17:397–407, 1987

Yudofsky SC, Kopecky JH, Kumik M, et al: The Overt Agitation Severity Scale for the objective rating of agitation. J Neuropsychiatry Clin Neurosci 9:541–548, 1997

Additional Readings

Fava M: Psychopharmacologic treatment of pathologic aggression. Psychiatr Clin North Am 20:427–451, 1997

Roger M, Gerard D, Leger JM: Value of tiapride for agitation in the elderly. Encephale 24:462–468, 1998

Tariot PN, Erb R, Leibovici A, et al: Carbamazepine treatment of agitation in nursing home patients with dementia: a preliminary study. J Am Geriatr Soc 42:1160–1166, 1998

12

Pain and Analgesics

Pain management is receiving more attention from physicians and their patients who want better treatment. The Joint Commission on Accreditation of Healthcare Organizations (JCAHO) now mandates that physicians consider pain as "the fifth vital sign." Unfortunately, the assessment and treatment of pain are difficult, and most psychiatrists have little interest or expertise in the field. A recent article on American Board of Psychiatry and Neurology subspecialty certification within psychiatry indicated that there are 5,327 certified child and adolescent psychiatrists and 2,595 certified geriatric psychiatrists; only 28 psychiatrists are certified in pain management. No psychiatry-based programs in pain management exist (Juul et al. 2004). In this chapter, we present essential information for assessment and management of pain complaints.

Pain is a frequent complaint and commonly prompts patients to seek medical attention. In a random sample of 1,265 people in the general population surveyed for the presence of significant or recurrent pain during a 6-month period, 37% reported no pain, 34% had pain in one location, 20% had pain in two locations, and 9% reported pain in three or more locations (Dworkin et al. 1990). It is often forgotten that every class of psychiatric medication is used in the management of pain, and many pain syndromes are responsive to psychiatric medications.

The psychiatrist's role in the assessment of patients with pain includes looking for pain syndromes that are responsive to psychotropic medications, comorbid psychiatric conditions, and psychological factors that amplify pain symptoms. The evaluation also includes review of current and past pain medications (e.g., effects, dosing schedule, side effects, drug interactions, misuse, abuse) and other treatments.

When pain has an acute onset, is well localized, and fits a recognized pathophysiological pattern, the patient usually receives analgesia from the physician. As long as the analgesia is adequate and the patient is not a suspected "addict," a psychiatrist is rarely consulted. In contrast, patients who have pain that is chronic, poorly localized, and resistant to treatment or that does not fit into a recognized pathophysiological pattern are often referred to a psychiatrist. The consultation request may read, "Rule out functional pain." Bouckoms and Hackett (1991) correctly pointed out that this "request to separate psyche from soma is often a symbolic write-off" (p. 39). The patient typically does not want to see a psychiatrist and is often angry about the referral. The spoken, or more typically unspoken, thought of the patient is, "I have real pain; it's not in my imagination!"

Pain is not purely "functional" or "organic"; it is a combination of both. Pain has two major components: the sensation (nociception) and the perception of that sensation. The perceptual component is influenced by emotional, cognitive, and psychosocial factors; these are as important as, if not sometimes more important than, the sensation. For example, two-thirds of the soldiers shot on the beachhead at Anzio, Italy, during World War II did not require morphine. Most denied pain despite serious injury (Beecher 1955). The gunshot wound meant immediate relief from combat and an honorable exit from the war for the wounded soldier.

Pain is very often undertreated. In a study of inpatient burn patients who received as-needed pain medications, 23% reported severe ("horrible") pain, and 30% reported extremely severe ("excruciating") pain during debridement and physiotherapy; at rest, 13% endorsed severe pain, and 20% endorsed extremely severe pain (Melzack 1990). At a cancer center, 42% of the patients with metastatic cancer received inadequate pain management. Physicians underestimated the pain their patients endured, even though opioid treatment of terminal cancer pain is widely accepted (Cleeland et al. 1994). In a survey of 1,320 physicians, 30% of the respondents endorsed occasionally or frequently underdosing outpatients with cancer pain out of fear of regulatory investigation; 50% endorsed occasionally or frequently prescribing a lower quantity of medication, and more than 50% acknowledged occasionally or frequently prescribing fewer refills (Guglielmo 2000). Numerous misconceptions on the part of the physician and the patient lead to undertreatment of pain (Table 12–1).

Pain Terminology

Knowledge of pain terminology and characteristics is essential for differential diagnosis and the selection of treatment modalities. Table 12–2 defines the terms commonly used by physicians to describe pain.

Nociceptive (Peripheral) Versus Central Pain

Nociceptive Pain

Nociceptive or peripheral pain is activated by stimulation of specialized nerve endings in the skin, subcutaneous tissues, muscles, bones, or viscera. When skin or underlying tissues are disrupted, the pain produced is well localized and sharp. The source of the lesion is easily found unless the pain is referred to another area of the body. In referred pain, recognition of the pain pattern is necessary (e.g., angina may be referred to the T1–T4 dermatomes, resulting in arm pain). Pain that occurs when viscera are stretched is less well localized. It may be sharp, colicky, or aching in quality.

Central Pain (Neuropathic or Deafferentation Pain)

Central pain involves neuronal structures proximal to the nociceptors. Therefore, it can occur without an obvious nociceptive source. Central pain is usually poorly localized, and the patient often has difficulty describing the pain. Examples of central pain include reflex sympathetic dystrophy, phantom limb pain, thalamic pain, posttherapeutic pain, and causalgia. Central nervous system (CNS) or central pain occurs in 20%–50% of chronic pain states (Bouckoms and Hackett 1991). The clinical characteristics of central pain are listed in Table 12–3.

Table 12–1.   Common misconceptions about pain

Physicians	Patients
Physical or behavioral signs of pain are more accurate than a patient self-report.	Severe or chronic pain cannot be effectively controlled.
Pain cannot exist in the absence of tissue damage.	Opioids are addictive.
	Pain is evidence of disease progression.
Pain without an obvious cause, or that is more severe than expected, is psychogenic.	It is admirable to ignore pain.
	Pain is an unavoidable result of aging and disease.
"Equal" noxious stimuli should produce the same level of pain in everyone.	Pain is a deserved punishment.
Experience teaches pain tolerance.	Opioids are a last resort ("I must be dying.").
Withhold all analgesics until the cause is established.	Residual pain is the result of limitations in medical science.
Patients who know pain medications, frequently visit emergency departments, or take opioids for a long time are "addicts."	Pain complaints indicate weakness, addiction, and/or lack of gratitude.
Opioid use will cause addiction.	
Patients who respond to a placebo are malingering.	
Patients readily express their pain to health care providers.	
Patients who overreport pain are probably addicted to drugs.	
Older and cognitively impaired patients do not perceive pain as intensely as younger patients.	
A patient who sleeps cannot have much pain.	
Patients with certain cultural, ethnic, or socioeconomic backgrounds consistently underreport or overreport their pain.	
The primary goal of chronic pain management is to minimize the dose of medication.	

Table 12–2. Pain terminology

Nociceptors	Nerve endings in the skin, tissue, and viscera activated by potentially damaging stimuli.
Central (neuropathic) pain	Results from injury to, or changes in, somatosensory pathways. It may persist without demonstrable nociceptive stimuli. (See Table 12–3 for clinical characteristics of central pain.)
Allodynia	The perception of a nonnociceptive stimulus (e.g., light touch) as painful.
Causalgia	A continuous burning pain usually following nerve injury. It may be associated with allodynia, sympathetic dysfunction, and glossy skin.
Deafferentation	Central pain that follows direct injury to the peripheral or central nervous system. Associated sensations include causalgia, dysesthesia, formication, and/or allodynia.
Dysesthesia	An unpleasant sensation (e.g., pins and needles).
Hyperesthesia	An excessive sensitivity to touch, pain, and other sensations.
Hyperalgesia	An exaggerated sensitivity to touch, pain, and other sensations.
Hyperpathia	An increased sensitivity to painful stimuli.
Hypoesthesia	A decreased sensitivity to touch, pain, and other sensations.
Hypoalgesia	A decreased sensitivity to painful stimuli.
Neuralgia	Pain in the distribution of a single nerve, usually the result of trauma or irritation.

Acute, Continuous, and Chronic Pain

Acute Pain

Acute pain is easily recognized. The patient is in obvious discomfort and usually manifests sympathetic nervous system hyperactivity. For example, a patient with renal colic will cry out in pain and writhe on the gurney. The flank pain is excruciating and often radiates into the groin or testicles. The patient is pale, diaphoretic, and nauseated and often vomits. This clinical picture is recognized by medical students and physicians alike. When acute pain is encountered, the source is identified, treatment is instituted, and analgesics are given, when appropriate.

Continuous Pain

Continuous pain occurs in cancer and other chronic disease states. Patients with continuous pain have a recognized nociceptive source, such as metastatic

Table 12–3.   Characteristics of central pain

Burning sensation

Change in sensory threshold: anesthesia, allodynia, hyperalgesia, or
   hyperesthesia

Delayed onset for days to weeks following injury

Dysesthesia

Lancinating (paroxysmal exacerbations)

Poor efficacy of narcotics

Nonanatomical distribution (may have trigger zones)

Source.   Adapted from Bouckoms 1988.

bone lesions from cancer. Narcotics, pain blocks, and ablative surgical procedure are used as necessary.

Hyman and Cassem (1989) offer several helpful management suggestions:

1. Give analgesics on a regular basis, not as needed (not prn). Write the or-
    der either for a routine regimen or so the patient has the option to decline
    (e.g., "Offer the patient 10 mg of morphine every 4 hours for pain"). In
    either instance, the patient does not have to "beg" for medication, and
    the staff is not placed in the position of labeling the patient's regular re-
    quests for narcotics as drug-seeking or addictive behavior.
2. Observe patients for constipation; 95% of the patients taking regular
    narcotics become constipated. Stool softeners, bulking agents, hydration,
    and laxatives are needed.
3. Monitor patients for tolerance to narcotics, which usually but not always
    occurs. Although the degree of tolerance that develops is variable, an
    increase of approximately 50% is sometimes necessary during the first
    2 weeks of treatment. Thereafter, smaller incremental increases in the
    narcotic may be required.
4. Do not consider narcotic addiction in a terminally ill patient. Even in the
    non–terminally ill patient, the risk of addiction is less than 1%.
5. Give two to three times the regular narcotic dose at bedtime so that the
    patient can sleep through the night.

6. If bone or inflammatory pain is present, give antiprostaglandin drugs (e.g., aspirin, nonsteroidal anti-inflammatory drugs such as ibuprofen).
7. Begin narcotics by the oral or suppository route. Later, if the pain worsens, intravenous, epidural, intrathecal, or cerebroventricular morphine is sometimes required.
8. Use pain adjuvants, behavioral treatment methods, and exercise to reduce narcotic requirements.

Other medication approaches to analgesia deserve mention: 1) the use of sustained-release morphine preparations, such as MS Contin and Roxanol-SR, which have a duration of action of 8–12 hours (for breakthrough pain, additional standard morphine preparations should be given); 2) the use of patient-controlled analgesia devices, which allow the patient, by pushing a button, to self-administer intravenous analgesics at doses and intervals preset by the physician (patient acceptance is very high, probably higher than efficacy); and 3) the use of epidural anesthesia or narcotics, which are extremely effective.

Chronic Pain

Chronic pain is defined as pain that has persisted for more than 6 months. The original nociceptive stimulus is either gone or cannot account for the pain. The pain has become centralized through mechanisms that are not understood. The mechanisms for the creation and maintenance of chronic pain are complex, involving stress analgesia, endogenous pain inhibition, and psychosocial contributors. The patient with chronic pain accommodates neurophysiologically and psychologically to pain and no longer behaves as if he or she is in acute pain. When this happens, even surgical interruption of specific pain pathways will not eliminate the suffering (Bouckoms and Hackett 1991).

Unfortunately, medical personnel apply their knowledge of and experience with acute pain to the patient who has chronic pain. The staff becomes suspicious because the patient with chronic pain reports severe distress but does not behave as if he or she has severe pain. The nurses see the patient laughing during a television show or engaging in a lively discussion with a hospital roommate. The staff concludes that the patient does not have "real" pain. To "prove" that the pain is "functional," a misguided physician or nurse may give the patient a saline injection (placebo) instead of a narcotic. If the patient responds positively to the placebo, the medical staff now believes that they have proven the pain is not real. Unfortunately, such a trial destroys any hope of developing a doctor-patient alliance; it does establish that the patient is a placebo responder.

To evaluate a patient who complains of pain continuously and chronically, the physician needs

- A detailed history of the pain complaint(s)
- An understanding of pain characteristics (types of pain and descriptors used) (the patient should complete a pain drawing to obtain a graphic, often dramatic depiction of the pain [Figure 12–1])
- A physical examination
- An analysis of impairment of social, physical, and occupational functioning
- A list of, and the patient's response to, current and past treatments
- A thorough understanding of the patient's history (i.e., a review of the often voluminous medical records, as well as psychiatric and psychosocial history)
- An examination of the temporal relation between significant past events and the onset or exacerbation of pain

Pain Behavior, Suffering, and Psychiatric Diagnoses

Pain, because it is a symptom, is imperceptible to the observer; it is experienced only by the patient. Pain behaviors, however, are "signs" that the physician can use to assess the patient's status. Nociception is the stimulus from the damaged tissue, and pain is the perceived sensation (the "Owwww!"). For some patients, particularly those with chronic pain, a suffering component develops (a moaning "Ohhhhhhhh!" or "Oyyyyyyyy!"). Suffering is the negative emotional response to the pain. Psychiatric diagnoses frequently accompany pain behavior and suffering. Depression, somatoform disorders, and anxiety disorders especially should be considered.

Psychiatric diagnoses to look for in chronic pain patients are listed in Table 12–4. Patients with psychotic disorders also may present with pain. The bizarre nature of the pain and the patient's thought processes will indicate whether psychosis is present. Malingering and factitious disorders also can

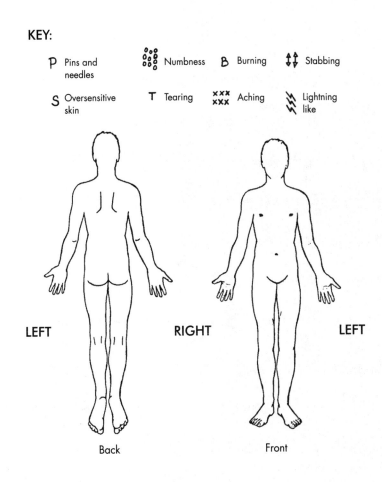

Figure 12–1. Pain drawing.

Instructions: Mark this drawing to indicate where you hurt. For example, if you have a stabbing-type pain only in the front part of your right shoulder, you would draw ↕↕ on the front of the figure's right shoulder exactly where your pain occurs. Use the key above to indicate the type of pains you are having.

Table 12–4. Psychiatric syndromes to look for in patients with chronic pain

Major depressive disorder
Dysthymic disorder
Generalized anxiety disorder
Substance abuse or dependence
Psychoactive substance withdrawal (especially narcotics)
Delusional disorder, somatic type
Somatoform disorders
    Somatization disorder
    Pain disorder
    Hypochondriasis
    Conversion disorder
Pain-prone patient (Engle 1959)
Factitious disorder
Malingering

present with a complaint of pain and associated pain behaviors (see Chapter 8, "Somatoform and Related Disorders," in this volume). Personality disorders can present with pain behavior in the absence of demonstrable pathological problems. The patient with an antisocial personality disorder may use pain to evade prosecution or to manipulate health care personnel to obtain narcotics and other drugs (malingering). Patients with borderline personality disorder may involve physicians in pathological relationships in which pain relief is the overt goal. Engle (1959) described these patients as "pain-prone."

Depression

Major depressive disorder is present in 30% or more of patients with chronic pain. Some authors, such as Lindsay and Wyckoff (1981), reported that as many as 87% of 300 patients referred to a pain center were depressed (Feighner diagnostic criteria). These authors also examined 196 patients referred for depression and found that 59% had pain complaints. Patients with depression and pain often will deny depression and depressed mood ("Doc, I'm not depressed. If I didn't have the pain, everything would be fine."). The key to diagnosis is a thorough investigation of all the signs and symptoms of depression (depressed mood, anhedonia, sleep disturbance, decreased interest, impaired concentration, anergy, guilt, psychomotor retardation or agitation, and suicidal ideation or preoccupation with death).

Anxiety

Anxiety and fear intensify pain. Unfortunately, patients often are not aware of the heightened anxiety and instead report an increase in pain. Low-dose neuroleptics (e.g., perphenazine, 2 mg, twice a day) or benzodiazepines are sometimes useful adjuvants to pain medications in the highly anxious patient (Drasner et al. 1992). Most patients with chronic pain have pain-related anxiety. When present, it predicts a dysfunctional adjustment to chronic pain (McCracken et al. 1999). Cognitive therapy can help patients to identify cause-and-effect misattributions related to their pain and anxiety symptoms. For example, when patients have fearful thoughts about when the next pain flare-up will occur, substituting more adaptive thoughts prevents the fears from becoming self-fulfilling prophecies.

Somatoform Disorders

Patients with somatoform disorders (see Chapter 8, "Somatoform and Related Disorders," in this volume) periodically complain of chronic pain. In fact, individuals with somatization disorder must have four pain symptoms during the course of their disturbance to meet DSM-IV-TR (American Psychiatric Association 2000) diagnostic criteria. Three other somatoform disorders to consider are hypochondriasis, conversion disorder, and pain disorder.

Measurement of Pain

The only way to determine whether a patient is in pain and the severity of that pain is to ask him or her. Changes in vital signs often but not always accompany acute pain and do not accompany chronic pain, so clinicians cannot rely on vital signs to determine the presence or severity of a patient's pain. Patients with pain, even severe pain, can be distracted from thinking about their pain and may even sleep. Hypnosis, which is arguably a form of therapeutic distraction, is used to effectively relieve pain, even severe pain. Because a patient "looks comfortable" does not mean that he or she does not have pain. Bottom line: pain is subjective; no objective measures exist. However, pain can be quantified with several assessment tools. The simplest method is to ask the patient to rate his or her pain intensity on a scale of 0 (no pain) to 10 (the worst pain imaginable). Other methods are listed in the following subsections.

Visual Analog Scale

The Visual Analog Scale (VAS) is a commonly used clinical and research scale. Patients rate their pain on a 100-mm scale from 0 to 10, with 0 being no pain and 10 being "extreme pain" or "the worst pain you've ever experienced." The VAS is commonly used in research studies, in which a 50% reduction in a patient's report of pain is considered significant.

Pain Drawing

A pain drawing (Figure 12–1) offers the patient an opportunity to present the pain graphically. The drawings are clinically valuable and show both the quality and the distribution of a patient's pain complaints. These drawings should be part of the evaluation of a patient with pain.

Other Useful Scales

Numerous other pain scales exist, including a color scale and facial expression scale. The color scale consists of a colored stripe that changes from white (no pain) through shades of pink to dark red (worst possible pain). The clinician should ask the patient to point to the area on the scale that shows his or her level of pain. A number scale next to the colored stripe quantifies pain severity. Several facial expression scales are used with children, adults who do not speak English, patients on respirators, and elderly patients who are demented or infirmed. The Faces Pain Scale for Adults and Children (Bieri et al. 1990) consists of eight images of faces with various expressions (e.g., smiling, frowning, grimacing). The patient selects the face that is consistent with his or her current level of pain.

Additional Aids to Diagnosis

Aids are available to help the psychiatrist identify whether significant psychological issues are present and to delineate the nature of these issues. An appropriate treatment plan can then follow.

Minnesota Multiphasic Personality Inventory

The Minnesota Multiphasic Personality Inventory–2 (MMPI-2; Butcher et al. 1989) is a useful diagnostic aid if used in combination with other information gathered during an examination. It is also helpful if obvious and subtle subscale scores are available. Occasionally, a physician will send a consultation note that states, "Give MMPI" (e.g., orthopedic surgeons often make this request for patients with chronic low back pain). The use of psychological tests alone to make psychiatric diagnoses is inappropriate. A blind interpretation of a patient's MMPI score without clinical correlation often leads to misdiagnosis because the patient with medical illness will endorse items on the MMPI/MMPI-2 that elevate the (Hy) hysteria and (Hs) hypochondriasis scales (Mapou et al. 2002).

Projective Tests

Projective tests such as the Rorschach inkblot test or Thematic Apperception Test may identify unconscious issues that play an important role in the perpetuation of pain.

Sadomasochistic Index (Pain-Prone)

Engle (1959), in his classic paper, "'Psychogenic' Pain and the Pain-Prone Patient," beautifully described patients who are predisposed to develop chronic pain because of their upbringings and personalities. These pain-prone patients share a common trait: a high sadomasochistic index. The histories of these patients are replete with punishing, abusive relationships, and their interpersonal interactions are often angry and bitter. Such patients are not consciously aware of the sadomasochistic nature of their relationships. Therefore, evaluation of patients' past and present relationships for this malignant sadomasochistic quality helps to identify such pain-prone individuals.

Physical Examination of the Patient With Pain

A physical examination is essential in a patient who has chronic pain (Deyo et al. 1992) and also may aid diagnosis in a patient who has acute pain. Psychiatrists who are unwilling to touch patients during an evaluation cannot properly treat patients with pain. "The physical examination involves a traditional neurological examination, during which the clinician looks for abnormal pain behavior, inconsistencies, and vague or changeable findings" (Holmgren et al. 2002, p. 1004). A physical examination also should include examination of the pain site and observation for sympathetic nervous system dysfunction (skin flushing, unusual sweating). The clinician should look for signs of central pain (see Table 12–3), such as pinprick felt as light touch, allodynia (perceived pain from nonnoxious stimuli), paroxysmal bouts of pain, hyperpathia, or allesthesia (sensation in one limb referred to the other).

Pharmacotherapy and Adjunctive Treatments for Pain

Pain and Placebo Effect

The placebo effect and "true" effects are *not* independent, consistent, or related to personality. Prior conditioning, active versus inactive placebo, and expectation all can vary the placebo response within and among individuals. Unfortunately, physicians and occasionally nurses still "test" a patient with pain by surreptitious substitution of saline for a strong analgesic. The intention is to test whether the patient's pain is "real." This is not helpful, and it usually destroys the physician-patient relationship by establishing the physician as an agent of deception. A positive placebo response (i.e., analgesia with saline) does not prove that the pain is bogus, that the person is an addict or malingerer, or that the patient would not benefit from an active medication. A significant percentage of healthy individuals have a positive placebo response. The more effective the previous medication, the more effective a subsequent placebo is likely to be; this is an expected, typical conditioned response. Placebo trials should be performed only with the cooperation of informed patients (Wall 1992). In fact, in 2000, the World Medical Association declared that the use of placebo medications in nearly all clinical trials is unethical when a treatment for that disease exists ("Direct-to-Consumer Ads Have Their Positive Side" 2000).

Analgesics

The initial choice of an analgesic for acute pain is typically based on the severity of pain reported by the patient (Table 12–5). Acute, very severe nociceptive pain, in the absence of a surgically or medically correctable cause, is best relieved by opiates. Opiates are not as efficacious in patients with central or chronic pain, whereas nonpharmacological treatment and other medications, such as antidepressants (e.g., duloxetine), anticonvulsants (e.g., clonazepam), neuropeptides (e.g., calcitonin in the case of phantom limb pain), α-adrenergic blockade, or clonidine, may prove more helpful (Maciewicz et al. 1985). The addition of nonpharmacological and pharmacological pain adjuvants such as stimulants, particularly in the terminally ill patient with continuous pain, may allow a reduction in opiate use and decrease side effects such as sedation.

Table 12–5. Pain severity and analgesic choice

Pain severity	Analgesic choice	Examples
Mild (pain score 1–3)[a]	Acetaminophen, nonsteroidal anti-inflammatory agents	Tylenol, ibuprofen (Motrin), naproxen (Naprosyn)
Moderate (pain score 4–6)[a]	Intravenous ketorolac, oral acetaminophen/opioid combinations	Toradol, Vicodin, Tylox, Tylenol with Codeine No. 3
Severe (pain score 7–10)[a]	Opioid	Morphine, hydromorphone (Dilaudid), fentanyl

[a]The patient is asked to rate his or her pain as follows: "Using a scale from 0 (no pain) to 10 (the worst pain that you have ever experienced or can imagine), where is your pain right now?"

Opiates (Narcotics)

Even though opiates are very effective in the treatment of nociceptive pain, they are underused in hospital settings. The reasons for undertreatment are physicians' underestimation of effective doses, overestimation of duration of action, and fears of addiction. Use of more than one narcotic is seldom necessary. Thus, a complicated regimen can almost always be simplified. A consulting psychiatrist who understands opiate pharmacology has the opportunity to improve patient treatment (Table 12–6).

Dependence

Physical dependence and tolerance (i.e., the dosage needed to achieve the same effect increases) may develop within the first weeks of opiate use. Physical dependence is usually manifest by withdrawal symptoms if the drug is discon-

Table 12–6.   Comparison of opiate potency and dosage

Drug (trade name)	Equal analgesic dose (mg) parenteral (im/iv)	Oral equivalent dose (mg)	Duration of analgesic (hours)
Opioid agonists			
Morphine[a]	10	30	4–5
Morphine sustained release (MS Contin, Oramorph SR)	—	30	8–12
Morphine sustained release (Kadian)	—	30	24
Hydromorphone (Dilaudid)	1.5	7.5	4–5
Codeine	120	200	4–6
Hydrocodone (Vicodin, Lortab)	—	30	4–6
Heroin	4	60	3–5
Fentanyl (Sublimaze, Duragesic)	0.1	—	1–2
Oxycodone (Percodan, Percocet, Tylox, Roxicet, Roxicodone)	—	20	4–6
Oxycodone controlled release (Oxycontin)	—	20	8–12
Levorphanol (Levo-Dromoran)	2	4	4–5
Meperidine (Demerol)	75–100	300	2–4
Methadone (Dolophine)	10	20	3–8
Propoxyphene (Darvon, Darvocet)	—	180–240	4

Table 12–6.   Comparison of opiate potency and dosage *(continued)*

Drug (trade name)	Equal analgesic dose (mg) parenteral (im/iv)	Oral equivalent dose (mg)	Duration of analgesic (hours)
Opioid agonists-antagonists[b]			
Butorphanol (Stadol)	2	—	2.5–3.5
Nalbuphine (Nubain)	12	—	4–6
Pentazocine (Talwin)	60	180	2–3

Note.   im = intramuscular; iv = intravenous.
[a]Divide total morphine use for 24 hours by 2 or 3, and give that number of milligrams of MS Contin two or three times a day, respectively.
[b]May precipitate withdrawal symptoms if patient has used pure opioid agonist(s) extensively. Abuse possible, but the potential for it is less.
Source.   Adapted from Bouckoms 1988, pp. 47–62; Hyman and Cassem 1989, pp. 1–17; Jaffe and Martin 1990, pp. 485–521.

tinued abruptly. The latter is preventable by gradually tapering the opiate. Narcotics that have partial antagonist properties (i.e., butorphanol, nalbuphine, pentazocine) can precipitate withdrawal in a patient taking another opiate.

Addiction and Pseudoaddiction

Addiction is a frequently misused term; it is a behavior disorder. It implies an overwhelming involvement with the use of a drug; extraordinary efforts to secure a supply, such as robbery; and a high likelihood of relapse following withdrawal. Porter reported that of 11,882 patients who received narcotics during hospitalization, 4 cases of abuse (0.03%) developed in patients with no history of problems (Jaffe and Martin 1990). Therefore, fear of abuse does not justify the routine undertreatment of pain. The proper selection of patients for opiate therapy is the key. Opiates should be used judiciously in patients with a history of abuse, an untreated affective illness, or a limited response to opiates in the past. When an acute injury occurs in a patient with a history of drug abuse or addiction, the amount of opiate needed by most patients undergoing a similar trauma should be used, and the medication should be tapered at a normal or typical pace.

Pseudoaddiction occurs when the underlying problem is untreated pain. The undertreated patient understandably becomes preoccupied with pain medications, may be demanding and irritable, and watches the clock intently anticipating his or her next dose. The medical staff often label such patients as drug seeking and may even withhold needed analgesics. The psychiatrist is often consulted in such cases to deal with (i.e., punish) the "addict." Fortunately, such cases are usually relatively easily resolved by talking to the patient, documenting pain severity, and reviewing the medication records. The patient's pain and mood improve markedly with increased opioid dosing.

Adverse Effects

Few side effects of opiates are serious. The only absolute contraindication is a documented allergy. (Note: many patients report an allergy to opiates, but they are not actually allergic. They have experienced a side effect, such as nausea and vomiting or hallucinations, not an allergic response.) Relative contraindications are severe bronchial asthma, increased intracranial pressure, and hypoxia (Bouckoms 1988). Common side effects are nausea, slight respiratory depression, sedation, and constipation (Table 12–7). Hypotension can

Table 12–7. Common narcotics-related problems and their solutions

Problem	Effects of problem	Solutions
As-needed (prn) dosing	Steep dose-response curve makes pain relief erratic (e.g., if one dose is missed, it can take 24 hours to return to therapeutic analgesia).	Avoid prn dosing.
Large individual variations in kinetics: Variation in release 5× variation in absorption 8× variation in volume of distribution 8× variation in elimination half-life	Failure to reach steady state	Sample solutions: MS Contin does not release morphine evenly, so 12-hour dosing intervals will have more peaks and troughs than oral morphine given every 4 hours; hence, give supplemental oral morphine doses until steady state is reached. Do not break, chew, or crush MS Contin tablets because release becomes more erratic if tablets are not ingested intact.
Underdosing	Ignorance and fear cause underdosing; safe administration of 450 mg/hour of iv morphine and 800 mg/day of oral morphine has been reported.	Dose adequately; avoid the three most common errors of underdosing when 1) switching from parenteral to oral forms of a narcotic, 2) beginning MS Contin, or 3) beginning fentanyl patches.
Active metabolites	Morphine-6-glucuronide (M6G), the most potent analgesic morphine sulfate metabolite, has a duration of action of 38–103 hours; M6G:MS ratio is 2:1 following a single dose of morphine and up to 20:1 during chronic use; the ratio reaches 45:1 during intrathecal administration.	Prescribe doses according to individual response. M6G levels may be more important in the spinal cord than in the brain. Measure M6G if possible.

Table 12–7.   Common narcotics-related problems and their solutions *(continued)*

Problem	Effects of problem	Solutions
Toxicity	Confusion, disorientation, hypomania, paranoia, hallucinations, seizures, muscle twitches, and agitation can occur with narcotics, especially meperidine, even at normal doses; normeperidine toxicity should be expected when meperidine is given iv, when renal function is impaired, or when dose exceeds 300 mg/day for more than 4 days.[a,b] Hydromorphone can produce myoclonus, even when other evidence of toxicity, such as sedation, is not evident. When GFR is poor and hydromorphone doses are high, toxicity may occur, even when equivalent doses of morphine were previously used without signs of toxicity.[c] Methadone doses necessary for analgesia on day 2 can accumulate and cause significant respiratory depression by day 5.	Morphine does not often cause toxicity; hence, it is the analgesic of choice for severe pain.
Errors in conversion from one route of administration to another (e.g., im to oral)	Lack of pain relief when switching from parenteral to oral (e.g., failure to triple the dose of morphine when switching from im to oral).	Transdermal fentanyl takes 24 hours to reach steady state; hence, augmentation with narcotics is necessary during the first 24 hours. Because methadone's analgesic half-life is 6 hours, methadone for analgesic effect is given more frequently than when used to treat drug addiction.

Table 12–7. Common narcotics-related problems and their solutions *(continued)*

Problem	Effects of problem	Solutions
Renal impairment	Decreased renal clearance that occurs with aging may increase narcotics level 2–3 times in a 70-year-old compared with a 20-year-old patient.	Decrease dose of narcotic in elderly patients. Morphine, despite increased levels of morphine sulfate and its metabolites in elderly patients, is generally well tolerated. Hydromorphone and metabolites accumulate less than morphine in patients with decreased GFR.
Opiate-insensitive pain	Neuropathic pain, especially with low doses of narcotics, does not respond.	Perform single-blind test giving morphine, 10 mg iv bolus; positive result is relief of ongoing pain or >3 cm decrease on VAS; if no result, give morphine, 20 mg iv bolus; if no result, give naloxone, 0.4 mg iv bolus, to confirm lack of opiate effect.
Delivery of drug is not consistent or adequate	Erratic clinical response	Consider alternative methods of delivery: iv, intrathecal, epidural, ventricular, or transdermal.[d]
Tolerance or excessive sedation	Efficacy decreases or side effects make narcotic intolerable.	Narcotic adjuvants (e.g., methylphenidate or antidepressants).[e,f]

Note. iv=intravenous; GFR=glomerular filtration rate; im=intramuscular; VAS=Visual Analog Scale.
[a]Bruera et al. 1992; [b]Jellema 1987; [c]Babul and Darke 1992; [d]Portenoy et al. 1990; [e]Bouckoms 1981; [f]Bruera et al. 1989.
Source. Reprinted from Holmgren A, Wise MG, Bouckoms AJ: "Pain Management," in *The American Psychiatric Publishing Textbook of Consultation-Liaison Psychiatry: Psychiatry in the Medically Ill,* 2nd Edition. Edited by Wise MG, Rundell JR. Washington, DC, American Psychiatric Publishing, 2002, p. 994. Copyright 2002, American Psychiatric Publishing. Used with permission.

occur, and hallucinations and confusional states can develop, particularly with meperidine (its metabolite normeperidine is neurotoxic) but less frequently with morphine.

Pharmacological Adjuvants

Pharmacological adjuvants improve the efficacy of analgesics. Psychostimulants (amphetamines, methylphenidate), serotonin-norepinephrine reuptake inhibitor(SNRI) antidepressants, anticonvulsants, benzodiazepines, antihistamines, neuroleptics, prostaglandin inhibitors, and nitrous oxide are effective adjuvants (Bouckoms 1988). Among antidepressants, duloxetine, venlafaxine (at higher doses), amitriptyline, or desipramine is recommended, whereas selective serotonin reuptake inhibitors such as fluoxetine are probably no more effective than placebo in a nondepressed patient who has chronic or persistent pain (Max et al. 1992). Trazodone is a frequently used adjuvant; in addition to effects on the pain syndrome itself, it significantly improves sleep and appetite.

Treatment and Management of Chronic Pain

An integrative approach to treatment planning is essential. Therefore, the psychiatrist must communicate directly with the patient and with the other treating clinicians. The psychiatrist should focus with the patient on modulating pain and increasing function rather than on a "cure" (Holmgren et al. 2002). We do not discuss in detail the diverse medications used in chronic pain treatment (e.g., steroids, nonsteroidal anti-inflammatory drugs, dextromethorphan, mexiletine, muscle relaxants, clonidine, calcium channel blockers, antihistamines, topical medications). Analgesics and surgical procedures are rarely curative in such patients. Treatment fads to alleviate chronic pain come and go (Deyo 1991), and patients who have chronic pain are desperate for relief.

Table 12–8 summarizes management principles for patients with chronic pain syndromes. Table 12–9 defines behavioral and psychotherapeutic techniques that are effective treatments of chronic pain and help to decrease or obviate the need for medications.

Table 12–8. Management principles for patients with chronic pain

Evaluate the patient with a multidisciplinary team, and treat the patient with active case management to prevent doctor shopping.

Ask how the pain and the condition causing the pain have affected the patient's life. The answer to that question frequently identifies potential psychosocial arenas for intervention.

Minimize medication use, and eliminate narcotics (in most cases).

Do not rely on "rest" as the centerpiece of management.

Ask patients to set goals focused around improved physical and psychosocial functioning.

Use physical therapy and behavioral treatment methods (see Table 12–9), which can markedly reduce or eliminate the need for analgesic medications.

Treat depression and anxiety disorders when present (use SNRIs), and work to decrease psychosocial stressors that may sustain pain or increase suffering.

Mobilize the patient, and work to improve function. The treatment plan's primary aim is to restore activity.

Reinforce increased activity (e.g., exercise), not maladaptive pain behaviors (e.g., groaning, medication-seeking).

Do no harm. Use surgical procedures only when clear evidence of reversible pathology exists.

Note. SNRI=serotonin-norepinephrine reuptake inhibitor.

References

American Psychiatric Association: Diagnostic and Statistical Manual of Mental Disorders, 4th Edition, Text Revision. Washington, DC, American Psychiatric Association, 2000

Babul N, Darke AC: Putative role of hydromorphone metabolites in myoclonus (letter). Pain 51:260–261, 1992

Beecher HK: The powerful placebo. JAMA 159:1602–1606, 1955

Bieri D, Reeve R, Champion G, et al: The Faces Pain Scale for the self assessment of severity of pain experienced by children: development, initial validation, and preliminary investigation for ratio scale properties. Pain 41:139–150, 1990

Bouckoms A: The role of psychotropics, anticonvulsants, and prostaglandin inhibitors. Drug Therapy 6(11):41–48, 1981

Bouckoms AJ: Pharmacologic treatment of severe pain and suffering in the critically ill patient, in Problems in Critical Care: Psychiatric Aspects of Critical Care Medicine. Edited by Wise MG. Philadelphia, PA, JB Lippincott, 1988, pp 47–62

Table 12–9.　Behavioral treatment methods for pain

Biofeedback	Computer-assisted measurement of physiological changes—previously thought to be involuntary—which brings them under voluntary control. Measurements can include surface electromyelography, temperature, galvanic skin response, respiration, pulse transit time, and distal plesmography.
Autogenic training	Mental exercises designed to produce relaxation imagery through suggestion that is sometimes coupled with relaxation and exercises.
Progressive muscle relaxation	A systematic approach to relaxation exercises involving the tensing and relaxing of muscle groups.
Hypnosis	A state of enhanced focus or awareness that can lead to increased levels of suggestibility. In some patients, this can reduce or block painful sensations.
Cognitive-behavioral therapy	Monitoring negative thoughts; recognizing the relation among thoughts, affects, and behaviors; and altering or replacing dysfunctional thoughts with more reality-oriented ones.

Source.　Adapted from Smith and Beers 1997, p. 281.

Bouckoms A, Hackett TP: The pain patient: evaluation and treatment, in Massachusetts General Hospital Handbook of General Hospital Psychiatry, 3rd Edition. Edited by Cassem NH. St. Louis, MO, Mosby-Year Book, 1991, pp 39–68

Bruera E, Brenneis C, Paterson AHG, et al: Use of methylphenidate as an adjuvant to narcotic analgesics in patients with advanced cancer. J Pain Symptom Manage 4:3–6, 1989

Bruera E, Schoeller T, Montejo G: Organic hallucinosis in patients receiving high doses of opiates for cancer pain. Pain 48:397–399, 1992

Butcher JN, Dahlstrom WG, Graham JR, et al: Manual for Administration and Scoring, Minnesota Multiphasic Personality Inventory—2: MMPI-2. Minneapolis, University of Minnesota, 1989

Cleeland CS, Gonin R, Hatfield AK, et al: Pain and its treatment in outpatients with metastatic cancer. N Engl J Med 330:592–596, 1994

Deyo RA: Fads in the treatment of low back pain. N Engl J Med 325:1039–1040, 1991

Deyo RA, Cherkin DC, Loeser JD, et al: Morbidity and mortality in association with operations on the lumbar spine: the influence of age, diagnosis, and procedure. J Bone Joint Surg Am 74:536–543, 1992

Direct-to-consumer ads have their positive side. Psychiatric News, February 4, 2000

Drasner K, Katz JA, Schapera A: Control of pain and anxiety, in Principles of Critical Care. Edited by Hall JB, Schmidt GA, Wood LDH. New York, McGraw-Hill, 1992, pp 958–973

Dworkin SF, Von Korff M, LeResche L: Multiple pains and psychiatric disturbance: an epidemiologic investigation. Arch Gen Psychiatry 47:239–244, 1990

Engle GL: "Psychogenic" pain and the pain-prone patient. Am J Med 26:899–918, 1959

Guglielmo WJ: Treating pain: can doctors put their fears to rest? Med Econ 77:46–48, 53–54, 57–58 passim, 2000

Holmgren A, Wise MG, Bouckoms AJ: Pain management, in The American Psychiatric Publishing Textbook of Consultation-Liaison Psychiatry: Psychiatry in the Medically Ill, 2nd Edition. Edited by Wise MG, Rundell JR. Washington, DC, American Psychiatric Publishing, 2002, pp 989–1013

Hyman SE, Cassem NH: Pain, in Scientific American Medicine (Current Topics in Medicine, Chapter II). Edited by Rubenstein E, Federman DD. New York, Scientific American, 1989, pp 1–17

Jaffe JH, Martin WR: Opioid analgesics and antagonists, in The Pharmacological Basis of Therapeutics, 8th Edition. Edited by Gilman AG, Rall TW, Nies AS, et al. New York, Pergamon, 1990, pp 485–521

Jellema JG: Hallucinations during sustained-release morphine and methadone administration (letter). Lancet 2:392, 1987

Juul D, Scheiber SC, Kramer TA: Subspecialty certification by the American Board of Psychiatry and Neurology. Acad Psychiatry 28:12–17, 2004

Lindsay PG, Wyckoff M: The depression-pain syndrome and its response to antidepressants. Psychosomatics 22:571–573, 1981

Maciewicz R, Bouckoms A, Martin JB: Drug therapy of neuropathic pain. Clin J Pain 1:39–49, 1985

Mapou RL, Law WA, Spector J, et al: Neuropsychological and psychological assessment, in The American Psychiatric Publishing Textbook of Consultation-Liaison Psychiatry: Psychiatry in the Medically Ill, 2nd Edition. Edited by Wise MG, Rundell JR. Washington, DC, American Psychiatric Publishing, 2002, pp 77–105

Max MB, Lynch SA, Muir J, et al: Effects of desipramine, amitriptyline, and fluoxetine on pain in diabetic neuropathy. N Engl J Med 326:1250–1256, 1992

McCracken LM, Spertus IL, Janeck A, et al: Behavioral dimensions of adjustment in persons with chronic pain: pain-related anxiety and acceptance. Pain 80:283–289, 1999

Melzack R: The tragedy of needless pain. Sci Am 262:27–33, 1990

Portenoy R, Foley K, Inturrisi R: The nature of opioid responsiveness and its implications for neuropathic pain: new hypothesis derived from studies of opioids infusions. Pain 43:273–286, 1990

Smith G, Beers D: Pain, in Behavioral Medicine in Primary Care: A Practical Guide. Edited by Feldman MD, Christensen JF. Stamford, CT, Appleton & Lange, 1997, pp 277–283

Additional Readings

Fields H, Liebeskind J (eds): Pharmacological Approaches to the Treatment of Chronic Pain: Concepts and Critical Issues. New York, IASP Press, 1994

Fishbain DA: Types of pain treatment facilities and referral selection criteria. Arch Fam Med 4:58–66, 1995

Joint Commission on Accreditation of Healthcare Organizations and National Pharmaceutic Council: Improving the Quality of Pain Management Through Measurement and Action. Oakbrook Terrace, IL, Joint Commission Resources, March 2003

National Pharmaceutic Council and Joint Commission on Accreditation of Healthcare Organizations: Pain: Current Understanding of Assessment, Management and Treatments. Oakbrook Terrace, IL, Joint Commission Resources, December 2001

Wall PD: The placebo effect: an unpopular topic. Pain 51:1–3, 1992

13

Personality, Response to Illness, and Medical Psychotherapy

Personality is a consistent and to some extent predictable set of behaviors that characterize a person's management of day-to-day living. These long-term traits are generally stable and usually ego-syntonic. However, stress can disturb the usual balance between needs, drives, external reality, and conscience. For example, medical illness and hospitalization present the patient with a strange, stressful, and demanding environment that may destabilize personality function. Most individuals are highly resilient and cope well with an illness or injury. When personality issues complicate the treatment of an illness or hinder the patient's cooperation with the medical or nursing staff, the consultation-liaison psychiatrist is often consulted.

Personality and Response to Illness

Psychological Regression

A person with an acute, serious illness who is admitted to a hospital may psychologically regress. This regression may be catalyzed by a loss of control of

239

Table 13–1. Individual defenses: common responses to illness

High adaptive level (optimal adaptation in handling stress)
  Affiliation
  Altruism
  Anticipation
  Humor
  Self-assertion
  Self-observation
  Sublimation
  Suppression
Mental inhibitions level (keeps threats and fears out of awareness)
  Displacement
  Dissociation
  Intellectualization
  Isolation of affect
  Reaction formation
  Repression
  Undoing
Minor image-distorting level (distortions used to regulate self-esteem)
  Devaluation
  Idealization
  Omnipotence
Disavowal level (removal from awareness or misattribution)
  Denial
  Projection
  Rationalization
Major image-distorting level (gross distortion or misattribution)
  Autistic fantasy
  Projective identification
  Splitting of self-image or image of others
Action level (deals with stressors by action or withdrawal)
  Acting out
  Apathetic withdrawal
  Complaining
  Help-rejecting
  Passive aggression

Table 13–1. Individual defenses: common responses
to illness *(continued)*

Level of defensive dysregulation (pronounced break with reality)
  Delusional projection
  Psychotic denial
  Psychotic distortion

Source. Adapted from American Psychiatric Association: *Diagnostic and Statistical Manual of Mental Disorders,* 4th Edition, Text Revision. Washington, DC, American Psychiatric Association, 2000, pp. 808–809. Copyright 2000, American Psychiatric Association. Used with permission.

basic body functions, such as eating, sleeping, and bladder and bowel control. The degree to which this is a problem depends on the severity of stress, the patient's baseline level of psychological functioning, and the quality of social supports. A regressed hospitalized patient would be unduly dependent on or demanding of the staff. A patient's behavior during times of severe stress does not necessarily reflect long-term personality dysfunction or the presence of a personality disorder.

Levels of Ego Defenses

Understanding the patient's defense or coping mechanisms is one way to identify his or her behavioral tendencies both during times of severe stress and, more importantly, during times of less stress. If the consultation-liaison psychiatrist's interventions can reduce anxiety and discomfort, the patient should be able to return to more typical, hopefully mature, defenses. DSM-IV-TR (American Psychiatric Association 2000) contains a method for the assessment of defense mechanisms and coping styles—the Defensive Functioning Scale. The Defensive Functioning Scale organizes these defense mechanisms (Table 13–1) from the highest (most adaptive) to the lowest (least adaptive) level.

Denial and displacement are common defenses seen in psychosomatic medicine patients. A patient in denial who avoids any expression of fear or dysphoria about a serious prognosis may complicate the course of the illness. A patient who displaces may change subjects when asked to talk about the illness or injury. A patient's characteristic defense mechanisms may stir powerful feelings in his or her providers and treatment team; these feelings may stimulate the consultation and may provide important diagnostic information for the consulting psychiatrist.

Personality and General Medical Conditions

Personality can interact with somatic illness in many ways. Maladaptive behaviors can directly increase the risk of diseases. For example, alcohol abuse can lead to liver disease, or failure to use a seat belt can lead to traumatic injury. Alternatively, chronic medical conditions, such as chronic pain or life-threatening chronic illness, can lead to maladaptive chronic behavior patterns (e.g., expectation of disappointment and rejection). Finally, neurological and medical conditions can produce profound personality change.

When an adult experiences a change in personality, the clinician should consider potential medical and toxic etiologies. Central nervous system (CNS) insults may either change personality traits or magnify preexisting ones. Various CNS lesions or conditions can cause secondary personality syndromes (see Table 13–2). The family of a patient with a secondary personality syndrome often reports that the patient is "not himself." Appropriate social behavior often disappears. Apathy, suspiciousness, affective instability, poor impulse control, and a change in demeanor also can occur.

Frontal lobe injuries, tumors, abscesses, and other lesions predispose patients to personality change or dysfunction. CNS frontal lobe lesions are common because of the vulnerability of the prefrontal cortex and frontal cortex to injury; in many cases, cognitive abilities are relatively preserved. Table 13–3 lists the clinical features of patients with frontal lobe personality syndromes.

Personality Disorder

Definition

"Personality traits—characteristic behavioral response patterns—are the typical ways that an individual thinks, feels, and relates to others. When these patterns are fixed, inflexible, unresponsive to changes in the environment, and maladaptive, they can result in psychological and social dysfunction" (Ursano et al. 2002, p. 116). Such behavior patterns may constitute a personality disorder. DSM-IV-TR includes 11 personality disorders: paranoid, schizoid, schizotypal, antisocial, borderline, histrionic, narcissistic, avoidant, dependent, obsessive-compulsive, and not otherwise specified.

Table 13–2. Medical causes of personality change

Alcoholic dementia

Alzheimer's disease (may be late manifestation)

Central nervous system tumors

Encephalitis

Frontal lobe disease (especially degenerative/ablative)

Head trauma

Human immunodeficiency virus infection

Huntington's disease

Medication adverse effects (e.g., steroids, thyroid medications, psychotropic medications)

Meningitis (acute and chronic)

Neurosurgical procedures

Neurosyphilis

Parkinson's disease

Pick's disease

Poisons

Postconcussional syndrome

Psychosurgery

Stroke

Subarachnoid hemorrhage

Subcortical dementia (often a major manifestation)

Temporal lobe disease (especially irritative/seizure)

Clinical Characteristics

Personality disorders are established by late adolescence or early adulthood. Behaviors associated with personality disorders are ego-syntonic. The behaviors feel "natural," and the individual may not understand why his or her actions upset others. The diagnosis of a personality disorder is based on long-term historical data, not on behavior at one point in time, especially a stressful time such as hospitalization with a life-threatening illness. Patients with personality disorders frequently lack empathy and usually believe that the environment must change when problems arise. CNS (especially frontal lobe) disease, head trauma, stressors, and situations that induce psychological regression can exacerbate personality dysfunction.

Table 13–3.   Clinical characteristics of frontal lobe syndromes

Disinhibition
Talkativeness
Pranks and joking
Lack of concern for future
Sexual indiscretion
Unconcern for feelings of others
Concentration or attention impairment
Cognitive function largely intact
Lack of initiative
Slowed psychomotor activity
Hyperactive tendon reflexes (may be present)
Tactlessness
Childish excitement
Diminished social control
Lack of concern for consequences of actions
Mood elevation
Inability to carry out planned activities
Lack of spontaneity
Grasp reflex
Babinski's sign (may be present)

Patients with personality disorders also affect the physician's and staff's abilities to respond appropriately, leading to nontherapeutic behaviors, such as avoiding the patient, not responding to a change in symptoms, or assigning the patient's care to the least skilled member of the team. In this way, countertransference can influence the patient's clinical outcome.

Differential Diagnosis

Included in the differential diagnosis of a personality disorder are all Axis I psychiatric disorders, personality traits, stress-related psychological regression, and secondary personality syndromes. Other characterological disturbances exist besides the official list of Axis II conditions in DSM-IV-TR (Ursano et al. 2002). Many of these conditions, such as alexithymia and type A behavior pattern, are of interest to consultation psychiatrists. As an example, alexithymia is an impaired ability to perceive or express emotions. In a severe form, it might qualify as a personality disorder because the individual's characteristic way of dealing with feelings is maladaptive and inflexible. Patients with alexithymia focus on nonemotional aspects of disease, such as pain or physical dysfunction, rather than on their emotions and internal distress. However, the operational definition makes reliable measurement of alexithymia difficult. In various studies, alexithymia was highly prevalent in patients with psychosomatic conditions, chronic psychogenic pain, and psychological conditions affecting a physiological disorder (Taylor et al. 1990). Some conditions, such as dysthymic disorder, cyclothymic disorder, and dissociative identity disorder (formerly called multiple personality disorder), are categorized by DSM-IV-TR as Axis I disorders, even though they are more characteristic of a personality disorder. DSM-IV-TR also provides criteria sets for depressive personality disorder and passive-aggressive personality disorder for further study to determine whether they are valid and discernible personality disorders.

Treatment and Management

General Considerations

Patients with a personality disorder rarely seek treatment; patterns of behavior are ingrained, stable, and "comfortable." More commonly, someone else, such as a family member or hospital staff, wants the patient's behavior to change, especially when the behavior complicates medical management. The psychiatric consult that is requested is not desired by the patient, who will likely see himself or herself as a victim, not the problem.

After receiving a consult on a patient with personality or coping style problems, the psychiatrist must 1) identify and attempt to reverse any remediable organic factors (Table 13–2), 2) carefully consider whether other psychiatric disorders are present, 3) establish baseline and current levels of personality functioning and past responses to stressors, and 4) try to understand the meaning of the illness and hospitalization to the patient. Optimal management of maladaptive stress responses is not possible without an understanding of how the patient sees himself or herself with this illness at this time (Groves and Kucharski 1991). In other words, why this patient and why now? Armed with these data, the consultant can recommend the most appropriate psychopharmacological, psychotherapeutic, and ward management interventions.

Pharmacotherapy

Neuroleptics. Patients with borderline, schizotypal, or paranoid personality disorders sometimes experience micropsychotic episodes, especially when stressed and regressed. These episodes frequently respond to low doses of neuroleptic medication. Drug treatment also may improve impulse control, mood, and severe, disabling anxiety.

Antidepressants. Antidepressant medications are indicated when clinical major depressive disorder occurs in a patient with a personality disorder. Antidepressants also can decrease affective instability in patients with borderline personality disorder. When such patients are taking antidepressants, the potential for overdose is often high, and a nonlethal medication should be used.

Lithium. Lithium helps to decrease affective symptoms and emotional lability in some patients with personality disorder. Patients with impulse control difficulty also may benefit from lithium.

Antianxiety agents and sedative-hypnotics. Antianxiety and sedative-hypnotic medications should be prescribed with caution and avoided when possible because patients with personality disorders are at risk for substance abuse, disinhibition, and overdose. However, judicious use of low-dose benzodiazepines for acute anxiety is sometimes necessary.

Other medications. Carbamazepine or propranolol may be effective in many patients with aggressive and assaultive behavior caused by secondary personality syndrome, explosive type (Patterson 1987). Patients with impulsive features (borderline, histrionic, antisocial, narcissistic, and dependent personality disorders) are at risk for suicidal gestures. Therefore, medications should be prescribed cautiously and in limited quantities at discharge. Antisocial patients often show drug-seeking behavior.

Group Psychotherapy

Group treatments are very useful for patients who tend to express affects through somatic representation. Such groups tend to facilitate communication with several people who may share similar diagnoses, characteristics, interests, anxieties, and misperceptions about illness (Lipsitt 2002). Patients learn from one another, depend less on the therapist, share stressful experiences, and sometimes model behavior after the therapist or other group members. Groups may be psychoeducational; supportive; expressive; homogeneous or heterogeneous (regarding illness); closed or open-ended; and inpatient, day hospital, or outpatient.

Clinic and Ward Management

Staff issues. Patients with personality syndromes or regressive behaviors often engender anxiety, anger, rage, resentment, an urge to punish, or avoidance behavior in the staff. The consultant may defuse a tense situation by educating the staff members about the patient's personality and why they feel or react as they do. This approach usually decreases the intensity of affect among hospital personnel and is hoped to translate into decreased affect in the patient. Giving the staff articles such as "Taking Care of the Hateful Patient" (Groves 1978) is helpful.

Patient issues. When staff-patient conflict exists, the consultant should objectively consider whether the patient has legitimate complaints. If legitimate problems exist, the consultant should help correct them. For some patients, especially patients with obsessive-compulsive personality styles, consultants should work with the treatment team to resurrect the patient's intellectual defenses. Giving the patient as much control as possible over treatment and activity decisions may decrease anxiety and unreasonable demands.

More frequently, however, patients require appropriate boundaries, structure, and limit setting. External control helps the primitively functioning or regressed patient retain internal control. Boundaries and limit setting are not punitive; they provide structure for the patient. Borderline, histrionic, antisocial, dependent, and narcissistic personality disorder patients are most likely to require such structure.

Transference and countertransference. Illness, hospitalization, pain, and fear increase the frequency and intensity of transference reactions. The physician is seen as a reliable parent or as an authority figure from the past. Alternatively, the physician is viewed with fear and suspicion as a disappointing figure from the past (Ursano et al. 1998). Manifestations of the transference to the physician and the medical staff may prompt the request for a psychiatric consultation. During the assessment, the patient also may develop similar transference feelings toward the consultation-liaison psychiatrist. Usually, however, the patient's transference feelings toward the consultation-liaison psychiatrist are less intense because the consultant has had much less contact with the patient. To assess countertransference, the psychiatrist uses his or her reactions to a patient as information to help understand what the treatment team experiences; this information can help the consultation-liaison psychiatrist make effective recommendations (Ursano et al. 2002).

Medical Psychotherapy

Definition

Medical psychotherapy is defined as "that which is intentionally (as contrasted with coincidentally) exercised on patients with medical illness by physicians with psychiatric training" (Lipsitt 2002, p. 1028). The ultimate aim of medical psychotherapy is to apply biopsychosocial interventions systematically to encourage psychotherapeutic change. Attempts to remove psychological defenses are almost always counterproductive. The consulting psychiatrist must remember that patients under the stress of hospitalization and severe illness use less "mature" but nevertheless adaptive defenses. Even if they cause problems for the ward or clinic, these defenses are the patient's best available coping tools and, unless dangerous, should initially be supported. A frontal assault on defenses usually makes matters worse, causing intense fear, despair, anger, or even psychosis.

Selection Process

Traditional selection criteria do not apply in inpatient or even some outpatient psychosomatic medicine settings. The consulting psychiatrist goes to the patient; the patient does not select the consulting psychiatrist. Patients typically have not identified a particular emotional issue for which they need help; the attending physician, house officer, or nurse requests the consultation. In fact, in inpatient settings, the patient rarely knows about the psychiatric consultation until the psychiatrist presents at the bedside. Patients in the psychosomatic medicine setting therefore seldom have the motivation for or receptivity to psychotherapy in its usual sense (Lipsitt 2002).

Setting

Although consultation psychiatrists provide their services in a variety of outpatient facilities, the setting of the medical psychotherapist is often the bedside, a hospital or clinic conference room, an intensive care unit, or—in special circumstances—even a hallway; medical psychotherapy rarely occurs in a well-furnished, quiet office. Hospitalized patients wear hospital garb and have little privacy.

The stereotypical 50-minute hour is nowhere more challenged than in medical settings, where encounters may last anywhere from a few minutes to more than 1 hour (Lipsitt 2002). Initial consultations or psychotherapy evaluations are often done in installments that are dictated by the patient's and staff members' schedules.

Associative Anamnesis

One interview technique especially suited to psychosomatic medicine work is associative anamnesis (Deutsch and Murphy 1955), which was derived in part from the psychoanalytic free associative process. Deutsch and Murphy found that both physiological and psychological data could be obtained by allowing the patient considerable latitude in speaking about his or her symptoms. They noted that the patient "drifts into a communication in which he inattentively mixes emotional and symptom material" (p. 20). In this way, they said, "it is possible to observe the somatic and the psychic components more nearly simultaneously" (p. 19). Through repetition of key somatic or affective words (the interviewer is not passive), "the patient is stimulated to give the needed information" (p. 20).

Formulation

The consultation psychiatrist must use data from a variety of sources to derive a formulation. The formulation, as much as if not more than the DSM-IV-TR diagnosis, is the consultation psychiatrist's road map to intervention (Lipsitt 2002).

Table 13–4 summarizes essential elements of the medical psychotherapy formulation.

Table 13–4. Elements of medical psychotherapy formulation

Character structure ("personality diagnosis")

Presenting problem (reason for request of consultation)

Patient's narrative (life story), including perceptions and attributions of current illness

Identified life event(s) or crisis that precipitated response

Defenses used by patient to negotiate stresses of medical illness, surgery, and hospitalization

Patterns from past are predictors of patient's response to caregivers and treatment interventions

Leads to guidelines for

   Psychotherapeutic intervention

   Physicians and other staff about

      Physician-patient relationship

      Relevance of patient's behavior to current illness

      Consulting psychiatrist's role in the care of the patient

Source. Adapted from Lipsitt DR: "Psychotherapy," in *The American Psychiatric Publishing Textbook of Consultation-Liaison Psychiatry: Psychiatry in the Medically Ill,* 2nd Edition. Edited by Wise MG, Rundell JR. Washington, DC, American Psychiatric Publishing, 2002, p. 1041. Copyright 2002, American Psychiatric Publishing. Used with permission.

References

American Psychiatric Association: Diagnostic and Statistical Manual of Mental Disorders, 4th Edition, Text Revision. Washington, DC, American Psychiatric Association, 2000

Deutsch F, Murphy W: The Clinical Interview. New York, International Universities Press, 1955

Groves JE: Taking care of the hateful patient. N Engl J Med 298:883–887, 1978

Groves JE, Kucharski A: Brief psychotherapy, in Massachusetts General Hospital Handbook of General Hospital Psychiatry. Edited by Cassem NH. St. Louis, MO, Mosby-Year Book, 1991, pp 321–341

Lipsitt DR: Psychotherapy, in The American Psychiatric Publishing Textbook of Consultation-Liaison Psychiatry: Psychiatry in the Medically Ill, 2nd Edition. Edited by Wise MG, Rundell JR. Washington, DC, American Psychiatric Publishing, 2002, pp 1027–1051

Patterson JF: Carbamazepine for assaultive patients with organic brain disease. Psychosomatics 28:579–581, 1987

Taylor GJ, Bagby RM, Ryan DP, et al: Validation of the alexithymia construct: a measurement-based approach. Can J Psychiatry 35:290–297, 1990

Ursano RJ, Sonnenberg SM, Lazar S: Concise Guide to Psychodynamic Psychotherapy: Principles and Techniques in the Era of Managed Care, 2nd Edition. Washington, DC, American Psychiatric Press, 1998

Ursano RJ, Epstein RS, Lazar SG: Behavioral responses to illness: personality and personality disorders, in The American Psychiatric Publishing Textbook of Consultation-Liaison Psychiatry: Psychiatry in the Medically Ill, 2nd Edition. Edited by Wise MG, Rundell JR. Washington, DC, American Psychiatric Publishing, 2002, pp 107–125

Additional Readings

Bloom BL: Focused single-session therapy: initial development and evaluation, in Forms of Brief Therapy. Edited by Budman S. New York, Guilford, 1981, pp 131–175

Horowitz MJ: Stress Response Syndromes. New York, Jason Aronson, 1976

Lipsitt DR: The patient-physician relationship in the treatment of hypochondriasis, in Hypochondriasis: Modern Perspectives on an Ancient Malady. Edited by Starcevic V, Lipsitt DR. New York, Oxford University Press, 2001, pp 265–290

Pyszczynski T, Greenberg J, Solomon S: A dual-process model of defense against conscious and unconscious death-related thoughts. Psychol Rev 106:835–845, 1999

Vaillant GE: Theoretical hierarchy of adaptive ego mechanisms. Arch Gen Psychiatry 24:107–118, 1971

Yamanda S, Greene G, Bauman K, et al: A biopsychosocial approach to finding common ground in the clinical encounter. Acad Med 75:643–648, 2000

14

Medicolegal Issues
in Consultation

We begin this chapter with a legal disclaimer—we are not lawyers! The views expressed in this chapter come from consultation psychiatrists who have dealt for many years with cases that raise thorny legal and ethical issues. Laws vary from state to state, legal precedents change, and hospitals have their own policies (e.g., do not resuscitate [DNR]). Therefore, clinicians must become familiar with pertinent general legal concepts, state laws, and hospital policies. Remember that it is always better for the physician to practice good medicine than to attempt to be a lawyer and practice bad medicine (Groves and Vaccarino 1987). There is no substitute for good faith, common sense, excellent documentation, and a high standard of medical care (Shouton et al. 1991); however, in difficult situations, it is occasionally necessary to consult a lawyer who understands medical practice and malpractice.

When a medicolegal issue arises, or could arise at some future time, very detailed documentation in the patient's medical record is of paramount importance. Fear that the patient will read the record should not preclude documentation. In fact, the consultation and notes should be written with the

Table 14–1.   Four elements needed to establish malpractice

1. Would a reasonable, careful, and prudent physician behave in the same or similar way (i.e., determine standard of care)?

2. Did the physician breach that standard of care in this specific case?

3. Was the patient injured?

4. Did the physician's unreasonable, careless, or inappropriate behavior cause that injury?

Source.   Adapted from Shouton et al. 1991.

expectation that the patient will read the medical record. Remember that a person who claims medical malpractice must prove four things (Table 14–1): 1) the standard of care can be established; 2) the physician breached the standard of care, 3) the patient sustained an injury, and 4) the physician's behavior caused the injury.

The terminology used in this chapter may or may not be familiar. For that reason, Table 14–2 contains a brief explanation of terms used; each definition is discussed in more detail in the following sections.

Confidentiality

A patient has the right to have confidential communications withheld from outside parties unless he or she gives authorization to release that information. Consultation work is unique in that the patient is not the customer. Once a consult is generated, the answer is given to the consultee, not the patient. Therefore, a patient-physician relationship does not exist. The consulting physician can accept or reject the opinion and recommendations of the consulting psychiatrist. The psychiatrist is unlikely to be found liable for adverse outcomes when his or her suggestions are not followed; however, he or she will likely be named in the suit along with everyone else. If the psychiatrist provides follow-up visits, and definitely if the psychiatrist writes orders, a patient-physician relationship likely exists and so does liability (Simon 2002). In any case, the psychiatrists should inform the patient about the flow of information at the beginning of a consultation.

Psychiatrists do not have carte blanche authorization when speaking to hospital staff members about all matters revealed by the patient (Simon 2002). Psychiatrists should only provide information sufficient to enable the staff to

Table 14–2. Definitions of terms

Confidentiality—the ethical and legal duty to not disclose information obtained in the course of evaluating or treating the patient without the patient's express or implied permission.

Competency—a court determination that a patient has the mental capacity to understand the nature of an act.

Capacity—a psychiatrist's determination, through examination, that a patient has the ability to understand and participate in medical and treatment decisions.

Informed consent—voluntary agreement by a competent person after full disclosure of facts needed to make a decision.

Right to refuse treatment—the right to determine what is or is not done to one's body (also called the right of self-determination).

Advance directives—health care documents (i.e., living will, durable power of attorney, or health care proxy) executed by competent individuals that state health care decisions and designate substitute health care decision makers in the event of future incompetence.

Guardianship—One who is appointed by the court and is legally responsible for the care and management of an incompetent person (sometimes called conservatorship).

Seclusion and restraint—treatment interventions that involve isolating the patient and/or physical or chemical immobilization.

function effectively on behalf of the patient. Rarely is it necessary to disclose intimate details about the patient's life; common statutory exceptions to confidentiality are summarized in Table 14–3.

In the strictest sense of the law, a psychiatrist performing a consultation should not speak to a patient's family or significant other without the patient's permission. Fortunately, the patient's refusal to allow the physician to contact the family or significant other is uncommon. If the patient refuses, the patient's reasons should be documented in a clear note in the medical record. The reverse phenomenon also can occur; the family or significant other may not want the patient told about his or her diagnosis and prognosis. The most understandable reason for this request is to protect the patient from the emotional trauma of a terminal diagnosis. With reassurance and the realization that secrecy is impossible and is almost always destructive rather than helpful, full communication is usually restored. Sometimes the request for secrecy is symptomatic of long-standing maladaptive relationships within the family. A

Table 14–3.   Common statutory exceptions to confidentiality between psychiatrist and patient

Child abuse

Competency proceedings

Court-ordered examination

Danger to self or others

Patient as a litigant

Intent to commit a crime or harmful act

Civil commitment proceedings

Communication with other treatment providers

Source.   Adapted from Simon RI: "Legal and Ethical Issues," in *The American Psychiatric Publishing Textbook of Consultation-Liaison Psychiatry: Psychiatry in the Medically Ill,* 2nd Edition. Edited by Wise MG, Rundell JR. Washington, DC, American Psychiatric Publishing, 2002, pp. 167–189. Copyright 2002, American Psychiatric Publishing. Used with permission.

brief consultation is unlikely to correct this situation; however, a useful focus is to help the staff deal with and provide care for a patient who has difficult family members.

Competency Versus Capacity

"In general, *competency* refers to some minimal mental, cognitive, or behavioral ability, trait, or capability required to perform a particular legally recognized act or to assume a legal role" (Simon 2002, p. 172). In this regard, it is clinically useful to differentiate between the terms *incompetence* and *incapacity.* Competency versus incompetency is a judicial decision, whereas incapacity refers to a clinical determination that is made by the consulting psychiatrist (Leo 1999; Mishkin 1989). Consultations to "evaluate competency" are actually evaluations for capacity; nevertheless, the term *competency* is in such wide use in clinical medicine that it is difficult to avoid using the term when discussing cases with consultees.

Incapacity does not prevent treatment. It merely means that the clinician must obtain substitute consent. The consultation question "Is the patient competent?" requires immediate clarification by asking, "Competent for what?" The determination of "competency" is not an all-or-none phenomenon. For example, a patient may be judged incompetent by the court to manage his or her financial affairs but still may be considered competent to refuse a medical procedure.

"Competency" evaluations constitute from 4% to 25% of the consults on a psychiatric consultation service; that number is increasing (Leo 1999). These consults are often urgent requests; most patients are found "competent" (Farnsworth 1990; Mebane and Rauch 1990). Most are requested because a patient refuses treatment or disposition (e.g., transfer from the hospital to a nursing home) or threatens to leave the hospital against medical advice (AMA) (Farnsworth 1990; Mebane and Rauch 1990). Masand et al. (1998) prospectively studied 88 consecutive requests for competency assessment and found that 38% involved the patient's ability to care for self, 27% of the patients had refused medical care, 18% of the patients wanted to sign out AMA, 18% of the physicians questioned the ability of the patient to give informed consent, and 14% involved other reasons. More rarely, physicians request evaluations to confirm a patient's capacity to give informed consent. Because the patient's mental status can change from one hour to the next, repetitive examinations are often necessary.

Roth and colleagues (1977) proposed a standard of competency that is important for the consultation psychiatrist to understand and apply. It is based on two variables: the treatment's risk-benefit ratio and the patient's decision regarding treatment (Figure 14–1). For example, a patient has a gangrenous leg, and amputation is proposed to save his life. The danger (potential risks) of this procedure to the patient is relatively low, and the benefits are high. Therefore, if the patient refuses amputation (cell B), a rigorous (high) threshold to establish competency is applied. Failure to pass this competency test, indicating that the patient lacks capacity, would lead the psychiatrist to recommend that the physician and the patient's family or significant other pursue court action to appoint a surrogate decision maker. If the patient consents to amputation (cell A), a lenient (low) threshold to establish competency is used. In contrast, in a clinical situation in which the surgical procedure is quite risky (e.g., heart transplant), a lenient (low) threshold to establish competency is applied to the patient who refuses the treatment (cell C). Consent to a heart transplant requires a stringent (high) threshold to establish competency because of the high mortality and morbidity associated with the procedure (cell D).

Treatment risk-benefit ratio

Patient's decision	Favorable outcome likely (i.e., relatively low risk and/or high potential benefit)	Unfavorable or question-able outcome quite possible (i.e., high risk)
Patient consents	**A** Low threshold for competency	**D** High threshold for competency
Patient refuses	**B** High threshold for competency	**C** Low threshold for competency

Figure 14–1.   Factors used to select competency threshold.

Source.   Adapted from Roth LH, Meisel A, Lidz CW: "Tests of Competency to Consent to Treatment." *American Journal of Psychiatry* 124:279–284, 1977. Copyright 1977, American Psychiatric Association. Used with permission.

The assessment of capacity to refuse treatment is not a simple process, and exact documentation is essential (i.e., write exact quotations in the medical record whenever possible), especially if the patient is refusing potentially life-saving or life-altering treatment. In some cases, the clinician may want a witness present who can verify that the details of the interview were reported accurately in the medical record. Impairment on mental status examinations (e.g., a Mini-Mental State Exam score of 10) is insufficient to declare a patient incompetent to make medical decisions. Such tests measure cognitive ability, not the ability to make decisions (Leo 1999). Table 14–4 describes the evaluation of a patient's capacity to make treatment decisions. When collecting this information, the clinician should use open-ended questions (e.g., "Tell me about your current medical condition"), avoid questions that require only "yes" or "no" answers, and pursue or clarify vague answers. For example, if the patient's only reply is, "I'm seriously ill" in response to the aforementioned question about the patient's condition, the clinician might ask the patient to describe the serious illness.

When the chance of future incompetency is high (e.g., Alzheimer's disease, cancer with brain metastasis), the psychiatrist should urge the patient and family, or significant other, to make immediate legal arrangements. The

Table 14–4. Assessment of capacity to make treatment decisions

Does the patient understand his or her

 Current medical condition?

 Expected course?

 Recommended treatment?

 Risks and benefits of treatment?

 Likely course without treatment?

 Treatment alternatives?

 Risks and benefits of alternative treatment(s)?

Source. Adapted from Leo 1999.

patient, while still competent, can prepare a living will or a durable power of attorney (Howe 1988; Leo 1999). The latter is a legal means of appointing a surrogate individual to make medical decisions when the patient is unable to do so.

Informed Consent and the Right to Refuse Medical Treatment

Informed consent requires an informed patient (i.e., one who can understand the information provided and is capable of making a reasoned judgment about the treatment or procedure). According to Simon (2002), there are four basic exceptions to the requirement of obtaining informed consent:

1. *Emergencies:* When the physician administers appropriate treatment in a medically emergent situation in which the patient or other people are endangered, and it has proved impossible to obtain either the patient's consent or that of someone authorized to provide consent for the patient, the law typically "presumes" that consent was granted.
2. *Incompetency:* Only a competent person can provide informed consent. When the patient does not have the capacity to provide consent, it is obtained from a substitute decision maker.
3. *Therapeutic privilege:* This exception is the most difficult to apply. Informed consent is not required if a psychiatrist determines that a complete disclosure of possible risks and alternatives might have a deleterious effect on the patient's health and welfare. This determination and its

rationale must be carefully documented; in such cases, it is prudent to obtain a second opinion from a respected colleague.

4. *Waiver:* A patient may voluntarily waive his or her right to information (e.g., the patient does not want information on possible negative surgical outcomes).

Signing Out Against Medical Advice

Leaving a hospital or emergency department AMA is the right of any competent patient, so long as he or she understands the nature and consequences of the act (Groves and Vaccarino 1987). The standard of competency will vary depending on the risk-benefit ratio in a particular situation (see Figure 14–1). A threat or an attempt to sign out AMA often signifies a communication problem between the patient (who may have a personality disorder or may not be coping well or both) and the staff. Patients who leave AMA often return to the hospital if the physician has not explicitly denied further care.

If the patient is not a danger to self or others and is competent, the psychiatrist cannot do much more than try to deal with the discharge as a treatment issue. A patient is not required to sign the hospital's AMA form before departure. If he or she refuses to sign the form, the clinician should simply write on the form, "Patient refused to sign form" or "Patient departed without signing the AMA form," and then sign and date the document. Regardless of whether the patient signs an AMA form, the situation is documented in the medical record, along with the annotated AMA form, detailing the recommendations made to the patient about further hospitalization and the possible risks of premature discharge.

Do-Not-Resuscitate (DNR) Orders

Patients who require cardiopulmonary resuscitation (CPR) usually have not thought about or expressed a preference about its use, and there is no time to think about the consequences of reviving a patient at the time of a cardiac arrest. A competent patient has the right to reject or insist on resuscitative treatment; that right is rarely overruled (Simon 2002). One exception is when the rights of a spouse or child are considered more important than the patient's decision (Miles et al. 1982). In certain situations, DNR status does not always mean resuscitation will not be attempted. When emergency medical services

(EMS) were called to long-term care facilities, resuscitation was attempted in 21% of residences who had requested DNR status (Becker et al. 2003). Also, when a cardiopulmonary arrest occurs during hemodialysis, resuscitation may be attempted even when a DNR order exists (Ross 2003). When a competent patient either requests or declines resuscitation and later becomes incompetent, a court may be required to reverse the patient's original decision (Miles et al. 1982). In some states, the family or significant other, physician, and/or hospital ethics committee can intervene to resuscitate the patient if a chance of recovery exists. If a patient has a major mental disorder (e.g., severe depression) and rejects resuscitation because he or she desires death as an "appropriate deserved" outcome, the patient is considered incompetent (Simon 2002). The consultant in the latter case would recommend that the family or significant other seek guardianship.

Do-not-resuscitate orders are written on the physician's order sheet, and the date, time, and reasons for the DNR order are documented in the chart. Hospital CPR policies make DNR decisions discretionary (Simon 2002). Hemphill and colleagues (2004) studied all admissions for intracerebral hemorrhage in nonfederal hospitals in California over 2 years ($N=8,233$). The percentage of patients with DNR orders varied from 0% to 70% across hospitals. Hemphill et al. concluded, "Being treated in a hospital that used DNR orders 10% more often than another hospital with a similar case mix increased a patient's odds of dying during hospitalization by 13% ($P<0.001$)" (p. 1130). Psychiatrists should become familiar with the specific hospital's policy before a DNR order is written.

Advance Directives

The Patient Self-Determination Act requires all hospitals, nursing homes, hospices, managed care organizations, and home health care agencies to advise patients or family members of their right to accept or refuse medical care in the form of an advance directive (Simon 2002). A living will is an example of an advance directive. This law also states that a hospital must, if the hospital wishes to receive Medicare and Medicaid payments, 1) develop policies about advance directives, 2) ask all patients admitted to the hospital if they have advance directives and enter those into the chart, 3) give patients information about advance directives, and 4) educate the staff and community about advance directives (Greco et al. 1991).

Unlike advance directives, the ordinary power of attorney created for the management of business and financial matters becomes null and void when the person who created it becomes incompetent. Only a durable power of attorney empowers an agent to make health care decisions. This document is much broader and more flexible than a living will, which covers just the period of a diagnosed terminal illness and specifies only that no extraordinary treatment be used to prolong life. To clarify the status of the durable power of attorney for health care decisions, several states have passed health care proxy laws. The health care proxy is a legal instrument like the durable power of attorney but is specifically created for the delegation of health care decisions.

Unfortunately, durable power of attorney agreements or health care proxies are easily revoked, even when reasonable evidence indicates that the patient is incompetent (Simon 2002). If the patient is grossly confused and is an immediate danger to self and others, the physician is on firm medical and legal ground to temporarily override the patient's treatment refusal. Otherwise, it is generally better to seek a court order for treatment than to risk legal entanglement by attempting to enforce the advance directive's original terms.

Guardianship

Under the American system of law, an individual is presumed competent unless adjudicated incompetent. Thus, incompetence is a legal determination made by a court of law on the basis of evidence that the individual's mental capacity is significantly impaired. For individuals who are judicially determined as unable to act for themselves, guardianship establishes a substitute decision maker (Leo 1999). In general,

> the appointment of a guardian is limited to situations in which the individual's decision-making capacity is so impaired that he or she is unable to care for personal safety or provide necessities such as food, shelter, clothing, and medical care (*In re Boyer* 1981). The standard of proof required for a judicial determination of incompetency is clear and convincing evidence. Although the law does not assign percentages to proof, clear and convincing evidence is in the range of 75% certainty. (Simon 2002, p. 177)

In many jurisdictions, there are two separate types of guardianship. A *specific* guardian is authorized to make decisions about a particular subject area, such as major or emergency medical procedures. A *general* guardian, by contrast, has total control over the disabled individual's person, estate, or both (Sales et al. 1982).

The process required to adjudicate incompetence is burdensome, costly, and lengthy and frequently interferes with treatment. The family is often unwilling to face court proceedings, declare their family member incompetent, and disclose sensitive family matters. To be successful, the family must understand that this is a time-consuming and taxing process (Burruss et al. 2000). Clear advantages are associated with having a surrogate or family member be the decision maker (Leo 1999). First, it maintains the integrity of the family unit and relies on those who are most likely to know the patient's wishes. Second, it is more efficient and less costly. There are some disadvantages, however. It can be legally risky to decide that a patient is incompetent and rely on the consent of a family member. Some family members may be more impaired than the patient, and relatives may not be available or want to get involved. Some patients recover competency within a short time. As soon as the patient recovers sufficient mental capacity, consent for further treatment should be obtained directly from the patient.

Involuntary Hospitalization

"Three main substantive criteria serve as the foundation for all statutory commitment requirements. These criteria require that the individual is 1) mentally ill, 2) dangerous to self or others, and/or 3) unable to provide for basic needs" (i.e., gravely disabled) (Simon 2002, p. 179). Clinicians do not legally commit patients; only a court can do that. The psychiatrist merely initiates a medical certification that brings the patient before the court, which usually occurs after a brief evaluation in the hospital (Simon 2002). Commitment laws vary greatly from state to state. A psychiatrist providing consultations to other physicians needs to become knowledgeable about local commitment laws and procedures, as well as local mental health treatment resources.

The psychiatrist, or the staff at the general hospital, may want to transfer a medically ill patient involuntarily to a psychiatric unit. For a few reasons, this is usually not possible. Fewer and fewer general hospitals have psychiatric units, and those that do are unwilling to accept medically ill patients. If the patient requires an intravenous line, he or she is typically too ill for a psychiatric facility. For these reasons, the solution is often to have the consultation psychiatrist take an active role in behavioral or psychiatric management of the patient in the general hospital setting. This helps decrease the medical staff's anxiety and can strengthen the relationship that the psychiatrist has with medical staff colleagues. A few medical settings have medical-psychiatric units, which are an ideal solution for the medical staff, the psychiatrist, and the patient.

Restraints

"Stringent legal regulation of seclusion and restraint has increased during the past decade, as have legal challenges on the use of seclusion and restraint in institutionalized mentally ill and mentally retarded patients" (Simon 2002, p. 180). These challenges make the legal issues surrounding seclusion and restraint especially complex for the consultation psychiatrist. It is enlightening to review contraindications to the use of restraints in a psychiatric facility (Simon 2002)—extremely unstable medical or psychiatric conditions and delirium or dementia. These are usually the indications for restraints in a general hospital setting! A common scenario in a general hospital is an agitated, paranoid, combative, confused (read delirious) patient who is seriously medically ill and in an intensive care unit (ICU); chemical and physical restraints are needed. Unrestrained delirious ICU patients can and do remove oxygen masks and pull out endotracheal tubes, arterial lines, intravenous lines, and, in one instance known to the authors, an intra-aortic balloon pump. Moreover, confused, medically ill patients will sometimes hit medical staff, climb over bed rails, and fall onto the floor. Such falls can result in fractures and subdural hematomas. Courts hold that restraints and seclusion are appropriate only when a patient presents a risk of harm to self or others, and a less restrictive alternative is not available (Simon 2002).

Restraint and seclusion must be implemented by a written order from an appropriate medical official. A physician on call at night can give a verbal order for restraint, as long as the patient is examined soon thereafter and an order is written. The examining physician must document the reasons for restraint (i.e., details of the patient's behavior), details of the examination, and types of restraint needed (e.g., two-point, waist-belt, vest, medication). Orders must be confined to specific, time-limited periods, and the patient's physical and mental condition must be regularly reviewed and documented. Extension of the original order must be reviewed and reauthorized.

Prescribing "Unapproved" Medications

The Food and Drug Administration (FDA) establishes the package label for all prescription drugs. This label contains information about use, dosages, method of administration, frequency, duration, relevant risks, contraindications, side effects, and precautions in prescribing the drug. The FDA evaluates only the clinical indications requested by the drug company. Failure to indicate other uses typically means that the FDA did not receive a request to review those data. The FDA applies the principle that good medical practice requires that a physician prescribe medication according to the best information available. Prescribing an FDA-approved medication for an unapproved purpose does not violate federal law (Macbeth et al. 1994). However, the physician who deviates from the package insert may have to explain such a departure should a lawsuit arise.

Consultation psychiatrists frequently prescribe medications for uses not approved by the FDA. For example, no drug is currently approved by the FDA for the treatment of delirium. However, several drugs are used, including neuroleptics and benzodiazepines, in the case of alcohol withdrawal. Nevertheless, prescribing drugs for nonapproved uses should be based on sound knowledge of the drugs, firm scientific rationale, and medical data. The psychiatrist should have texts or journal articles available to substantiate that a nonapproved use is accepted practice.

According to Simon (2002), the need for obtaining informed consent is heightened when a medication is prescribed for an unapproved use. This presents unique problems for consultation psychiatrists who almost daily see patients with serious medical illness, delirium, and/or dementia. The situation is often emergent, and the patient may lack capacity (is incompetent and cannot give informed consent). Intravenous haloperidol—not FDA approved for intravenous use, for delirium, or for the large doses sometimes used—has been used effectively thousands and thousands of times for more than 25 years. If the psychiatrist approaches the patient's family to obtain consent for intravenous haloperidol, the recommendation may be quickly rejected, "Why is a psychiatrist seeing my mother?!! She is not crazy!" or "You are not going to experiment on my mother with mind-altering drugs!" One method to deal with this difficult situation is to preemptively work with ICU staff and medical staff to develop an accepted, approved hospital or ICU protocol for delirious patients based on a review of the literature. That way, the medical or ICU staff can approach the family and reassure them that "this is what we do in cases such as this."

References

Becker LJ, Yeargin K, Rea TD, et al: Resuscitation of residents with do not resuscitate orders in long-term care facilities. Prehosp Emerg Care 7:303–306, 2003

Burruss JW, Kunik ME, Molinari V, et al: Guardianship applications for elderly patients: why do they fail? Psychiatr Serv 51:522–524, 2000

Farnsworth MG: Competency evaluations in a general hospital. Psychosomatics 31:60–66, 1990

Greco PJ, Schulman KA, Lavizzo-Mourey R, et al: The patient self-determination act and the future of advance directives. Ann Intern Med 115:639–643, 1991

Groves JE, Vaccarino JM: Legal aspects of consultation, in Massachusetts General Hospital Handbook of General Hospital Psychiatry. Edited by Hackett IP, Cassem NH. Littleton, MA, PSG Publishing, 1987, pp 591–604

Hemphill JC 3rd, Newman J, Zhao S, et al: Hospital usage of early do-not-resuscitate orders and outcome after intracerebral hemorrhage. Stroke 35:1130–1134, 2004

Howe EG: Forensic issues in critical care medicine, in Problems in Critical Care. Edited by Wise MG. Philadelphia, PA, JB Lippincott, 1988, pp 171–187

Leo RJ: Competency and the capacity to make treatment decisions: a primer for primary care physicians. Prim Care Companion J Clin Psychiatry 1:131–141, 1999

Lothen-Kline C, Howard DE, Hamburger EK, et al: Truth and consequences: ethics, confidentiality, and disclosure in adolescent longitudinal prevention research. J Adolesc Health 33:385–394, 2003

Macbeth JE, Wheeler AM, Sither JW, et al: Legal and Risk Management Issues in the Practice of Psychiatry. Washington, DC, Psychiatrists Purchasing Group, 1994

Masand PS, Bouckoms AJ, Fischel SV, et al: A prospective multicenter study of competency evaluations by psychiatric consultation services. Psychosomatics 39:55–60, 1998

Mebane AH, Rauch HB: When do physicians request competency evaluations? Psychosomatics 31:40–46, 1990

Miles SH, Cranford R, Schultz AL: The do-not-resuscitate order in a teaching hospital. Ann Intern Med 96:660–664, 1982

Mishkin B: Determining the capacity for making health care decisions, in Issues in Geriatric Psychiatry (Advances in Psychosomatic Medicine Series, Vol 19). Edited by Billig N, Rabins PV. Basel, Switzerland, Karger, 1989, pp 151–166

Ross LF: Do not resuscitate orders and iatrogenic arrest during dialysis: should "No" mean "No"? Semin Dial 16:395–398, 2003

Roth LH, Meisel A, Lidz CW: Tests of competency to consent to treatment. Am J Psychiatry 134:279–284, 1977

Sales BD, Powell DM, Van Duizend R: Disabled Persons and the Law: Law, Society, and Policy Services, Vol 1. New York, Plenum, 1982, p 461

Shouton R, Groves JE, Vaccarino JM: Legal aspects of consultation, in Massachusetts General Hospital Handbook of General Hospital Psychiatry, 3rd Edition. Edited by Cassem NH. St. Louis, MO, Mosby-Year Book, 1991, pp 619–638

Simon RI: Legal and ethical issues, in The American Psychiatric Publishing Textbook of Consultation-Liaison Psychiatry: Psychiatry in the Medically Ill, 2nd Edition. Edited by Wise MG, Rundell JR. Washington, DC, American Psychiatric Publishing, 2002, pp 167–189

Additional Readings

Appelbaum PS: Privacy in psychiatric treatment: threats and responses. Am J Psychiatry 159:1809–1818, 2002

Cantor MD, Braddock CH 3rd, Derse AR: Do-not resuscitate orders and medical futility. Arch Intern Med 163:2689–2694, 2003

Simon RI: Clinical Psychiatry and the Law, 3rd Edition. Washington, DC, American Psychiatric Publishing, 2001

15

Suicidality

For physicians, few events evoke more anguish than the loss of a patient by suicide. Unlike many psychiatric symptoms or syndromes, suicidal statements or behaviors usually lead to prompt psychiatric referral. Unfortunately, considerable research has yet to identify specific indicators that would assist a population-based prevention program in making significant inroads into the baseline *population* suicide rate (Kessler et al. 1999). However, a clinically useful systematic approach to the assessment and management of suicidality among potentially suicidal *individuals* is possible.

Epidemiology

Completed Suicides

General Population

Suicide is the eighth leading cause of death in the United States. At a rate of 11 per 100,000 per year, it accounts for 1.3% of deaths from all causes (Ventura et al. 1998). The most successful suicide method is shooting. The elderly account for one-fourth of suicides, although they account for only 10% of the population. Suicides among whites occur at twice the rate in nonwhites, except for Native Americans. Clear warning signs precede 80% of suicides; 82% see a physician within 6 months and 53% within 1 month of a completed suicide. The rate of suicide is twice as high in families of suicide victims as in families with comparison subjects who die of other causes (Runeson and Asberg 2003).

Table 15–1 summarizes suicide risk factors in the general population. The male-to-female ratio for suicide is 3:1. Over the course of the life cycle, men and women also have different patterns of suicide. For men, suicide rates gradually rise during adolescence, increase sharply in early adulthood, and parallel advancing age up to the 75- to 84-year age bracket, at which time they reach a rate of 22.0 suicides per 100,000 (Schneidman 1989). Men tend to use more violent means, such as shooting, hanging, and jumping. For women, suicide rates peak in midlife, then decline. Marriage, especially if there are children, significantly lessens the risk of suicide. Marital separation, however, represents a higher risk than having never been married. Divorced men have four times the suicide rate of married men, and divorced women have three times the rate of married women.

Medical-Surgical Patients

Physical disease is an independent suicide risk factor, present in 25%–75% of people who commit suicide (Kontaxakis et al. 1988). In nearly all suicides among medical-surgical patients, the patients had a history of recent loss of emotional support; anger was the predominant affect. Table 15–2 summarizes clinical observations associated with suicide among medical-surgical patients.

The reported suicide rate in most hospitals is lower than in the general population, varying between 3.2 and 15.0 per 100,000 per year (Sanders 1988). Access to means of suicide is more difficult in hospitals, and patients who give clear warning signs are usually promptly attended to. Jumping is the most successful suicide method in general hospital patients. Most general hospital patients who commit suicide have chronic, painful, or disfiguring illnesses (Sanders 1988). They also have a high frequency of psychiatric illness, particularly mood disorders and alcohol use disorders. Interpersonal problems with family members and ward staff are common.

Table 15–1. Suicide risk factors in the general population

Psychiatric

Major depression—at least 40% of all suicides (particularly endogenous depression); risk is increased further if comorbid panic attacks are present

Alcohol dependence—25% of all suicides (rate 50–75 times that in the general population)

Drug addiction—10% die by suicide

Personality disorders—especially borderline and obsessive-compulsive

Schizophrenia—especially with hallucinations that command self-harm

Organic psychoses

History of suicide attempt(s)—especially if attempts were serious

Family history of suicide

Poor physical health—renal dialysis, cancer, human immunodeficiency virus infection, cardiorespiratory disease, terminal illness, disfiguring illness

Psychological

History of recent loss (spouse, child, parent, job, financial)

History of parental loss during childhood

Important dates—anniversaries, holidays, etc.

Family instability

Early life history of deprivation or abuse

Family exhausted with patient's illness

Giving away valued possessions

Social

Social isolation—loss of social supports

Sex—males three times the rate of females

Race—whites twice the rate of nonwhites, except in urban areas, where rate is the same; Native Americans have higher rates than other ethnic groups

Age—in men, rates rise with age greater than 45; in women, peak risk is about age 55, then the rate declines

Religion—Protestants and atheists have higher rates than Jews and Catholics

Geography—urban rates higher than rural rates

Marital status—divorced > single > widowed > married

Socioeconomic—high rates at both ends of spectrum; retired and unemployed at high risk

Table 15–2. Factors associated with suicide in medical-surgical patients

Chronic illness

Debilitating illness

Painful illness

Low pain tolerance

Renal dialysis

Cardiorespiratory disease

AIDS, AIDS-related complex, and HIV infection

Disrupted physician-patient relationship

Interpersonal problems with family or staff

Medical staff may appear more important to the patient than family is

Coexisting psychiatric illness, especially depression, substance use disorders, and personality disorder

Impulsivity

Alcohol, barbiturate, sedative-hypnotic, or narcotic withdrawal

Loss of emotional support

Poor social supports

Attempted Suicides

General Population

The ratio of suicide attempts to completions is about 10:1. In contrast to the 3:1 male-to-female ratio in completed suicides, a 3:1 female-to-male ratio exists for suicide attempts. Suicide attempts are a common reason for admissions to general hospitals. For example, 1%–2% of all admissions to emergency departments and 1%–5% of all admissions to medical intensive care units are drug overdoses (Bostwick 2002). The elderly attempt suicide less frequently than those younger than 65 but are successful more often.

Drugs used in nonlethal suicide attempts are commonly available: benzodiazepines, alcohol, nonnarcotic analgesics, antidepressants, barbiturates, and antihistamines. Overdoses of acetaminophen, with its potential liver toxicity and over-the-counter availability, are particularly likely to result in a medical-surgical or psychiatric admission (Litman 1989).

Medical-Surgical Patients

Although not well studied, the rate of attempted suicide in general hospital settings is estimated at 24 per 100,000 per year (Sanders 1988). The most frequent psychiatric diagnosis in attempters, in contrast to the depression and alcoholism in hospitalized suicide completers, is personality disorder. Again, a recent history of loss of emotional support is common. Wrist-slashing and drug overdose are the most common nonlethal suicide attempt methods in hospitals.

Clinical Features and Risk Factors

Whereas Table 15–1 summarizes psychiatric, psychological, and social risk factors for suicide, Table 15–3 describes a short, useful mnemonic—SAD PERSONS—to help with rapid bedside evaluation of suicide risk (Patterson et al. 1983).

Table 15–3. SAD PERSONS Scale

One point is scored for each positive factor

Scores:	0–2 = little risk
	3–4 = follow closely
	5–6 = strongly consider psychiatric hospitalization
	7–10 = very high risk; hospitalize or commit

Sex	Male—more men complete, more women attempt
Age	Elderly or adolescents
Depression	Especially with hopelessness
Previous attempt	Especially if potentially lethal
Ethanol abuse	Or other drugs
Rational thinking loss	Command hallucinations, organic brain syndrome
Social support deficit	Or perception of poor supports
Organized plan	Will, available means
No spouse	Separated, divorced, widowed, single
Sickness	Especially chronic and debilitating illnesses

Source. Adapted from Patterson et al. 1983.

Psychiatric Disorders Associated With Increased Suicide Risk

According to psychological autopsies, 95% of the patients who completed suicides had psychiatric diagnoses, including 40% with mood disorders, 20%–25% with alcoholism, 10%–15% with schizophrenia, and 20%–25% with personality disorders (Litman 1989). Of the patients with mood disorders, 15% will eventually commit suicide (Guze and Robins 1970), and 10% of the patients with schizophrenia will eventually kill themselves (Miles 1977), with the risk for both highest early in the illness course. More recent data suggest that the lifetime risk of suicide may be lower: 6% for mood disorders, 7% for alcohol dependence, and 4% for schizophrenia (Inskip et al. 1998).

History of a suicide attempt is an important predictor of future suicide risk. One of every 100 suicide attempt survivors will die by suicide within 1 year of the index attempt, a suicide risk approximately 100 times that of the general population (Hawton 1992). Suicide is often a response to a loss, real or metaphorical. Fantasies of revenge, punishment, reconciliation with a rejecting object, relief from the pain of loss, or reunion with a dead loved one may be evident (Furst and Ostow 1979). Holidays and anniversaries of important days in the life and death of the deceased loved one also increase suicide risk.

Medical Disorders Associated With Increased Suicide Risk

Reviews of death certificates indicate that about 5% of suicide completers have a terminal illness (Murphy 1986); however, this rate may underrepresent the true prevalence. Many physicians misstate causes of death on death certificates to help patients' families avoid adverse financial and psychosocial consequences. Suicide rates higher than those in the general population are reported in cardiorespiratory patients, Alzheimer's disease patients, patients on renal dialysis, cancer patients, and patients infected with human immunodeficiency virus (HIV) (Bostwick 2002). The fear of pain, disfigurement, and loss of function from cancer, HIV disease, and chronic renal failure can precipitate suicide, particularly early in the patient's course. The high relative risk just after diagnosis corresponds to a time of greatest fear (Bostwick 2002).

Approach to the Patient

Epidemiological Risk Assessment

The proper assessment of suicidality requires a great deal of data. Much of the data can be collected, even from an uncooperative patient, by reviewing the medical record, interviewing the family, and talking to acquaintances and hospital staff. Simple demographic data such as age, sex, race, marital status, and religion provide other important epidemiological information.

Individual Risk Assessment

If suicide risk assessment were based on only epidemiological data, then many false-positive cases would result. Ultimately, the psychiatric examination of the *individual* patient leads to estimation of risk and a treatment plan. Asking a patient about suicidal ideation and plans does not increase suicide risk. Table 15–4 summarizes several important lines of inquiry. The psychiatrist should always inquire about recent real and perceived losses, including relationships, health, functional abilities, and physical integrity.

Treatment and Management

Identifying the Risk Level

Initial management decisions may be difficult because patients are often ambivalent about suicide. There is a gradation of risk. Most patients examined are at "some risk." Information from a third party often helps the clinician gain other perspectives on the patient's situation. The clinician should always err on the side of safety. The response of both patient and third party to the treatment plan gives some indication of the patient's resilience and of the social resources available to aid in recovery from the suicidal crisis.

Protecting the Patient

The physician must be particularly vigilant in the emergency department, which is an easy place for a suicidal patient to obtain the means for self-harm (Anderson and Tesar 1991). If the patient's suicide potential is questionable, he or she should be hospitalized, voluntarily or involuntarily. Once the patient is admitted to the hospital, his or her room should be secured (Bostwick

Table 15–4. Lines of questioning during examination of a potentially suicidal medical patient

Is the patient discouraged about his or her medical condition?

Does the patient believe that life is worth living?

Does the patient wish to die?

Does the patient have a plan?

What is the method planned?

Is there anything that would change his or her mind?

Does the patient have a history of recent substance abuse?

What medical illnesses are present?

What psychiatric diagnoses are present?

Does the patient have a history of suicide attempts?

Does the patient have a family history of suicide attempts?

Does the patient have a history of impulsivity?

What is the level of psychological defensive functioning?

Has the patient made a will recently?

Does the patient have a history of recent losses, and how do they relate to past losses?

Does the patient talk of plans for the future?

What is the nature of the patient's social support system?

2002). The staff must 1) remove anything that a patient could potentially use to injure himself or herself, such as sharp objects or material that could be fashioned into a noose; 2) search luggage and possessions; 3) monitor all objects coming into the room (e.g., the cutlery on the dinner tray) that are potential weapons; and 4) provide constant observation initially by using a sitter. The physician must carefully document the clinical diagnosis and treatment plan in the patient's chart; there is no room for communication error. Frequent updates and reassessments of suicide potential and the treatment plan are necessary.

Treating or Removing Risk Factors

Treatment of Psychiatric Disorders

Depressed patients should be given antidepressant medications. If the depressed suicidal patient is imminently suicidal, medically unable to tolerate antidepressants, or delusional, the psychiatrist should proceed directly to electroconvulsive therapy. He or she should observe the patient for a period of increased suicide risk as energy improves but hopelessness remains. Substance abuse issues should not be overlooked. Alcohol abuse is underdiagnosed among the medically ill, including patients in the general hospital. The psychiatrist should ask about command hallucinations and treat psychotic symptoms with neuroleptic medications. Any remediable causes of cognitive impairment must be removed.

Medical Psychotherapy

Brief psychotherapy is quite helpful in some patients, especially when dealing with themes of loss. The psychiatrist should approach such patients with an accepting, supportive, empathic, and concerned manner and attempt to develop a therapeutic alliance. The patient's family should be involved, whenever possible. The clinician should make an effort to reestablish or strengthen the patient's connections to friends or community social service agencies.

Ward or Outpatient Management

Hospitals have suicide precaution guidelines, which should be placed in the chart and communicated to the ward staff. Suicide risk level must be continuously reassessed. Staff must be aware of "hidden murderers" (i.e., individuals whose actions encourage a suicide attempt, such as an exhausted family member who "accidentally" leaves a knife on the patient's meal tray or leaves a window open); these may include family, hospital personnel, or even psychotherapists (Maltsberger and Buie 1974).

The clinician should treat agitation and overt suicidal behavior promptly with physical restraints, chemical restraints, or both. Physical restraints are often required if a patient is unpredictable or impulsive.

The consultant's chart notes should identify the level of suicide risk, clearly state the plan, and report the interval at which the consultant will return to continue the assessment and recommend modifications to the plan (Bostwick 2002). The consultant also should arrange follow-up care for the patient before discharge and detail it in the chart so that it is part of the inpatient's discharge plan.

In the emergency department or outpatient clinic setting, Davidson (1993) suggested that outpatient management is acceptable if the suicidal patient has 1) satisfactory impulse control, 2) no psychosis or intoxication,

3) no specific plan or easily accessible means, 4) accessible social supports to which he or she is willing to turn, and 5) a capacity for establishing rapport with the consultant.

References

Anderson WH, Tesar G: The emergency room, in Massachusetts General Hospital Handbook of General Hospital Psychiatry, 3rd Edition. Edited by Cassem NH. St. Louis, MO, Mosby-Year Book, 1991, pp 445–464

Bostwick JM: Suicidality, in The American Psychiatric Publishing Textbook of Consultation-Liaison Psychiatry: Psychiatry in the Medically Ill, 2nd Edition. Edited by Wise MG, Rundell JR. Washington, DC, American Psychiatric Publishing, 2002, pp 127–148

Davidson L: Suicide and aggression in the medical setting, in Psychiatric Care of the Medical Patient. Edited by Stoudemire A, Fogel BS. New York, Oxford University Press, 1993, pp 71–86

Furst S, Ostow M: The psychodynamics of suicide, in Suicide: Theory and Clinical Aspects. Edited by Hankoff LD, Einsidler B. Littleton, MA, PSG Publishing, 1979, pp 165–178

Guze SB, Robins E: Suicide and primary affective disorders. Br J Psychiatry 117:437–438, 1970

Hawton K: Suicide and attempted suicide, in Handbook of Affective Disorders, 2nd Edition. Edited by Paykel ES. New York, Guilford, 1992, pp 635–650

Inskip HM, Harris EC, Barradough B: Lifetime risk of suicide for affective disorder, alcoholism and schizophrenia. Br J Psychiatry 172:35–37, 1998

Kessler RC, Borges H, Walters EE: Prevalence of and risk factors for lifetime suicide attempts in the National Comorbidity Survey. Arch Gen Psychiatry 56:617–626, 1999

Kontaxakis VP, Christodoulou GN, Mavreas VG, et al: Attempted suicide in psychiatric outpatients with concurrent physical illness. Psychother Psychosom 50:201–206, 1988

Litman RE: Suicides: what do they have in mind?, in Suicide: Understanding and Responding. Edited by Jacobs D, Brown HN. Madison, CT, International Universities Press, 1989, pp 143–154

Maltsberger JT, Buie DH: Countertransference hate in the treatment of suicidal patients. Arch Gen Psychiatry 30:625–633, 1974

Miles CP: Conditions predisposing to suicide: a review. J Nerv Ment Dis 164:231–246, 1977

Murphy GE: Suicide and attempted suicide, in The Medical Basis of Psychiatry. Edited by Winokur G, Clayton PJ. Philadelphia, PA, WB Saunders, 1986, pp 562–579

Patterson WM, Dohn HH, Bird J, et al: Evaluation of suicidal patients: the SAD PERSONS scale. Psychosomatics 24:343–349, 1983

Runeson B, Asberg M: Family history of suicide among suicide victims. Am J Psychiatry 160:1525–1526, 2003

Sanders R: Suicidal behavior in critical care medicine: conceptual issues and management strategies, in Problems in Critical Care Medicine. Edited by Wise MG. Philadelphia, PA, JB Lippincott, 1988, pp 116–133

Schneidman ES: Overview: a multidimensional approach to suicide, in Suicide: Understanding and Responding. Edited by Jacobs D, Brown HN. Madison, CT, International Universities Press, 1989, pp 1–30

Ventura SJ, Anderson RN, Martin JA, et al: Births and deaths: preliminary data for 1997. Natl Vital Stat Rep 47:1–41, 1998

Additional Readings

Adams KS: Suicide and attempted suicide. Med Clin North Am 34:3200–3208, 1983

Berger D: Suicide risk in the general hospital. Psychiatry Clin Neurosci 49 (suppl 1): 585–589, 1995

Bostwick JM, Pankratz VS: Affective disorders and suicide risk: a reexamination. Am J Psychiatry 157:1925–1932, 2000

Burt RA: The Supreme Court speaks—not assisted suicide but a constitutional right to palliative care. N Engl J Med 337:1234–1236, 1997

Kaplan A, Klein R: Women and suicide, in Suicide: Understanding and Responding. Edited by Jacobs D, Brown HN. Madison, CT, International Universities Press, 1989, pp 257–282

Morgan AC: Special issues of assessment and treatment of suicide risk in the elderly, in Suicide: Understanding and Responding. Edited by Jacobs D, Brown HN. Madison, CT, International Universities Press, 1989, pp 239–255

Simon GE, VonKorff M: Suicide mortality among patients treated for depression in an insured population. Am J Epidemiol 147:155–160, 1998

16

Geriatric Psychiatry

Epidemiology

In 1900, people age 65 years and older made up only 4% of the total population; people age 65 years and older now make up 13% of the total population. The subgroup of elderly persons age 85 years and older is growing at an even faster pace, constituting 10% of those age 65 years and older in 1990 and a predicted 22% in 2050 (Unützer et al. 2002). The group age 85 years and older has the greatest frequency of chronic physical illnesses, dependency, and long-term care needs. By 2050, the number of persons with Alzheimer's disease will have tripled (Hebert et al. 2003). This means that psychiatrists who perform consultations for other physicians will increasingly function as geriatric psychiatrists.

Psychiatric Disorders

Delirium

Because of neuronal loss with aging and the likelihood of other risk factors, geriatric patients have an increased prevalence of delirium. Early signs include agitation, beclouded consciousness, sleep disturbance, irritability, hypoactivity or hyperactivity, disorientation, impaired short-term memory, perceptual disturbances, and fear or anxiety. As cognitive dysfunction progresses, disordered attention and concentration become prominent. (See Chapter 3, "Delirium," in this clinical manual for a complete discussion of delirium.)

Dementia

Dementia is a major public health challenge. The most common dementia, dementia of the Alzheimer's type, occurs in 3% of individuals ages 65–74 years, 19% of individuals ages 75–84 years, and 47% of individuals older than 85 (Unützer et al. 2002). Patients with dementia expend 3.3 times more Medicare cost than do nondemented patients; hospitalization was 54% of that cost (Bynum et al. 2004). The majority of elderly patients with dementia develop behavioral and psychological symptoms of dementia (BPSD) (e.g., psychosis, aggression, sleep disturbance, agitation, mood disorders) at some stage (Lawlor 2004), and their clinical picture can mimic delirium if a longitudinal historical perspective is not taken. The clinician should use accessory sources of information in the assessment of cognitive function and the patient's ability to perform activities of daily living.

Depression

Geriatric depression often presents differently from depression in young adults (Mueller et al. 2004; National Institutes of Health Consensus Development Panel on Depression in Late Life 1992; Small 1991) (Table 16–1). When compared with younger patient with MDD, individuals who were ages 65–79 years at the time of index episode were more likely to be divorced/widowed/separated, to have primary depression, and to have a history of medical illness, particularly cardiovascular disease or cancer (Mueller et al. 2004). They are more likely to minimize or deny depression, complain about memory problems, and become preoccupied with somatic symptoms. Symptoms such as loss of appetite, anhedonia, anergy, and insomnia are more prominent than depressed mood in elderly patients (Unützer et al. 2002). Elderly white men have very high suicide rates (Vyrostek 2004); men older than 75 commit suicide at a rate higher than any other age group (Figure 16–1).

Table 16–1. Clinical features of geriatric depression

Compared with young adult depressed patients, geriatric patients who are clinically depressed are

More likely to

Minimize or deny depressed mood

Become preoccupied with somatic symptoms

Complain about memory

Be divorced, widowed, or separated

Have primary depression

Less likely to

Express guilt

Seek help from a psychiatrist

Accept a psychological explanation for their illness

Source. Adapted from Small GW, Gunay I: "Geriatric Medicine," in *The American Psychiatric Press Textbook of Consultation-Liaison Psychiatry.* Edited by Rundell JR, Wise MG. Washington, DC, American Psychiatric Press, 1996, pp. 878–898; Mueller TI, Kohn R, Leventhal N, et al.: "The Course of Depression in Elderly Patients." *American Journal of Geriatric Psychiatry* 12:22–29, 2004.

Anxiety

The prevalence of anxiety disorders declines with age, although recognition in the elderly is complicated by depression, cognitive impairment, and physical illness (Sable and Jeste 2001). About 5.5% of individuals age 65 years and older have an anxiety disorder, whereas 11% of elderly men and 25% of elderly woman take anxiolytic medications (Sadavoy et al. 1991). This disparity is partially explained by the fact that most patients are prescribed psychotropics, especially anxiolytics, by primary care physicians, whereas psychiatrists are more likely to prescribe antidepressants, particularly in cases of mixed anxiety and depression (Sadavoy et al. 1991). In addition, complaints of insomnia are extremely common; in a primary care setting, anxiety disorders were found in 35% of the individuals who complained of insomnia (Kroenke et al. 1994). Benzodiazepines, which are often prescribed for anxiety and/or insomnia, are a risk factor for falls and fractures in the elderly, especially benzodiazepines that are oxidatively metabolized (Sgadari et al. 2000). Benzodiazepines metabolized by conjugation have a lower risk (e.g., lorazepam, oxazepam, and temazepam—mnemonic "LOT")

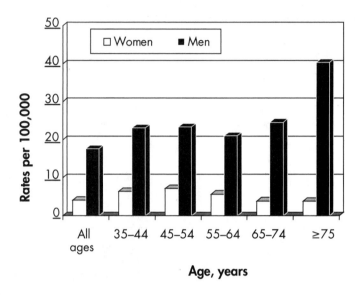

Figure 16–1.   Completed suicides by age.

Source.   Data from Vyrostek et al. 2004.

Psychosis

Even though psychotic symptoms occur in numerous illnesses in the elderly (i.e., primary psychotic disorders, mood disorders, and neurodegenerative disorders), evidence of effective treatments derived from randomized placebo-controlled trials is limited (Hoeh et al. 2003). Approximately 13% of all schizophrenic individuals have onset of the disorder in their 50s, 7% in their 60s, and only 3% after age 70 (Sadavoy et al. 1991). Delusional disorder (lifetime risk=0.05%–0.1%) usually presents in middle to late adulthood, with an average age at onset in men of 40–49 years and in women of 60–69 years (Sadavoy et al. 1991). Psychosis associated with dementia occurs in 30%–60% of patients with Alzheimer's dementia (Perez-Madrinan et al. 2004). Zubenko and colleagues (1991) found associations between the presence of psychosis and the densities of senile plaques and neurofibrillary tangles in the brains of patients with Alzheimer's disease. Perez-Madrinan and colleagues (2004) reported that patients with Alzheimer's disease and psychosis, particularly those with misidentification and hallucinations, show greater cognitive impairment and a more rapid cognitive decline than their counterparts without psychosis. Regardless of whether the psychiatric disorder is dementia with psychotic symptoms or primary psychosis, atypical antipsychotics are commonly used and seemingly effective, although tolerability differs among agents (Alexopoulos et al. 2004; Tariot et al. 2004).

Substance-Related Disorders

Elderly persons often underreport their alcohol consumption, and clinicians fail to recognize alcohol-related problems in elderly patients (Rigler 2000). Decreased lean body mass and total body water cause the total volume of distribution for alcohol to decline with age (Unützer et al. 2002). Cognitive and cerebellar functions after a standard alcohol load worsen with age.

Diagnostic Evaluation

Clinical History

The clinician must attend to the patient's physical symptoms and medical history, as well as to the patient's psychiatric history. Multiple medical conditions and multiple medications are the rule rather than the exception. Frequently, the signs and symptoms of medical and psychiatric disorders overlap. Because obtaining a history is sometimes difficult, a reliable collateral source saves time and contributes important clinical information.

Physical Examination

Sometimes, the consultation-liaison psychiatrist must perform a limited physical examination, particularly a neurological examination. Consultants occasionally discover a physical sign overlooked by the consultee. For example, an agitated, disturbed patient (e.g., a frail elderly patient with psychosis) can make the medical staff consultee anxious and thus cloud clinical assessment (Unützer et al. 2002).

Mental Status Examination

Depressed elderly patients who minimize dysphoria may divulge their depression nonverbally through facial expressions and sighs. A careful investigation of suicidal thinking and intent is essential because elderly people often choose lethal methods for suicide. Cognitive assessment of geriatric patients is also important. The consultant should follow the cortical mapping guidelines for cognitive examination discussed in Chapter 2, "Mental Status Examination and Other Tests of Brain Function," in this volume.

Laboratory Findings

Abnormal sodium and chloride levels can indicate dehydration that may, if untreated, progress to delirium, lethargy, or convulsions. Serum creatinine levels may overestimate glomerular filtration rate in elderly patients because decreased protein intake and decreased muscle mass cause a decline in creatinine production, which decreases serum creatinine levels. Therefore, normal serum levels for serum urea nitrogen and creatinine may conceal decreased renal function, and small elevations may represent significant dysfunction. Liver function, as reflected by hepatic function tests, should remain adequate throughout life. To assess renal clearance accurately, the National Kidney Foundation (NKF) and American Society of Nephrology (ASN) recommend estimating glomerular filtration rate (GFR) using the MDRD Study equation. This equation uses serum creatinine in combination with age, sex, and race to estimate GFR (Levey et al. 1999).

Treatment and Management

Treatment of Medical Problems

Most psychiatric problems in elderly patients occur either because of or concurrently with medical illnesses. Even though the consultee is in charge of the medical treatment, the consultant, when appropriate, must recommend further diagnostic evaluations or alternative medical treatments. Older patients are much more likely to follow up with psychiatric treatment if it is delivered in an integrated manner rather than in a referral to a specialty clinic. In a study by Bartels and colleagues (2004), 71% of the older patients engaged in treatment when mental health treatment was integrated with primary care compared with 49% of the older patients who were referred to mental health or substance abuse treatment clinics.

Age-Related Pharmacological Issues

Pharmacokinetic Factors

Aging potentially influences five main pharmacokinetic factors (Table 16–2): absorption, distribution, hepatic function, protein binding, and renal excretion. Although these factors may change with age, considerable interindividual variability exists.

Absorption.   It was commonly thought that gastric acid secretion declined with normal aging; however, recent studies show that the majority of people maintain gastric acid secretion late into life and only 5%–10% of older Caucasians have hypochlorhydria secondary to atrophic gastritis (McLean and Le Couteur 2004). Old age is associated with slowing of gastric emptying, decreased peristalsis, and slowing of colonic transit secondary to regional loss of neurons. These effects may be numerically impressive but not clinically significant (might effect t_{max} and C_{max} rather than the AUC [area under the curve]) (McLean and Le Couteur 2004). In elderly patients, drug-drug interactions are more likely to influence absorption. For example, antacids may delay absorption of psychotropic drugs and therefore delay their onset of action. Anticholinergic drugs, such as amitriptyline, also slow absorption and gastric motility and ultimately delay onset of action of other drugs. In addition, medications such as cholestyramine can inhibit absorption and decrease effectiveness.

Distribution.   Lean muscle mass and total body water decrease with age by 10%–15%, whereas total body fat tends to increase by 20%–40% (McLean and Le Couteur 2004). For fat-soluble (lipophilic) drugs, this means an increased volume of distribution, more accumulation, and a prolonged elimination half-life (McLean and Le Couteur 2004). Because psychotropic drugs, except lithium, are highly lipophilic, they may remain in an elderly patient's system for days or even weeks after the medication is discontinued (Salzman 1992).

Hepatic function.   Lipophilic drugs are converted to water-soluble compounds, mainly by hepatic enzymes, before elimination by the kidney; there-

Table 16–2.   Pharmacokinetic changes associated with psychotropic drugs and aging

Factor	Age effect	Consequence
Absorption	↓ Gastric acidity	In absence of gastric pathology or drug-drug interactions, not clinically significant
	↓ GI motility	
	↓ GI blood flow	
	↓ GI surface area	
Distribution	↑ Volume of distribution for lipophilic drugs (due to increased fat)	May prolong elimination half-life for lipophilic drugs
	↓ Volume of distribution for hydrophilic drugs, such as lithium (due to decreased body water)	May lead to ↑ drug levels for hydrophilic drugs, and so dose must be reduced
Hepatic function	↓ Hepatic blood flow	↑ Circulating, unmetabolized, and partially metabolized drug
	↓ Hepatic enzyme activity	*First-pass effect:* Prolonged time required for elimination
	↓ Demethylation	Prolonged exposure to unmetabolized drug
	↓ Hydroxylation	
Protein binding	↓ Albumin	Unclear effects
	↑ α_1 glycoprotein	Unclear effects
Renal excretion	↓ Renal blood flow	↓ Lithium clearance
	↓ Glomerular filtration rate	↑ Toxicity
	↓ Tubular excretion rate	↓ Clearance of antidepressant hydroxyl metabolite, potentially causing ↑ cardiotoxicity; ↑ Elimination half-life of BZDs, especially those oxidatively metabolized; may result in falls, accidents, and fractures

Source.   Adapted and updated from Wise MG, Tierney J: "Psychopharmacology in the Elderly." *Journal of the Louisiana State Medical Society* 144:471–476, 1992; McLean AJ, Le Couteur DG: "Aging Biology and Geriatric Clinical Pharmacology." *Pharmacology Review* 56:163–184, 2004.

fore, the effects of age on the liver are particularly important to psychotropic drugs. Hepatic metabolism is dependent on hepatic blood flow and hepatic enzyme activity, two factors that tend to decrease with age. Hepatic blood flow may decrease by as much as 40% by age 65, and there may be a similar or slightly less reduction in liver mass (McLean and Le Couteur 2004). Demethylation and hydroxylation are the two metabolic mechanisms that inactivate many psychotropics; both tend to slow with age, although hydroxylation typically slows first. The summary effect of these hepatic changes may prolong the duration of action and elimination half-life of many psychotropic drugs by as much as two- to threefold (Sadavoy et al. 1991).

Protein binding. Except for lithium, most psychotropic drugs are highly protein-bound. This means that changes in protein concentrations may have significant effects on a psychotropic drug's pharmacological activity, metabolism, and elimination. Antidepressants mostly bind to sites available on α_1 glycoprotein, whereas benzodiazepines and neuroleptics bind mainly to albumin. Studies indicate that aging causes a decrease in serum albumin and a likely increase in α_1 glycoprotein, although the clinical significance of this is unclear (McLean and Le Couteur 2004). As McLean and Le Couteur note, "Overall, age-related effects on protein binding have minimal clinical significance" (p. 173). Malnutrition, medical illness, and drug-drug interactions can alter the unbound (active) fraction of a drug.

Renal excretion. Biotransformation to water-soluble metabolites is important in the renal clearance of psychotropic drugs. Elderly individuals may have decreased renal blood flow, decreased glomerular filtration rate, and decreased tubular excretion rate. Age-related decline in glomerular filtration rate is often considered the most important pharmacokinetic change in old age, primarily because some renally eliminated drugs, such as gentamicin, digoxin, and lithium, have a narrow therapeutic window and are frequently monitored (i.e., levels are seen). GFR does decrease in old age, but in the absence of disease, it may not decrease as much as previously suspected. On average, GFR declines less than 1 mL/min/year after middle age; in many healthy people, GFR may not decline at all. The effects of comorbidity (e.g., hypertension, diabetes) and polypharmacy (e.g., coadministration of lithium with thiazide diuretics, ACE inhibitors, and/or nonsteroidal anti-inflammatory drugs) are a more important influence on lithium concentrations (Sproule et al. 2000).

A 30%–50% dose reduction with close attention to blood levels is recommended (Sproule et al. 2000). The clearance of tricyclic antidepressants' hydroxyl metabolites also decreases, which is potentially toxic to the cardiac conduction system (Salzman 1992).

Pharmacodynamic Factors

Aging has multiple effects on pharmacodynamics. As Unützer et al. (2002) note:

> Pharmacodynamics…change with age. Neurotransmitter synthesis and turnover, receptor binding, and synaptic neurotransmission change in many brain areas as people age. The precise clinical significance of such changes is unknown, but available evidence suggests that elderly persons have greater receptor-site sensitivity for many drugs, particularly benzodiazepines (e.g., diazepam). By contrast, changes in β-adrenergic function result in lower sensitivity to β-adrenergic stimulation and blockade. (p. 862)

Polypharmacy

The use of multiple drugs affects all pharmacokinetic and pharmacodynamic processes. About as many older individuals take over-the-counter drugs as take prescribed drugs, with an average number of 1.8 over-the-counter drugs taken per day (Hanlin et al. 2001). Because elderly persons are likely to use more than one medication, drug-drug interactions are a critical issue in management. Metabolism of psychotropic drugs is often complicated by chronic medical illnesses and medications that alter gastrointestinal, hepatic, or renal function. Because potential combinations of various drugs and diseases are too numerous to study systemically (Unützer et al. 2002), comprehensive data are unavailable.

Electroconvulsive Therapy

Electroconvulsive therapy is generally the safest and most effective treatment for severe depression in medically compromised elderly patients and is the treatment of choice for psychotic depression (Unützer et al. 2002). Patients with multiple medical problems and those older than 75 years are at increased risk for adverse effects, but modification of the treatment regimen helps to minimize risks. Short-term memory effects are common but short-lived in elderly patients. Overall, cognitive dysfunction should improve with electroconvulsive therapy (Stoudemire et al. 1991).

Psychotherapy

One of the problems constantly facing the older patient is loss—loss of physical function, loss of friends and loved ones through death or disability, and, possibly, loss of economic and social status. Bereavement and grief are common. Elderly people, especially the very old, do not seem to have much anxiety about death (Sadavoy et al. 1991). However, they often have fears of pain, abandonment, and disability. Appropriate, reality-based reassurance is often helpful.

As with most medically ill patients seen by the consultation-liaison psychiatrist, the elderly patient has his or her psychological defenses stripped away by the medical illness and cumulative losses. As long as the elderly patient has reasonable cognitive function, there is no reason that he or she cannot benefit from psychotherapeutic techniques used with other medically ill patients. Therefore, crisis intervention is no different with elderly people: help the patient adjust to the situation, correct the patient's distortions about the events at hand, and help the patient use intrapsychic strengths and mobilize external supports.

Caregivers for elderly patients often need support and respites from caregiving duties, and they may need psychiatric treatment because clinical depression occurs so commonly.

Elder Abuse

The 1998 National Elder Abuse Incidence Study (U.S. Department of Health and Human Services 1998) found that 551,011 persons, age 60 years and older, experienced abuse, neglect, and/or self-neglect in a 1-year period. Almost 80% of new incidents of abuse, neglect, and/or self-neglect were not reported; persons age 80 years and older were two to three times more likely to suffer abuse and neglect than the younger old population. Among known perpetrators of abuse and neglect, the perpetrator was a family member in 90% of cases (two-thirds of the perpetrators were adult children or spouses). According to Small and Gunay (1996, p. 886), "clinicians should consider the possibility of elder abuse when a caregiver 1) expresses frustration in providing care, 2) shows signs of psychological distress, 3) has a history of abuse or violence, or 4) has a history of alcohol or drug abuse."

Table 16–3. Suggested strategies for psychiatric consultation for geriatric patients

Collect history from multiple sources.

Have patient and/or family bring in all medications available to patient to include prescribed, over-the-counter, and alternative medicines. (Polypharmacy and multiple prescribing physicians are the rule, not the exception.)

Recognize unique clinical presentations of geriatric syndromes.

Search for medical and toxic causes of psychiatric syndromes.

Reduce polypharmacy whenever possible.

Follow conservative and rational pharmacological guidelines.

When you prescribe medications to a patient who has mild memory dysfunction, have patient use medication reminders (e.g., alarms); for patients with moderate to severe dysfunction, someone else must administer medications.

Identify adverse drug effects sooner rather than later.

Emphasize nonpharmacological interventions.

Source. Adapted from Small GW, Gunay I: "Geriatric Medicine," in *The American Psychiatric Press Textbook of Consultation-Liaison Psychiatry.* Edited by Rundell JR, Wise MG. Washington, DC, American Psychiatric Press, 1996, pp. 878–898. Copyright 1996, American Psychiatric Press. Used with permission.

Conclusion

Consultation-liaison psychiatrists will increasingly evaluate and treat geriatric patients, given the changing demographic patterns. Consultation for geriatric patients requires that consultation-liaison psychiatrists retain medical skills and knowledge of unique aspects of psychiatric syndromes in the elderly. Table 16–3 is a summary of suggested strategies for psychiatric consultation for geriatric patients.

References

Alexopoulos GS, Streim J, Carpenter D, et al: Expert Consensus Panel for Using Antipsychotic Drugs in Older Patients. J Clin Psychiatry 65 (suppl 2):5–99, 2004

Bartels SJ, Coakley EH, Zubritsky C, et al: Improving access to geriatric mental heath services: a random trial comparing treatment engagement with integrated versus enhanced referral care for depression, anxiety, and at-risk alcohol use. Am J Psychiatry 161:1455–1462, 2004

Bynum JP, Rabins PV, Weller W, et al: The relationship between a dementia diagnosis, chronic illness, Medicare expenditures, and hospital use. J Am Geriatr Soc 52:187–194, 2004

Hanlin JT, Fillenbaum GG, Ruby CM, et al: Epidemiology of over-the-counter drug use in community dwelling elderly: United States perspective. Drugs Aging 18:123–131, 2001

Hebert LE, Scherr PA, Bienias JL, et al: Alzheimer disease in the US population: prevalence estimates using the 2000 census. Arch Neurol 60:1119–1122, 2003

Hoeh N, Gyulai L, Weintraub D, et al: Pharmacologic management of psychosis in the elderly: a critical review. J Geriatr Psychiatry Neurol 16:213–218, 2003

K/DOQI clinical practice guidelines for chronic kidney disease: evaluation, classification, and stratification. Am J Kidney Dis 39:S1–S266, 2002

Kroenke K, Spitzer RL, Williams JBW, et al: Physical symptoms in primary care: predictors of psychiatric disorders and functional impairment. Arch Fam Med 3:774–779, 1994

Lawlor BA: Behavioral and psychological symptoms in dementia: the role of atypical antipsychotics. J Clin Psychiatry 65 (suppl 11):5–10, 2004

Levey AS, Bosch JP, Lewis JB, et al: A more accurate method to estimate glomerular filtration rate from serum creatinine: a new prediction equation. Modification of Diet in Renal Disease Study Group. Ann Intern Med 130:461–470, 1999

McLean AJ, Le Couteur DG: Aging biology and geriatric clinical pharmacology. Pharmacol Rev 56:163–184, 2004

Mueller TI, Kohn R, Leventhal N, et al: The course of depression in elderly patients. Am J Geriatr Psychiatry 12:22–29, 2004

National Institutes of Health Consensus Development Panel on Depression in Late Life: Diagnosis and treatment of depression in late life. JAMA 268:1018–1024, 1992

Perez-Madrinan G, Cook SE, Saxton JA, et al: Alzheimer disease with psychosis: excess cognitive impairment is restricted to the misidentification subtype. Am J Geriatr Psychiatry 12:449–456, 2004

Rigler SK: Alcoholism in the elderly. Am Fam Physician 61:1710–1716, 1883–1884, 1887–1888 passim, 2000

Sable JA, Jeste DV: Anxiety disorders in older adults. Curr Psychiatry Rep 3:302–307, 2001

Sadavoy J, Lazarus LW, Jarvik LF (eds): Comprehensive Review of Geriatric Psychiatry. Washington, DC, American Psychiatric Press, 1991

Salzman C: Clinical Geriatric Psychopharmacology, 2nd Edition. Baltimore, MD, Williams & Wilkins, 1992

Sgadari A, Lapane KL, Mor V, et al: Oxidative and nonoxidative benzodiazepines and the risk of femoral fracture: the systematic assessment of geriatric drug use via epidemiology study group. J Clin Psychopharmacol 20:234–239, 2000

Small GW: Recognition and treatment of depression in the elderly. J Clin Psychiatry 52 (suppl):11–22, 1991

Small GW, Gunay I: Geriatric medicine, in The American Psychiatric Press Textbook of Consultation-Liaison Psychiatry. Edited by Rundell JR, Wise MG. Washington, DC, American Psychiatric Press, 1996, pp 878–898

Sproule BA, Hardy BG, Shulman KI: Differential pharmacokinetics of lithium in elderly patients. Drugs Aging 16:165-177, 2000

Stoudemire A, Hill CD, Morris R, et al: Cognitive outcome following tricyclic and electroconvulsive treatment of major depression in the elderly. Am J Psychiatry 148:1336–1340, 1991

Tariot PN, Profenno LA, Ismail MS: Efficacy of atypical antipsychotics in elderly patients with dementia. J Clin Psychiatry 65 (suppl 11):11–15, 2004

Unützer J, Small GW, Gunay I: Geriatric medicine, in The American Psychiatric Publishing Textbook of Consultation-Liaison Psychiatry: Psychiatry in the Medically Ill, 2nd Edition. Edited by Wise MG, Rundell JR. Washington, DC, American Psychiatric Publishing, 2002, pp 853–869

U.S. Department of Health and Human Services, Administration on Aging: The National Elder Abuse Incidence Study, 1998. Available at: http://www.aoa.gov/eldfam/Elder_Rights/Elder_Abuse/ABuseReport_Full.pdf. Accessed January 31, 2005.

Vyrostek SB, Annest JL, Ryan GW: Surveillance for fatal and nonfatal injuries—United States, 2001. MMWR Surveill Summ 53:1–57, 2004

Zubenko GS, Moosy J, Martinez AJ, et al: Neuropathologic and neurochemical correlates of psychosis in primary dementia. Arch Neurol 48:619–624, 1991

Additional Readings

Hay DP, Klein DT, Hay LK, et al: Agitation in Patients With Dementia. Washington, DC, American Psychiatric Publishing, 2003

Mellow AM (ed): Geriatric Psychiatry (Review of Psychiatry Series; Oldham JM, Riba MB, series eds). Washington, DC, American Psychiatric Publishing, 2003

Rodriguez MM, Grossberg GT: Estrogen as a psychotherapeutic agent. Clin Geriatr Med 14:177–189, 1998

17

Special Psychosomatic Medicine Settings and Situations

Consultation-liaison psychiatrists practice in many different outpatient and inpatient psychosomatic medicine settings. Some consultation-liaison psychiatrists conduct most or all of their work in subspecialty settings, such as oncology units or human immunodeficiency virus/acquired immunodeficiency syndrome (HIV/AIDS) clinics. Although an exhaustive review of each of these settings is beyond the scope of this "pocket" guide, we highlight unique characteristics of subspecialty units and patient populations. Many "rules," pearls, and guidelines discussed in previous chapters are modified to fit special situations.

Pregnancy and the Postpartum Period

Psychopharmacology During Pregnancy

Medications may cause teratogenesis at all stages of pregnancy, although risk is greatest during the first trimester. In an ideal world, pregnant and breast-feeding women would never need to receive psychopharmacological agents. However, in the real world, clinicians must balance the risks of teratogenesis and effects on a breast-feeding child against the risks and effects of severe psychiatric illness on both the mother and the child. Women with mood disorders are at high risk for symptom exacerbation, especially during the immediate postpartum period. Each case is unique and must take into account stage of pregnancy, severity of psychiatric illness, degree of functional impairment when ill, quality of social supports, and compliance with medical follow-up and monitoring.

Teratogenic potential is neither proven nor disproven for neuroleptics, antidepressants, benzodiazepines, and sedative-hypnotics. It is accepted practice to avoid use of these medications during pregnancy, particularly during the first trimester. Clinicians substitute alternative therapies, including psychotherapy and electroconvulsive therapy (ECT), when possible.

Ample evidence indicates that mood-stabilizing medications can cause birth defects. Exposure up to 32 days after conception can affect neural tube development and closure, exposure 21–56 days after conception may affect heart formation, and exposure during days 42–63 may influence development of the lip and palate (Yonkers et al. 2004). In pregnant women, lithium should be used only when lifesaving benefits clearly outweigh this potential risk. There may be up to a 20- to 40-fold higher rate of cardiovascular malformations—most notably, Ebstein's anomaly in offspring exposed in utero—compared with the general population (Cohen et al. 1994). Carbamazepine and valproate should be avoided as well, particularly if the patient is taking more than one anticonvulsant—combination therapy increases the risk of teratogenesis (Yonkers et al. 2004). In contrast, lamotrigine, which was recently approved for maintenance treatment of bipolar disorder, appears to be associated with a lower rate of malformations and is a first-line treatment for epilepsy in women during their reproductive years (Karceski et al. 2001).

Because of the potential for physiological dependency in the newborn, it is prudent to taper and stop medications a few weeks before delivery. Infants born to mothers who are physically dependent on opiates or sedative-hypnotics may experience withdrawal.

If a woman taking psychiatric medication is trying to become pregnant, she may choose to continue taking the drug until she misses her first period; the longer she is medication-free, the higher the risk of relapse. Fortunately, ECT is a safe and effective option for psychotic and mood disorders that occur during pregnancy. Fetal cardiac monitoring should be used during ECT to detect and correct any arrhythmias that may develop from use of barbiturates and atropine; atropine should be avoided if possible (Yonkers et al. 2004).

Psychopharmacology and Breast-Feeding

Nursing mothers who take psychotropic medications will, with some exceptions, excrete those medications in breast milk. Generally, concentrations in breast milk are much lower than levels in the blood, so that total amounts ingested by a nursing infant are small. However, most clinicians advise mothers who are breast-feeding their infants to avoid most psychopharmacological medications and advise against breast-feeding if the psychiatric disorder is severe. Breast-feeding infants exposed to nortriptyline, paroxetine, or sertraline are unlikely to develop detectable or elevated plasma drug levels, whereas infants exposed to fluoxetine, and perhaps citalopram, appear to be at higher risk for developing elevated levels (Weissman et al. 2004).

Postpartum Psychiatric Disorders

Postpartum Mood Disorders

After labor and delivery, 60%–80% of women develop mild transient dysphoria ("blues"); 10% develop a major depressive episode (Stotland 2002). Postpartum depression usually occurs 1–2 weeks after delivery and may not occur until the second or third child. A woman who experiences postpartum depression is at increased risk for episodes with future births. Antidepressant medications should be administered, and the patient should be counseled to bottle-feed her infant. ECT is also an effective treatment for postpartum depression. Lithium postpartum prophylaxis has been found to reduce the rate of relapse from near 50% to less than 10% (Cohen et al. 1995).

Postpartum Psychosis

Postpartum psychosis, especially with aggression or fearful delusions about the infant, is a psychiatric emergency. Preventing infanticide is the priority. Postpartum psychoses may be associated with obstetrical events such as toxemia, malpresentations, hydramnios, and placental defects (Nadelson and Notman 1986). One-third of the patients who experience postpartum psychosis have similar difficulties in future pregnancies. No significant deleterious effects of maternal antipsychotics on the nursing infant have been found (Stotland 2002).

Fetal Alcohol Syndrome

Alcohol abuse by pregnant women can cause fetal alcohol syndrome. Cardinal features include growth retardation before and after birth, small head circumference, flattened facial features, mental retardation, low birth weight, developmental delays, and behavioral abnormalities.

Pediatric Psychosomatic Medicine

Consultation-liaison psychiatrists may find themselves providing consultation for children and adolescents because of the scarcity of child and adolescent psychiatrists with experience in psychosomatic medicine. The general psychiatrist involved in consultation work with children or adolescents cannot simply equate child and adolescent psychosomatic medicine with the adult consultation process. Pediatric consultation has several important differences, including the developmental perspective, the family focus, the process of consulting to pediatricians, and differences in the children's medical system.

Developmental Perspective

To perform psychiatric consultation with children, the psychiatrist must understand and maintain a developmental perspective. A developmental perspective implies recognition that the rapid physical and psychological changes taking place in a child or an adolescent alter the manifestations of disease, the effect of illness on the patient's life, and coping capacities (Fritz and Brown 2002). The fact that developmental steps exist for each stage of childhood and adolescence presents a major organizing paradigm to the consultant who seeks to assess the meaning of a symptom or a behavior. The stress of an illness or hospitalization frequently leads to regression, in which a child appears much less mature (i.e., temporarily loses some of the cognitive, emotional, or behavioral advances previously achieved). Such regression is disconcerting for parents, difficult for caregivers, and often uncomfortable for the child. The assessment and management of regressive behavior is a common reason that pediatricians request psychiatric consultation (Fritz and Brown 2002).

Family Focus

In contrast to many adult consultations, with the possible exception of a geriatric patient with cognitive dysfunction, the medical history and psychiatric history are virtually never obtained from only the pediatric patient; the examiner must interview a parent or an adult caregiver (Fritz and Brown 2002). Occasionally, the focus of a consultation is entirely on the parents' concerns or difficulties; here, the consultant can make an important contribution without direct involvement of the child. A consultation that would take approximately an hour and a half with an adult may take three times that long with a child.

Consultation Process

The consultant should advise the referring pediatrician how to prepare both the patient and the parents for psychiatric consultation. Information is often provided by not only the parents but also people outside the family, including a child's schoolteacher, caseworker, or therapist. Although this information is often difficult to obtain quickly, the consultant should use the authority of the hospital or clinic and create the degree of urgency necessary to obtain facts rapidly from these outside sources (Fritz and Brown 2002).

The consultant should assess the child's understanding of the medical situation, as well as the child's associated fears and expectations. "Regressive symptoms during hospitalization (e.g., immature behavior, clinging, enuresis) are extremely common in preschoolers, but the same behavior in a young adolescent is a cause for more concern" (Fritz and Brown 2002, p. 721). In addition to describing elements well known to every adult psychiatrist (e.g., affect, thought processes, and cognition), the consultant must observe and describe the quality of the child's relationship with parents and unit staff. Key elements to the mental status examination of children and adolescents include physical appearance, interpersonal interactions, capacities (intelligence, affect, motor, speech, attention), attitudes and feelings (toward illness, hospitalization, self, others, reasons for the consultation), and observations about play and fantasy (e.g., three wishes, dreams).

Administrative and Legal Issues

A child or an adolescent may request that the psychiatrist keep information from the parents or pediatrician. Adolescents, in particular, may request confidentiality as a condition for cooperation. In most cases, this request is appropriate to honor and must be explained to the parents. The age at which informed consent and the right to refuse treatment become the prerogative of the patient rather than the parent varies from state to state. In general, however, from mid-adolescence on, a consultant should err in the direction of assuming that the patient has the same legal rights and need for informed consent as an adult (Fritz and Brown 2002).

Psychopharmacology

Psychostimulants are used in treating attention-deficit/hyperactivity disorder (ADHD), which may occur in children following neurological events, such as head injury. Common side effects of psychostimulants include loss of appetite, irritability, abdominal pain, and insomnia. Clinicians have concerns about abuse potential of psychostimulants, which have affected their general acceptability.

Atomoxetine is a nonstimulant medication developed for the treatment of ADHD. It is a highly specific inhibitor of the norepinephrine transporter, with minimal affinity for other noradrenergic receptors or other neurotransmitter transporters or receptors (Michelson et al. 2002). Atomoxetine is superior to placebo in reducing ADHD symptoms and in improving social and family functioning in children, adolescents, and adults. There do not appear to be statistically significant differences in outcomes in early randomized, open-label studies comparing atomoxetine and methylphenidate (Kratochvil et al. 2002); atomoxetine can be effectively administered once daily, a big advantage for efficacy and compliance. The most common adverse effects are decreased appetite, an initial period of weight loss followed by an apparent normal growth rate, and mild increases in blood pressure and heart rate that plateau during treatment and then resolve on discontinuation (Kratochvil et al. 2002).

Antidepressants are used for major mood disorders, enuresis, anxiety disorders, and ADHD. Up to 5% of children and 8% of adolescents meet diagnostic criteria for depression, with the incidence increasing markedly after puberty (Wagner et al. 2004). In double-blind, placebo-controlled trials, fluoxetine, sertraline, and citalopram have shown efficacy in the treatment of major depression in children and adolescents, as has paroxetine for the treatment of depression in adolescents (Wagner et al. 2004). Tricyclic antidepressants are sometimes used in children to treat depression or ADHD. Similar to the adverse effects seen in adults, the most common side effects of tricyclics in children are anticholinergic and quinidine-like cardiac conduction delays. An electrocardiogram and vital signs are used to establish a baseline; the clinician also should observe for congenitally prolonged QT interval and then repeat these tests frequently during treatment.

Neuroleptics are used for psychotic disorders and severe agitation associated with brain disorders. Important adverse effects in children are similar to those seen in adults and include sedation, parkinsonism, dystonias, and neuroleptic malignant syndrome. Anxiolytics are used primarily for chronic anxiety disorders or anticipatory anxiety (e.g., prior to painful medical procedures). Sedation and blunting of cognition are especially common side effects in children. Behavioral disinhibition and dependence are serious but occur rarely. Analgesics are underused in pediatric settings.

Burns

Epidemiology

More than 2 million people experience burns serious enough to seek health care every year in the United States; 70,000 require hospitalizations, and 5,000 die (Warden and Heinbach 1991). Mortality risk depends on the severity of the burn and the age of the patient. Children and the elderly are at highest risk. Psychiatric disorders predispose people to severe burns: 14%–21% of hospitalized adult burn patients have substance-related disorders, 8%–12% have dementia, and 24%–39% have other psychiatric disorders (Fauerbach et al. 1996; MacArthur and Moore 1975). Burn patients are at high risk for developing psychiatric syndromes in the hospital, including delirium, substance withdrawal syndromes, and mood disorders.

Delirium

During the first 24–72 hours after a severe burn, the patient typically has a brief period of initial lucidity, which offers an opportunity to assess the patient's history, personality dynamics, and coping patterns. After that, between 30% and 70% of hospitalized patients with severe burns develop delirium, presumably caused by stress and burn-induced metabolic disturbances

(Andreasen et al. 1977). Correction of metabolic abnormalities and infections helps to reverse the psychiatric symptomatology. Neuroleptics are the best pharmacological treatment for the symptoms of delirium. Neuroleptics decrease fear, anxiety, agitation, pain, and insomnia. Haloperidol is a good choice because of its low incidence of cardiovascular and anticholinergic side effects.

Pain Management

Pain in burn patients is often undertreated (Raison et al. 2002). Although pain is a continuing and critical issue for the burn patient, it becomes especially important during dressing changes and debridement, which may produce acute, excruciating pain. Narcotics are the drugs of choice for treatment of this pain. Methadone is a good choice because of its excellent absorption and slow clearance. Caution should be exercised with meperidine because its metabolite, normeperidine, is a central nervous system (CNS) irritant that causes mental status changes. Neuroleptics, antidepressants, and psychostimulants are effective narcotic adjuvants. Dressing changes often require additional preemptive analgesia. Short-acting narcotics such as fentanyl citrate are useful and are given about 45–60 minutes before dressing changes or debridement.

Many clinicians use hypnosis to help patients control pain. Hypnosis is not considered a substitute for adequate pharmacological control of pain; its use is complicated by the hypnotizability of the patient, the severity of the pain, the busy and noisy setting of the burn unit, and the high frequency of secondary mental disorders (e.g., delirium).

Mood Syndromes

Clinicians should strongly consider the possibility of a medically induced secondary mood syndrome in depressed burn patients (Raison et al. 2002). Burn patients are at risk for many of the causes of secondary depression, particularly metabolic or electrolyte abnormalities and infection. Burn patients lose water at a rate several times faster than normal; hypovolemic shock is common. Following the shock phase is a period of intense catabolism and negative nitrogen balance. In addition, associated anorexia, weight loss, exhaustion, and lassitude may lead unsuspecting clinicians to overdiagnose depression.

Psychoactive Substance Use Withdrawal Syndromes

As many as one-fifth of burn patients have substance-related disorders. Some of these patients will experience withdrawal syndromes while initially hospitalized with severe burns. Unfortunately, the time courses for most withdrawal syndromes coincide with the critical periods of burn patients' medical courses. The clinician should expect and observe closely for signs of alcohol, opiate, barbiturate, and sedative-hypnotic withdrawal; withdrawal can greatly complicate medical care if not managed early and aggressively. The clinician should ask the family about the patient's substance use patterns; heavy or daily use indicates the need for pharmacological prophylaxis.

Psychosocial Issues in Burn Patients Likely to Die

Many patients with severe burns will die. They usually are told their prognosis early in the course of treatment while they are still lucid. The psychiatric consultant's role with these patients may include consultation on several issues: death, denial, dying, sense of loss, pain control, do-not-resuscitate orders, unfinished business, religious requests, and last wishes. Denial is common in severely burned patients, especially early on. The psychiatrist should not confront the denial, especially early after a burn. Conversely, he or she should answer direct questions (e.g., "Will I die?") kindly but honestly.

Psychiatric Issues in Recovery

As patients recover from their burns, many issues arise: changes in body image, difficulties with finances, problems with postdischarge care, negative reactions by family, limitations in occupations, and low self-esteem. Facial burns usually cause more psychological difficulty than do burns to other body areas. A patient should not be forced to view a deformity until he or she is ready; he or she may choose to wait several weeks before looking in a mirror. Brief psychotherapy, family discussions, and honest explanations help prepare the hospitalized burn patient for long-term consequences and the prolonged rehabilitation process. Giving the patient a decision-making role in the hospital helps reestablish a sense of control and reduces dependency. Potential areas for increased patient responsibility include eating schedules, visiting hours, dressing change times, physical therapy activities, sleep periods, and some medication decisions.

Longer-term psychotherapy is sometimes required to help severely burned patients adjust to permanent disfigurement and changes in body image and self-esteem. In one study, 35.3% of the burn patients met criteria for post-traumatic stress disorder at 2 months, 40% met the criteria at 6 months, and 45.2% met the criteria at 12 months postinjury (Perry et al. 1992). Cognitive or group psychotherapy can help lead the patient toward acceptance and psychological growth.

Cancer

Primary Psychiatric Disorders

Primary psychiatric disorders occur in 20%–58% of cancer patients. The prevalence of current major depressive disorder in cancer centers is 8%–14% (Fawzy et al. 2002). Antidepressant choice depends on target symptoms and the anticipated side effects in a given patient. In patients without cardiac conduction defects, tricyclic antidepressants are sometimes beneficial, especially if effects on sleep, appetite, and pain are sought. However, selective serotonin reuptake inhibitors (SSRIs) are the most widely prescribed antidepressants; it is fortunate that competitive cytochrome P450 enzyme inhibition is unlikely to affect most chemotherapy regimens (Fawzy et al. 2002). A trial of a psychostimulant, such as dextroamphetamine methylphenidate or pemoline, is appropriate for a rapid effect in systemically ill patients who are depressed, apathetic, and not eating.

Trazodone is widely used among oncology patients, especially when sedation is desired. Unfortunately, potential adverse effects include nausea and orthostatic hypotension. Nevertheless, the lack of anticholinergic side effects makes trazodone an attractive agent to use alone or in combination with SSRIs. SSRIs lack significant anticholinergic and sedative side effects. However, they can add to anorexia, jitteriness, and agitation (Fawzy et al. 2002). Most SSRIs inhibit metabolism by the cytochrome P450 enzyme system. Fortunately, this is unlikely to affect chemotherapy regimens.

Secondary Psychiatric Disorders

Secondary psychiatric disorders due to CNS metastases occur with many cancers, especially lung, breast, gastrointestinal, renal, and prostate (Lishman

1987). The likelihood of these syndromes becomes greater as a cancer progresses and as the number and intensity of treatments increase. Structural lesions of the brain can cause both focal and generalized neuropsychiatric signs. Psychiatric symptoms also occur secondary to chemotherapeutic agents (Table 17–1) or secondary to medications used for symptom control. Metoclopramide, for example, is used for gastroesophageal reflux and to prevent nausea. Because metoclopramide is a CNS dopamine antagonist, it can produce extrapyramidal symptoms that are misdiagnosed ("The patient has a conversion reaction").

Anticipatory Nausea and Vomiting

Patients who vomit with chemotherapy may develop a conditioned response, usually nausea and vomiting, to the hospital, nurse, or sight and smell of medical facilities. This clinical phenomenon can be prevented or managed in several ways, including use of optimal antiemetic treatment or hypnosis. If the patient develops a phobic response, the site of treatment should be changed and a benzodiazepine used before treatment (Fawzy et al. 2002). Systematic desensitization extinguishes the conditioned response. Cognitive distraction can block the perception of the conditioned stimulus and may eliminate the associated anxiety (Fawzy et al. 2002).

Pain Management

Occasionally, pain management is an issue during consultation. Fears of addiction have no place in the treatment of the cancer patient. Narcotics such as methadone are the treatment of choice. Neuroleptics, antidepressants, and psychostimulants help diminish psychiatric components of pain (suffering, fear, and insomnia) and are good narcotic adjuvants. When bone metastases are present, prostaglandin inhibitors such as aspirin and nonsteroidal anti-inflammatory drugs are very useful.

Delivering Bad News

Problems most frequently seen in cancer patients are anxiety, dysphoria, and anger about the illness and its implications for the future. Patients with cancer should be told the truth. In telling patients they have a malignant and possibly fatal cancer, Cassem (2004) suggested that physicians 1) rehearse the

Table 17–1.   Psychiatric manifestations of chemotherapeutic agents

Agent	Side effect
Hormones	
Tamoxifen	Hot flashes, sleep disorder, irritability
Aminoglutethimide	Initial syndrome of rash, malaise, fatigue
Fluoxymesterone	Irritability, increased libido, hirsutism
Corticosteroids	Dose-related manic and depressive features, psychosis, insomnia, hyperactivity
Chemotherapeutic agents	
Procarbazine	Somnolence, psychosis, delirium, disulfiram-like effect (do not mix with alcohol)
L-Asparaginase	Somnolence, lethargy, delirium; not dose related
Pyrimidine analogues (inhibit DNA synthesis)	
Cytosine arabinoside	Leukoencephalopathy may result from high dose: syndrome of personality change (drowsiness, dementia, psychomotor retardation, ataxia); cerebellar syndrome
5-Fluorouracil	Fatigue, rarely delirium or seizure
Folate antagonists	
Methotrexate	Neurological toxicity with high-dose or intrathecal regimens
Metaphase inhibitors	
Vincristine, vinblastine	Dysphoria, lethargy
Alkylating agents	
Ifosfamide	Lethargy, delirium, cerebellar signs, mimics alcohol intoxication
Biologicals	
Interferon	Mainly flulike syndrome, with fever, myalgias, malaise, which dissipates; diffuse encephalopathy noted at high doses; syndrome of fatigue, difficulty in concentration, psychomotor retardation, general disinterest
Interleukin-2 (IL-2)	Delirium (dose related); mainly flulike syndrome, with malaise, chills, anorexia, fatigue, depression

Source.   Adapted from Fawzy FI, Servis ME, Greenberg DB: "Oncology and Psychooncology," in *The American Psychiatric Publishing Textbook of Consultation-Liaison Psychiatry: Psychiatry in the Medically Ill,* 2nd Edition. Edited by Wise MG, Rundell JR. Washington, DC, American Psychiatric Publishing, 2002, pp. 657–678. Copyright 2002, American Psychiatric Publishing. Used with permission.

statement so it can be delivered calmly, 2) be brief—no more than three sentences, 3) encourage the patient to talk, and 4) reassure the patient that he or she will receive continued attention and care.

Death and Dying

People usually die as they have lived. Personality characteristics are often exaggerated with increased stress, and fewer mature defense mechanisms are used. The dying patient may or may not want to be alone and is generally comfortable talking about death. It is usually the family members, and sometimes the ward staff, who are reluctant to engage in such conversations. The importance of religious faith and the belief in an afterlife in dying patients should not be underestimated. The clinician should discuss do-not-resuscitate orders, wills, and comfort measures early. If the patient wants, time at home or private times with family while in the hospital should be arranged.

Depression

In a medically ill dying patient, the attribution of neurovegetative symptoms is often difficult. Almost all seriously ill patients have problems with sleep, energy, and appetite and may have some difficulty with concentration. The following characteristics help identify a depressed medically ill patient: sustained depressed mood, decreased psychomotor movements, suicidal ideation, helplessness, worthlessness, and hopelessness. The depressed patient also has anhedonia. The depressed dying patient with less than 3 weeks to live may respond to a rapid-acting psychostimulant, such as methylphenidate.

Anxiety

The threat of death can cause anxiety. If an individual does not mention fears of dying, the clinician should inquire either indirectly (e.g., "You look scared. How are you doing?") or directly (e.g., "Are you worried that you may die?"). If the patient believes that he or she is dying, the clinician should respond according to the reality of the situation. If the fear is unrealistic, reassurance and an explanation about the current situation usually will decrease anxiety and fear. If death is imminent, the clinician should ask the patient, "What frightens you the most about dying?" Three common fears are abandonment, uncontrollable pain, and shortness of breath (Cassem 2004). Anxiety disorders are commonly associated with neurological insults (Wise and Rundell 1999). Anxiety also may be substance induced; corticosteroids, metoclopramide, prochlorperazine, and bronchodilators can cause significant anxiety (Breitbart and Lintz 2002).

Antianxiety medications are very effective if symptomatic or disabling anxiety persists after psychological support and the opportunity for abreaction are provided. Benzodiazepines, however, also can result in lethargy and/or confusion. When terror or extreme fear is present, low doses of major tranquilizers (neuroleptics) often are more efficacious than benzodiazepines. Haloperidol (0.5–5.0 mg twice daily), thioridazine (10–25 mg three to four times a day), or olanzapine (2.5–10 mg twice daily) can reduce panic or extreme anxiety markedly (Breitbart and Lintz 2002).

Pain

In patients with advanced cancer, 60%–90% have pain (Foley 1985). In addition, depression and anxiety increase the experience of pain. In the evaluation process, the first step is to assess quality of pain, time course, fluctuations, and factors that exacerbate or relieve it. Mental status examination and medical and neurological evaluations are performed. Pain is also assessed repeatedly to balance the analgesic dosage against the level of pain and alertness. Pain is frequently undertreated in medically ill and dying patients.

Neurology and Neurosurgery

Head Injury

Because of the swirling movement of traumatic forces within the brain during acceleration and deceleration injuries, head trauma is likely to produce changes in the axial structure of the brain (Waziri 1986). Therefore, subcortical structures, such as the limbic system, are often affected. In addition, in closed head injuries, contrecoup lesions are more severe than lesions in portions of the brain closest to the source of trauma. The only exception to this is when the head is perfectly still at the time of impact (Lishman 1998), an uncommon event. Frequent neuropsychiatric findings in head trauma patients include emotional lability, irritability, personality change, fear, rage, impulsivity, memory loss, and apathy. Secondary depression and mania also can occur. Symptoms of postconcussional syndrome include headache, dizziness, tiredness, and insomnia. Memory dysfunction, concentration problems, perceptual changes, dysthymia, anxiety, irritability, and personality changes also may occur (Fricchione et al. 2002). Postconcussional syndrome is not correlated with head injury severity or degree of loss of consciousness.

In most head injuries, consciousness is impaired, ranging from a momentary daze to prolonged coma. Retrograde (before the trauma) and anterograde (after the trauma) amnesia commonly occur with significant head trauma. The degree of anterograde and retrograde amnesia each correlates positively with trauma severity and negatively with prognosis for full recovery. Generally, the period of retrograde amnesia shrinks faster than the period of anterograde amnesia. The degree and speed of recovery after head injury depend on many factors: premorbid neuropsychiatric state, amount of brain damage, location of brain damage, emotional effect of the injury, quality of medical care, compensation/litigation, and motivation (Lishman 1998).

CNS Infection

Usually, CNS infections present with nonfocal findings such as obtundation, irritability, or restlessness. When focal findings occur, an abscess should be suspected. Fever and focal signs may or may not be present; however, their absence typically delays the diagnosis of an abscess. CNS abscesses also may present with headaches, confusion, personality change, and memory loss. Chronic meningitis and neurosyphilis are becoming more common because of HIV infections. Chronic meningitis clinical features last for more than 6 weeks and include headache, fever, stiff neck, focal neurological deficits, behavioral dyscontrol, cognitive dysfunction, and confusion. Neurosyphilis may have a variety of neuropsychiatric presentations, most commonly progressive dementia, mania, depression, and psychosis. The physician should assess for the possibility of meningeal inflammation by flexing the neck and hip joints (Kernig's and Brudzinski's signs).

Primary and Metastatic CNS Tumors

Half of the patients with primary CNS tumors develop psychiatric symptoms. Focal findings are usually present, but nonspecific signs and symptoms, such as personality change and affective lability, also may occur. The nature of neuropsychiatric symptomatology depends on the location of the tumor, the degree to which intracranial pressure is increased, and the constitution of the individual. Neuropsychiatric findings are more likely when tumors are frontal, limbic, or temporal than when tumors are parietal or occipital.

Lung, breast, gastrointestinal, pancreatic, renal, and prostate cancers are the most likely to metastasize to the brain. CNS metastases eventually develop in 15%–25% of metastatic cancer patients, including 35%–45% of lung cancer patients (Lohr and Cadet 1987). CNS metastatic tumors are sometimes symptomatic before the primary tumor, especially when the primary tumor is in the lung. The posterior fossa is the site of 30% of CNS tumors, 22% are found in temporofrontal areas, 12% are in the parietal region, 10% are in the pituitary, and 4% are in the occipital lobes (Lohr and Cadet 1987). If discovered early, when a single CNS metastasis exists, neurosurgical intervention is often warranted.

Because psychiatric symptoms of brain tumors are nonfocal, the clinician must maintain a high index of suspicion in patients who have cancer. A brain tumor should be suspected in patients with psychiatric symptoms and 1) frequent or unremitting headaches, 2) vomiting, 3) seizures, 4) visual complaints, and 5) any focal neurological finding (Lohr and Cadet 1987).

Subcortical and Limbic System Disease

Parkinson's disease, Huntington's chorea, progressive supranuclear palsy, and some elements of HIV dementia are examples of conditions that principally involve subcortical and limbic areas of the brain. Neuropsychiatric symptoms, such as emotional lability, fear, rage, apathy, impulsiveness, hallucinations, and delusions, are therefore common, although they are diverse and nonspecific. In Parkinson's disease patients, 65% develop dementia by age 85; 40% can expect to have at least one episode of major depressive disorder (Fricchione et al. 2002).

Normal-Pressure Hydrocephalus

Of patients with dementia, 7% have normal-pressure hydrocephalus (NPH) (Martin and Black 1987). NPH is important to recognize because it is usually treatable. The classic NPH diagnostic triad is dementia, gait disturbance, and urinary incontinence.

Poststroke Depression

The major psychiatric sequela of stroke is depression, although anxiety disorders occur more commonly than appreciated (Wise and Rundell 1999). Wiart (1997) reported that poststroke depression occurs in 30%–50% of hemiplegic patients in the first 2 years after a stroke. Most cases are minor depression; up to 25% are severe depression. The average duration of major untreated poststroke depression is 1 year. Minor depression or dysthymic disorder may last longer, often more than 2 years. Poststroke depression is associated with higher mortality after stroke (Williams et al. 2004).

Lacunar strokes and infarcts also have psychiatric sequelae.

Lacunar infarcts are small lesions, often the result of hypertension, that occur in the deeper subcortical parts of the cerebrum and in the brain stem....They result from occlusion of the small penetrating branches of the large cerebral arteries. A wide range of mood changes may occur after lacunar strokes, including emotional incontinence and depression. (Fricchione et al. 2002, p. 681)

HIV Disease and AIDS

AIDS was the leading cause of death in the United States among men and women ages 25–44 years in 1994 (Centers for Disease Control and Prevention 1995). Since then, major gains have occurred in treating HIV disease as a result of the effectiveness of highly active antiretroviral therapy. AIDS is no longer one of the top three causes of death in the United States (Halman et al. 2002). Patients with HIV disease and HIV specialists now generally perceive HIV disease as a chronic medical condition rather than a relentlessly progressive infection.

The psychiatric treatment and management of HIV disease must take into consideration a wide range of ongoing etiological factors, including premorbid primary psychiatric disorders, disorders secondary to HIV-1 CNS infection, advanced systemic disease, and neuropsychiatric side effects of commonly used HIV/AIDS medications (Halman et al. 2002). Advanced systemic disease and HIV-1 CNS infection can constrain the pharmacotherapeutic options available to the psychiatric consultant. Psychotherapeutic interventions must take into account the perspectives of patients who come from communities that often have been marginalized, socially disenfranchised, and impoverished. Management plans frequently require liaison with community-based HIV/AIDS service organizations and highly diverse social and family support groups.

AIDS

More than 1 million Americans are likely infected with HIV. The end stage of this infection is AIDS. Neuropsychiatric complications in AIDS patients include memory deficits, concentration impairment, dementia, psychomotor slowing, motor deficits, apathy, withdrawal, depression, or psychosis. In the final stages of the disease, delirium, profound slowness, severe dementia, focal neurological signs, secondary neurological disorders (e.g., tumors, CNS toxoplasmosis), seizures, and agitation are common.

Neuropsychiatric findings in AIDS may be caused by primary effects of the virus itself, neurotoxic by-products of the immune responses to the virus, indirect consequences of systemic disease (e.g., hypoxia, malnutrition), or intracranial tumors or infections that occur as a result of the immunocompromised state. The most common CNS opportunistic conditions that present with changes in mental status include HIV dementia, toxoplasmosis, CNS lymphoma, cryptococcal meningitis, and progressive multifocal leukoencephalopathy (Halman et al. 2002). Unless the patient is near death from nonneurological causes, aggressive diagnostic workup is indicated when new neuropsychiatric symptoms emerge in AIDS patients. Treatment is possible for many AIDS-related CNS disorders, especially toxoplasmosis, herpes simplex infection, and CNS lymphoma.

The frequency with which mental status changes are due to medication side effects has increased. The use of more medications—medications more effective at crossing the blood-brain barrier and in combination with one another—in more systemically ill patients has resulted in neuropsychiatric syndromes. The most common psychiatric side effects are asthenia, insomnia, depression, delirium, mania, and irritability. Often, the symptoms are mild and nonspecific but some may become the focus of psychiatric consultation.

HIV Infection Without AIDS

Secondary mental syndromes can occur in HIV-infected patients without AIDS, although less commonly than in AIDS patients. Most early-stage patients have cerebrospinal abnormalities, including cerebrospinal pleocytosis, elevated protein, increased immunoglobulin, and oligoclonal bands. When neuropsychiatric findings occur in early HIV disease, they tend to involve subcortical, integrative, and executive functions: visuospatial integration, visuospatial memory, reaction time, verbal fluency, nonverbal fluency, problem solving, conceptual skills, set shifting, concentration, speed of mental processing, and mental flexibility. Language and related general intellectual skills are usually spared.

Psychopharmacological Issues

SSRIs are generally well tolerated and effective in HIV-related major depression, with a 57%–83% response rate and no deleterious effects on immune status (Halman et al. 2002). Studies of antidepressant efficacy among HIV-infected patients, however, are notable for substantial placebo response and attrition (Rabkin et al. 1999), suggesting that unknown factors are important in efficacious diagnosis and treatment of depression in HIV disease. For HIV/AIDS patients, the dosing principle of starting low and increasing slowly applies. Fluoxetine or paroxetine should be started at 10 mg/day and increased to the standard dosage after 7–10 days (Halman et al. 2002). Drug interactions can occur between SSRIs (especially fluvoxamine) and some antiretroviral therapies because of competition for cytochrome P450 3A3/3A4 metabolism, but these interactions are not usually clinically significant. Because citalopram has little interaction with these enzymes, it may have special utility in treating depression in HIV-positive patients receiving antiretroviral treatment.

At low doses, both dextroamphetamine and methylphenidate are effective for HIV-related major depression, as primary agents (Fernandez and Levy 1992) or as adjuvant agents, with response rates up to 80%. They are especially effective for anergia, apathy, and anorexia; some patients also report improved mood, attention, and concentration. Although stimulants are not usually first-line treatments for major depression, they should be especially considered as an adjunct or a substitute for conventional antidepressants in patients with a predominance of apathy compared with sadness and in patients who are unable to tolerate the side effects of conventional antidepressants.

Organ Transplantation

The consultation-liaison psychiatrist is often called on to fulfill many formal and informal functions as a member of the organ transplant team. The degree to which the psychiatrist is accepted as a member of the transplant team depends on 1) his or her ability to communicate effectively and succinctly with other team members, 2) the extent to which his or her clinical judgment is trusted, 3) his or her ability to effectively diffuse adverse transplant team member reactions to patients, and 4) the psychiatrist's ability to work collaboratively and effectively with other transplant team members (Skotzko and Strouse 2002).

Transplant Donors

Heart and liver transplants involve brain-dead donors, whereas renal transplants frequently involve living family donors. The consultation-liaison psychiatrist should evaluate potential interpersonal, marital, or family problems encountered by donor families. For example, is the family "black sheep" donating out of a conscious or an unconscious desire to improve his or her standing in the family system? Although the mortality rate for kidney donors is very low (calculated to be 0.03%), preoperative donor anxiety occurs (Surman and Prager 2004).

Transplant Recipients

In potential organ transplant recipients, the psychiatric consultant is sometimes asked to comment on whether psychiatric contraindications to transplantation exist. Psychiatric illness is only a minor factor in deciding whether a particular patient should receive a donor organ. Successful transplant outcomes have been reported in patients who have mental retardation, anxiety disorders, mood disorders, psychoactive substance use disorders, and personality disorders (Surman and Prager 2004). More important than psychiatric predisposition to successful postoperative psychosocial functioning are the success of the allograft and strength of social supports. Table 17–2 summarizes biopsychosocial criteria for psychiatric evaluation of potential transplant recipients.

Rating Scales

Two rating scales are available for the clinical assessment of psychosocial factors in transplant candidates: the Psychosocial Assessment of Candidates for

Table 17–2. Biopsychosocial screening criteria for solid organ transplantation

Absolute contraindications

Active substance abuse

Psychosis significantly limiting informed consent or compliance

Refusal of transplant and/or active suicidal ideation

Factitious disorder with physical symptoms

Noncompliance with the transplant system

Unwillingness to participate in necessary psychoeducational and psychiatric treatment

Relative contraindications

Dementia or other persistent cerebral dysfunction, if unable to arrange adequate psychosocial resources to supervise compliance *or* if dysfunction known to correlate with high risk of adverse posttransplant neuropsychiatric outcome (e.g., alcohol dementia, frontal lobe syndromes)

Treatment-refractory psychiatric illness, such as intractable, life-threatening mood disorder, schizophrenia, eating disorder, character disorder

Source. Adapted from Skotzko CE, Strouse TB: "Solid Organ Transplantation," in *The American Psychiatric Publishing Textbook of Consultation-Liaison Psychiatry: Psychiatry in the Medically Ill,* 2nd Edition. Edited by Wise MG, Rundell JR. Washington, DC, American Psychiatric Publishing, 2002, pp. 623–655. Copyright 2002, American Psychiatric Publishing. Used with permission.

Transplantion (PACT), developed by Olbrisch and colleagues (1989), and the Transplant Evaluation Rating Scale (TERS), developed by Twillman et al. (1993). "Both scales include weighted ratings for psychiatric diagnoses, substance abuse, health behaviors, adherence, social support, prior coping, and disease-specific coping. The TERS also rates affective and mental states" (Skotzko and Strouse 2002, p. 625). Both the PACT and the TERS have good interrater reliability and predictive power, with similar conceptual items being correlated with one another (Skotzko and Strouse 2002).

Perioperative Issues

Acute secondary mental disorders are common during the perioperative period. Common etiological factors for delirium in transplant recipients include the consequences to the brain of chronic organ failure, the residua of general anesthesia, lengthy transplant surgery, volume and electrolyte shifts associated with reperfusion of the new organ, cyclosporine loading, postoperative opiate treatment, early graft dysfunction, fever, coagulopathy, and infection (Abbasoglu et al. 1998; Plevak et al. 1989). Psychoactive substance withdrawal is also possible during the postoperative period.

The first signs of *cyclosporine neurotoxicity* are often seen in the intensive care unit (ICU) (Skotzko and Strouse 2002). After an early lucid period, patients are lethargic and confused and require reintubation despite previously adequate respiratory functioning (Craven 1991). Variable symptoms are seen, including seizures, cortical blindness, aphasia, paresthesia, neuropathy, delusions, and agitation. Obtundation, deeper coma, status epilepticus, and death rarely occur. Diffuse white matter changes are seen on magnetic resonance imaging, accompanied by symmetric electroencephalographic dysrhythmia. In some cases, cyclosporine holidays are associated with symptom remission and normalization of white matter changes (De Groen et al. 1987).

Critically Ill Patients and the ICU

Given the nature of their work, critical care physicians and nurses regularly encounter patients who have fear, anxiety, denial, anger, depression, dependency, or maladaptive personality features. A psychiatrist who is comfortable working in a critical care setting offers great assistance to both patients and medical colleagues. To perform optimally in a critical care setting, a psychiatrist must have sound medical skills and be credible. He or she must examine the patient with a mental status and a physical examination, including a basic neurological examination. The critically ill patient's mental status examination provides important information for decision making. If the patient has delirium or dementia, the focus of the differential diagnosis is to identify the etiological agent(s). The detection and correction of underlying cause(s) are often lifesaving in the seriously ill patient (see Chapter 3, "Delirium," and Chapter 4, "Dementia").

Mental Status Examination

Examining patients in the ICU is a challenge. First, the patient's level of consciousness should be noted. Next, the psychiatrist must establish a method of communication. If the patient cannot communicate verbally, he or she can write answers on a tablet. The psychiatrist can administer the entire Mini-Mental State Exam to any patient who can write (see Chapter 2, "Mental Status Examination and Other Tests of Brain Function"). Writing may show spatial disorientation, misspellings, inappropriate repetition of letters (perseveration), and linguistic errors.

For patients who are unable to speak or write, the psychiatrist may either use an eye blink method of communication (one blink=yes, two blinks=no) or have the patient squeeze the psychiatrist's finger with his or her hand (one squeeze=yes, two squeezes=no). Questions should be phrased to allow for a yes or no response (e.g., "Are you feeling frightened?"). To determine whether a patient is confused, the psychiatrist should also ask nonsense questions (e.g., "Do catfish fly?" "Do beagles yodel?"). If the patient looks surprised or amused and properly answers the question, a secondary mental syndrome is not as likely.

Changes in Medical-Surgical Management

Patients in ICUs have serious physical illnesses. A large proportion of the psychiatric symptoms and disorders seen in the ICU setting are secondary to these medical disorders and/or toxicity from their treatments. Consequently, the psychiatrist must consider whether changes in the medical management of a patient would alleviate the psychiatric symptoms. For example, it makes no sense (and would be ineffective) to treat delirium caused by hypoxia or hypoglycemia with neuroleptics alone. Whenever possible, delirium should be treated specifically (e.g., reversal of hypoxia with oxygen or hypoglycemia with glucose). A special note of temporal correlations between the onset of mental symptoms and changes in the medical-surgical management of the patient should be made. The ICU flowchart or laboratory summary sheet may indicate a metabolic or infectious problem that explains an altered mental status. The psychiatrist also should review the medication list, with special attention paid to medications added just prior to symptom onset or discontinued before symptom onset (i.e., a withdrawal reaction). These and other temporal correlations are often the primary (or only) clues available to help identify the cause of psychiatric symptoms in the ICU (Shuster and Stern 2002).

Psychopharmacological Treatment

Serious physical illness may increase the patient's sensitivity to drug effects. Symptomatic treatment alone may not solve the problem; it may even create new problems. A thorough knowledge of the pharmacological properties of psychotropic agents is crucial to their successful use in the ICU. Most psychotropics are metabolized in the liver and cleared through the liver or kidneys. Therefore, altered hepatic or renal function clearly influences the choice and dosing of psychotropic medications. Clinical experience shows that doses below the standard therapeutic range are often effective in patients with medical illness, especially when drug interactions or renal or hepatic impairment slows drug clearance (Shuster and Stern 2002). Some critically ill patients, however, require doses similar to those required in healthy adults. Higher doses are safely achieved by titrating beneficial effects to side effects.

Respirators

Patients often experience anxiety when a ventilator is removed. As Shuster and Stern (2002) note:

> Anxiety is particularly common when a patient is weaned from the ventilator. Several factors can play a role in the anxiety: patients may experience at least brief periods of relative hypoxia during weaning trials; prolonged ventilation usually leads to deconditioning of muscles of respiration, so patients become frightened by the unfamiliar difficulty they experience with breathing until these muscles are reconditioned; and patients often become psychologically dependent on the ventilator and fearful when the device is disconnected. (p. 765)

Intra-aortic Balloon Pump

An intra-aortic balloon pump renders a patient immobile. Because of the intra-aortic balloon pump, patients must remain on their backs. In addition, numerous intravenous and intra-arterial lines are typically present, restricting arm movement. These physical restrictions can cause severe anxiety. Lorazepam is usually a good choice to relieve anxiety. It can be given intravenously (1 or 2 mg) and has a low frequency of adverse effects in a critically ill patient population. When a patient's anxiety reaches panic proportions, administration of a high-potency neuroleptic at a low dose is often helpful.

Male Erectile Disorder (Impotence)

Many medical diseases and pharmacological agents are associated with male erectile disorder. The ability to have an erection requires normal functioning in four areas: 1) adequate arterial flow to and through the penis; 2) normal neurological function, particularly the autonomic nervous system; 3) normal hormonal function; and 4) normal erotogenic input. Erotogenic function is impeded by depression, anxiety, interpersonal issues, and fatigue.

History

The pattern of erectile function and dysfunction helps the clinician decide whether a medical evaluation is necessary. If the patient has erections in the morning, during sleep, during masturbation, with a sexual partner other than the spouse, or spontaneously when intercourse is not planned, a psychological reason for impotence is very likely. If the patient has never had erectile function or has lost erectile function, a toxic or medical etiology is possible, and an evaluation is indicated.

Medications can cause impotence (Table 17–3). It is diagnostically helpful to correlate the onset of sexual dysfunction with initiation of or increases in prescribed or over-the-counter medications (Brown et al. 2002).

Evaluation

The evaluation of erectile dysfunction includes a physical examination, with particular attention to neurological function. A full evaluation of impotence is expensive. It may include a sleep laboratory evaluation, which often is diagnostic. Strain gauges are connected to the penis and monitor whether nocturnal erections occur during rapid eye movement (REM) sleep. If full erections occur during REM sleep, a psychological etiology for impotence is probable. Other diagnostic studies may include Doppler blood flow studies, nerve conduction studies, tests of bladder function, and cavernosonograms. Laboratory studies may include glucose tolerance test, serum urea nitrogen and creatinine levels, liver function tests, and hormonal studies (e.g., thyroid, testosterone, prolactin, follicle-stimulating hormone, and luteinizing hormone).

Table 17–3. Medications that may cause male erectile disorder (impotence)

Alcohol	Amitriptyline	Amoxapine
Amphetamines	Amyl nitrite	Atenolol
Atropine	Baclofen	Barbiturates
Benztropine	Bromocriptine	Bupropion
Captopril	Carbamazepine	Chlorambucil
Chlorothiazide	Chlorpromazine	Cimetidine
Clidinium	Clofibrate	Clomipramine
Clonidine	Cyclophosphamide	Cytosine arabinoside
Desipramine	Dichlorphenamide	Digoxin
Diphenhydramine	Disopyramide	Disulfiram
Fenfluramine	Glycopyrrolate	Guanethidine
Haloperidol	Hydralazine	Hydrochlorothiazide
Hydroxyzine	Imipramine	Indomethacin
Interferon alfa	Isocarboxazid	Ketoconazole
Lithium	Maprotiline	Melphalan
Methadone	Methaqualone	Methotrexate
Methscopolamine	Methyldopa	Metoclopramide
Metoprolol	Mexiletine	Morphine
Nadolol	Naproxen	Nortriptyline
Pargyline	Phenelzine	Phentolamine
Phenytoin	Pimozide	Pindolol
Prazosin	Procarbazine	Progestins
Propranolol	Protriptyline	Scopolamine
SSRIs	Thiazide diuretics	Thioridazine
Thiothixene	Timolol	Tranylcypromine
Trihexyphenidyl	Trimipramine	Verapamil

Note. SSRI = selective serotonin reuptake inhibitor.
Source. Adapted from Brown GR, Gass G, Philbrick K: "Sexual Disorders and Dysfunctions," in *The American Psychiatric Publishing Textbook of Consultation-Liaison Psychiatry: Psychiatry in the Medically Ill,* 2nd Edition. Edited by Wise MG, Rundell JR. Washington, DC, American Psychiatric Publishing, 2002, pp. 455–475. Copyright 2002, American Psychiatric Publishing. Used with permission.

Treatment

Some causes of impotence are reversible (e.g., hyperthyroidism, alcohol, prescribed drugs), and others are usually irreversible (e.g., spinal cord injury, autonomic neuropathies such as those found in type 1 diabetes). In the latter case, a penile prosthesis may be considered. Psychological impotence may be caused by many factors. A thorough interview with the patient and sexual partner usually clarifies the underlying issues. If marital discord exists, marital therapy is recommended prior to referral for sexual therapy.

References

Abbasoglu O, Goldstein RM, Vodapally MS, et al: Liver transplantation in hyponatremic patients with emphasis on central pontine myelinolysis. Clin Transplant 12:263–269, 1998

Andreasen NJ, Hartford CE, Knott JR, et al: EEG changes associated with burn delirium. Dis Nerv Syst 38:27–31, 1977

Breitbart W, Lintz K: Psychiatric issues in the care of dying patients, in The American Psychiatric Publishing Textbook of Consultation-Liaison Psychiatry: Psychiatry in the Medically Ill, 2nd Edition. Edited by Wise MG, Rundell JR. Washington, DC, American Psychiatric Publishing, 2002, pp 771–804

Brown GR, Gass G, Philbrick K: Sexual disorders and dysfunctions, in The American Psychiatric Publishing Textbook of Consultation-Liaison Psychiatry: Psychiatry in the Medically Ill, 2nd Edition. Edited by Wise MG, Rundell JR. Washington, DC, American Psychiatric Publishing, 2002, pp 455–475

Cassem NH: End of life issues: principles of care and ethics, in Massachusetts General Hospital Handbook of General Hospital Psychiatry, 5th Edition. Edited by Stern TL, Fricchione GL, Cassem NH, et al. St. Louis, MO, Mosby, 2004, pp 365–387

Centers for Disease Control and Prevention: Update: acquired immunodeficiency syndrome—United States, 1994. MMWR Morb Mortal Wkly Rep 44:64–67, 1995

Cohen LS, Friedman JM, Jefferson JW, et al: A reevaluation of risk of in utero exposure to lithium. JAMA 271:146–150, 1994

Cohen LS, Sichel DA, Robertson LM, et al: Postpartum prophylaxis for women with bipolar disorder. Am J Psychiatry 152:1641–1645, 1995

Craven JL: Cyclosporine-associated organic mental disorders in liver transplant recipients. Psychosomatics 32:94–102, 1991

De Groen PC, Aksamit AJ, Rakela J, et al: Central nervous system toxicity after liver transplantation: the role of cyclosporine and cholesterol. N Engl J Med 317:861–866, 1987

Fauerbach JA, Lawrence J, Haythornthwaite J, et al: Preinjury psychiatric illness and postinjury adjustment in adult burn survivors. Psychosomatics 37:547–555, 1996

Fawzy FI, Servis ME, Greenberg DB: Oncology and psychooncology, in The American Psychiatric Publishing Textbook of Consultation-Liaison Psychiatry: Psychiatry in the Medically Ill, 2nd Edition. Edited by Wise MG, Rundell JR. Washington, DC, American Psychiatric Publishing, 2002, pp 657–678

Fernandez F, Levy JK: Psychopharmacotherapy of psychiatric syndromes in asymptomatic and symptomatic HIV infection. Psychiatr Med 9:377–394, 1992

Foley KM: The treatment of cancer pain. N Engl J Med 313:84–95, 1985

Fricchione G, el-Chemali Z, Weilburg JB, et al: Neurology and neurosurgery, in The American Psychiatric Publishing Textbook of Consultation-Liaison Psychiatry: Psychiatry in the Medically Ill, 2nd Edition. Edited by Wise MG, Rundell JR. Washington, DC, American Psychiatric Publishing, 2002, pp 679–700

Fritz GK, Brown LK: Pediatrics, in The American Psychiatric Publishing Textbook of Consultation-Liaison Psychiatry: Psychiatry in the Medically Ill, 2nd Edition. Edited by Wise MG, Rundell JR. Washington, DC, American Psychiatric Publishing, 2002, pp 717–727

Halman MH, Bialer P, Worth JL, et al: HIV Disease/AIDS, in The American Psychiatric Publishing Textbook of Consultation-Liaison Psychiatry: Psychiatry in the Medically Ill, 2nd Edition. Edited by Wise MG, Rundell JR. Washington, DC, American Psychiatric Publishing, 2002, pp 807–851

Karceski S, Morrell M, Carpenter D: The expert consensus guideline series: treatment of epilepsy. Epilepsy Behav 2:A1–A50, 2001

Kratochvil CJ, Heiligenstein JH, Dittmann R, et al: Atomoxetine and methylphenidate treatment in children with ADHD: a prospective, randomized, open-label trial. J Am Acad Child Adolesc Psychiatry 41:776–784, 2002

Lishman WA: Organic Psychiatry, 2nd Edition. Oxford, England, Blackwell Scientific, 1987

Lishman WA: Organic Psychiatry: The Psychological Consequences of Cerebral Disorder, 3rd Edition. Oxford, England, Blackwell Scientific, 1998

Lohr JB, Cadet JL: Neuropsychiatric aspects of brain tumors, in The American Psychiatric Press Textbook of Neuropsychiatry. Edited by Hales RE, Yudofsky SC. Washington, DC, American Psychiatric Press, 1987, pp 351–364

MacArthur JD, Moore FD: Epidemiology of burns. JAMA 231:259–263, 1975

Martin MJ, Black JL: Neuropsychiatric aspects of degenerative disease, in The American Psychiatric Press Textbook of Neuropsychiatry. Edited by Hales RE, Yudofsky SC. Washington, DC, American Psychiatric Press, 1987, pp 257–286

Michelson D, Allen AJ, Busner J, et al: Once-daily atomoxetine treatment for children and adolescents with attention deficit hyperactivity disorder: a randomized, placebo-controlled study. Am J Psychiatry 159:1896–1901, 2002

Nadelson CC, Notman MT: The psychiatric aspects of obstetrics and gynecology, in Consultation-Liaison Psychiatry and Behavioral Medicine. Edited by Houpt JL, Brodie HKH. Philadelphia, PA, JB Lippincott, 1986, pp 367–378

Olbrisch ME, Levenson J, Hamer R: The PACT: a rating scale for the study of clinical decision-making in psychosocial screening criteria for organ transplant candidates. Clin Transplant 3:164–169, 1989

Perry SW, Difede J, Musngi G, et al: Predictors of posttraumatic stress disorder after burn injury. Am J Psychiatry 149:931–935, 1992

Plevak DJ, Southorn PA, Narr BJ, et al: Intensive care unit experience in the Mayo Liver Transplantation Program: the first 100 cases. Mayo Clin Proc 64:433–445, 1989

Rabkin JG, Wagner GJ, Rabkin R: Fluoxetine treatment for depression in patients with HIV and AIDS: a randomized, placebo-controlled trial. Am J Psychiatry 156:101–107, 1999

Raison CL, Pasnau RO, Fawzy FI, et al: Surgery and surgical subspecialties, in The American Psychiatric Publishing Textbook of Consultation-Liaison Psychiatry: Psychiatry in the Medically Ill, 2nd Edition. Edited by Wise MG, Rundell JR. Washington, DC, American Psychiatric Publishing, 2002, pp 593–622

Shuster JL Jr, Stern TA: Intensive care units, in The American Psychiatric Publishing Textbook of Consultation-Liaison Psychiatry: Psychiatry in the Medically Ill, 2nd Edition. Edited by Wise MG, Rundell JR. Washington, DC, American Psychiatric Publishing, 2002, pp 753–770

Skotzko CE, Strouse TB: Solid organ transplantation, in The American Psychiatric Publishing Textbook of Consultation-Liaison Psychiatry: Psychiatry in the Medically Ill, 2nd Edition. Edited by Wise MG, Rundell JR. Washington, DC, American Psychiatric Publishing, 2002, pp 623–655

Stotland NL: Obstetrics and gynecology, in The American Psychiatric Publishing Textbook of Consultation-Liaison Psychiatry: Psychiatry in the Medically Ill, 2nd Edition. Edited by Wise MG, Rundell JR. Washington, DC, American Psychiatric Publishing, 2002, pp 701–716

Surman OS, Prager LM: Organ failure and transplantation, in Massachusetts General Hospital Handbook of General Hospital Psychiatry, 5th Edition. Edited by Stern TL, Fricchione GL, Cassem NH, et al. St. Louis, MO, Mosby, 2004, pp 641–670

Twillman RK, Manetto C, Wolcott DL: The Transplant Evaluation Rating Scale: a revision of the psychosocial levels system for evaluating organ transplant candidates. Psychosomatics 34:144–153, 1993

Wagner KD, Robb AS, Findling RL, et al: A randomized, placebo-controlled trial of citalopram for the treatment of major depression in children and adolescents. Am J Psychiatry 161:1079–1083, 2004

Warden GD, Heinbach DM: Burns, in Principles of Surgery, 7th Edition. Edited by Schwartz SI, Shires GT, Spencer FC, et al. New York, McGraw-Hill, 1991, pp 223–262

Waziri R: The amnestic syndrome, in The Medical Basis of Psychiatry. Edited by Winokur G, Clayton PJ. Philadelphia, PA, WB Saunders, 1986, pp 20–28

Weissman AM, Levy BT, Hartz AJ, et al: Pooled analysis of antidepressant levels in lactating mothers, breast milk, and nursing infants. Am J Psychiatry 161:1066–1078, 2004

Wiart L: Post-cerebrovascular stroke depression. Encephale 3:51–54, 1997

Williams LS, Ghose SS, Swindle RW: Depression and other mental health diagnoses increase mortality risk after ischemic stroke. Am J Psychiatry 161:1090–1095, 2004

Wise MG, Rundell JR: Anxiety and neurological disorders. Semin Clin Neuropsychiatry 4:98–102, 1999

Yonkers KA, Wisner KL, Stowe Z, et al: Management of bipolar disorder during pregnancy and the postpartum period. Am J Psychiatry 161:608–620, 2004

Additional Readings

Beck BJ, Worth JL: Patients with HIV infection and AIDS, in Massachusetts General Hospital Handbook of General Hospital Psychiatry, 5th Edition. Edited by Stern TL, Fricchione GL, Cassem NH, et al. St. Louis, MO, Mosby, 2004, pp 671–695

Classen PJ, Butler LD, Koopman C, et al: Supportive-expressive group therapy and distress in patients with metastatic breast cancer: a randomized clinical intervention trial. Arch Gen Psychiatry 58:494–501, 2001

Grady BJ: Telepsychiatry, in The American Psychiatric Publishing Textbook of Consultation-Liaison Psychiatry: Psychiatry in the Medically Ill, 2nd Edition. Edited by Wise MG, Rundell JR. Washington, DC, American Psychiatric Publishing, 2002, pp 927–936

Levinsky NG: Organ donation by unrelated donors. N Engl J Med 343:430–432, 2000

Prince JB, Wilens TE, Biederman J, et al: Psychopharmacology for children and adolescents, in Massachusetts General Hospital Handbook of General Hospital Psychiatry, 5th Edition. Edited by Stern TL, Fricchione GL, Cassem NH, et al. St. Louis, MO, Mosby, 2004, pp 411–445

Ross GW, Bowen JD: The diagnosis and differential diagnosis of dementia. Med Clin North Am 86:455–476, 2002

Tesar GE, Locala JA: The emergency department, in The American Psychiatric Publishing Textbook of Consultation-Liaison Psychiatry: Psychiatry in the Medically Ill, 2nd Edition. Edited by Wise MG, Rundell JR. Washington, DC, American Psychiatric Publishing, 2002, pp 889–916

Index

*Page numbers printed in **boldface** type refer to tables or figures.*